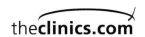

EMERGENCY MEDICINE CLINICS OF NORTH AMERICA

Medical Toxicology

GUEST EDITORS
Christopher P. Holstege, MD and
Mark A. Kirk, MD

CONSULTING EDITOR
Amal Mattu, MD

May 2007 • Volume 25 • Number 2

SAUNDERS

An Imprint of Elsevier, Inc.
PHILADELPHIA   LONDON   TORONTO   MONTREAL   SYDNEY   TOKYO

W.B. SAUNDERS COMPANY
A Division of Elsevier Inc.

1600 John F. Kennedy Boulevard, Suite 1800 • Philadelphia, Pennsylvania 19103-2899

http://www.theclinics.com

EMERGENCY MEDICINE CLINICS　　　　　　　　　　　　**Volume 25, Number 2**
OF NORTH AMERICA　　　　　　　　　　　　　　　　　　**ISSN 0733-8627**
May 2007　　　　　　　　　　　　　　**ISBN-13: 978-1-4160-4307-2**
Editor: Karen Sorensen　　　　　　　　　　　　**ISBN-10: 1-4160-4307-1**

The ideas and opinions expressed in *Emergency Medicine Clinics of North America* do not necessarily reflect those of the Publisher. The Publisher does not assume any responsibility for any injury and/or damage to persons or property arising out of or related to any use of the material contained in this periodical. The reader is advised to check the appropriate medical literature and the product information currently provided by the manufacturer of each drug to be administered to verify the dosage, the method and duration of administration, or contraindications. It is the responsibility of the treating physician or other health care professional, relying on independent experience and knowledge of the patient, to determine drug dosages and the best treatment for the patient. Mention of any product in this issue should not be construed as endorsement by the contributors, editors, or the Publisher of the product or manufacturers' claims.

Emergency Medicine Clinics of North America (ISSN 0733-8627) is published quarterly by Elsevier Inc., 360 Park Avenue South, New York, NY, 10010-1710. Months of issue are February, May, August, and November. Business and Editorial Offices: 1600 John F. Kennedy Boulevard, Suite 1800, Philadelphia, PA 19103-2899. Customer Service Office: 6277 Sea Harbor Drive, Orlando, FL 32887-4800. Periodicals postage paid at New York, NY, and additional mailing offices. Subscription prices are $193.00 per year (US individuals), $297.00 per year (US institutions), $259.00 per year (international individuals), $351.00 per year (international institutions), $237.00 per year (Canadian individuals), and $351.00 per year (Canadian institutions). International air speed delivery is included in all *Clinics'* subscription prices. All prices are subject to change without notice. POSTMASTER: Send address changes to *Emergency Medicine Clinics of North America*, Elsevier Periodicals Customer Service, 6277 Sea Harbor Drive, Orlando, FL 32887-4800. **Customer Service: 1-800-654-2452 (US). From outside of the US, call 1-407-345-4000. E-mail: hhspcs@harcourt.com.**

Emergency Medicine Clinics of North America is covered in *Index Medicus, Current Contents/Clinical Medicine, EMBASE/Excerpta Medica, BIOSIS, SciSearch, CINAHL, ISI/BIOMED,* and *Research Alert.*

Printed in the United States of America.

CONSULTING EDITOR

AMAL MATTU, MD, Program Director, Emergency Medicine Residency; and Associate Professor, Department of Emergency Medicine, University of Maryland School of Medicine, Baltimore, Maryland

GUEST EDITORS

CHRISTOPHER P. HOLSTEGE, MD, Director, Division of Medical Toxicology, Department of Emergency Medicine, University of Virginia; Blue Ridge Poison Center, University of Virginia Health System, Charlottesville, Virginia

MARK A. KIRK, MD, Director, Medical Toxicology Fellowship, Blue Ridge Poison Center, Division of Medical Toxicology, Department of Emergency Medicine, University of Virginia, Charlottesville, Virginia

CONTRIBUTORS

LAURA K. BECHTEL, PhD, Research Associate, Blue Ridge Poison Center, University of Virginia Health System; Division of Medical Toxicology, Department of Emergency Medicine, University of Virginia, Charlottesville, Virginia

MICHAEL L. DEATON, PhD, Professor, Integrated Science and Technology, James Madison University, Harrisonburg, Virginia

STEPHEN G. DOBMEIER, BSN, Managing Director, Blue Ridge Poison Center, University of Virginia Health System, Charlottesville, Virginia

DAVID L. ELDRIDGE, MD, Assistant Professor, Department of Pediatrics, Brody School of Medicine, East Carolina University, Greenville, North Carolina

TIMOTHY B. ERICKSON, MD, FACEP, FACMT, FAACT, Professor, Department of Emergency Medicine, Division of Clinical Toxicology, University of Illinois at Chicago, Toxikon Consortium, Chicago, Illinois

CHARLES J. FASANO, DO, Attending Physician, Department of Emergency Medicine, Albert Einstein Medical Center; Assistant Professor, Department of Emergency Medicine, Thomas Jefferson University, Philadelphia, Pennsylvania

BLAKE FROBERG, MD, Medical Toxicology Fellow, Indiana Poison Center, Methodist Hospital, Clarian Health Partners, Indiana University School of Medicine, Indianapolis, Indiana

R. BRENT FURBEE, MD, FACMT, Medical Director, Indiana Poison Center, Methodist Hospital, Clarian Health Partners, Indiana University School of Medicine, Indianapolis, Indiana

CHRISTOPHER P. HOLSTEGE, MD, Director, Division of Medical Toxicology, Department of Emergency Medicine, University of Virginia; Blue Ridge Poison Center, University of Virginia Health System, Charlottesville, Virginia

DANYAL IBRAHIM, MD, Medical Toxicology Fellow, Indiana Poison Center, Methodist Hospital, Clarian Health Partners, Indiana University School of Medicine, Indianapolis, Indiana

WILLIAM KERNS II, MD, FACEP, FACMT, Program Director, Division of Toxicology, Department of Emergency Medicine, Carolinas Medical Center, Charlotte, North Carolina

MARK A. KIRK, MD, Director, Medical Toxicology Fellowship, Blue Ridge Poison Center, Division of Medical Toxicology, Department of Emergency Medicine, University of Virginia, Charlottesville, Virginia

CHAD KORNEGAY, MD, Internal Medicine-Pediatrics Residency Program, Brody School of Medicine, East Carolina University, Greenville, North Carolina

DAVID T. LAWRENCE, DO, Medical Toxicology Fellow, Blue Ridge Poison Center, Division of Medical Toxicology, Department of Emergency Medicine, University of Virginia, Charlottesville, Virginia

JENNY J. LU, MD, Medical Toxicology Fellow, Department of Emergency Medicine, Division of Clinical Toxicology, University of Illinois at Chicago, Toxikon Consortium, Chicago, Illinois

JILL E. MICHELS, PharmD, Clinical Assistant Professor, Palmetto Poison Center, South Carolina College of Pharmacy, University of South Carolina, Columbia, South Carolina

GERALD F. O'MALLEY, DO, Director of Research, and Director, Division of Toxicology, Albert Einstein Medical Center; Clinical Associate Professor of Emergency Medicine, Thomas Jefferson University Hospital; Consulting Toxicologist, Children's Hospital of Philadelphia; Faculty Consultant, Philadelphia Poison Control Center, Philadelphia, Pennsylvania

RIKA N. O'MALLEY, MD, Resident Physician, Department of Emergency Medicine, Albert Einstein Medical Center, Philadelphia, Pennsylvania

TRACEY H. REILLY, MD, Medical Toxicology Fellow, Division of Medical Toxicology, Department of Emergency Medicine, University of Virginia, Charlottesville, Virginia

WILLIAM H. RICHARDSON III, MD, Department of Emergency Medicine, Palmetto Health Richland; Palmetto Poison Center, South Carolina College of Pharmacy, University of South Carolina, Columbia, South Carolina

ADAM K. ROWDEN, DO, Attending Physician, Department of Emergency Medicine, Albert Einstein Medical Center, Philadelphia, Pennsylvania

MATTHEW SALZMAN, MD, Attending Physician, Department of Emergency Medicine, Albert Einstein Medical Center, Philadelphia, Pennsylvania

CHERYL M. SLONE, MD, Department of Emergency Medicine, Palmetto Health Richland, Columbia, South Carolina

TREVONNE M. THOMPSON, MD, Medical Toxicology Fellow, Department of Emergency Medicine, Division of Clinical Toxicology, University of Illinois at Chicago, Toxikon Consortium, Chicago, Illinois

JASON VAN EYK, MD, Internal Medicine-Pediatrics Residency Program, Brody School of Medicine, East Carolina University, Greenville, North Carolina

BRAM P. WISPELWEY, Research Assistant, Critical Incident Analysis Group, Department of Psychiatry, University of Virginia, Charlottesville, Virginia

CONTENTS

> Toxic overdose can present with various clinical signs and symp-
> toms. These may be the only clues to diagnosis when the cause of
> toxicity is unknown at the time of initial assessment. The prognosis
> and clinical course of recovery of a patient poisoned by a specific
> agent depends largely on the quality of care delivered within the
> first few hours in the emergency setting. Usually the drug or toxin
> can be quickly identified by a careful history, a directed physical
> examination, and commonly available laboratory tests. Once the
> patient has been stabilized, the physician must consider how to
> minimize the bioavailability of toxin not yet absorbed, which
> antidotes (if any) to administer, and if other measures to enhance
> elimination are necessary.

> Pediatric patients present unique concerns in the field of medical
> toxicology. First, there are medicines that are potentially dangerous
> to small children, even when they are exposed to very small
> amounts. Clinicians should be wary of these drugs even when
> young patients present with accidental ingestions of apparently
> insignificant amounts. Next, over-the-counter laxatives and syrup

of ipecac, although not commonly considered abused substances, may be misused in both the setting of Munchausen's syndrome by proxy and in adolescents who have eating disorders. Their use should be considered in any gastrointestinal illness of uncertain origin. Finally, as the use of syrup of ipecac at home now has been discouraged by many, some have explored using activated charcoal at home as a new method of prehospital gastrointestinal decontamination. The literature examining activated charcoal and its use in this capacity is discussed.

FORTHCOMING ISSUES

RECENT ISSUES

EMERGENCY
MEDICINE
CLINICS OF
NORTH AMERICA

ELSEVIER
SAUNDERS

Emerg Med Clin N Am 25 (2007) xv–xvi

Foreword

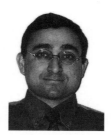

Amal Mattu, MD
Consulting Editor

Medical toxicology is a field that has grown steadily in importance during the past few decades, but its importance has never been greater than it is today. More than 2 million toxic exposures are reported annually to the American Academy of Poison Control Centers [1]. Intentional, accidental, and iatrogenic exposures are common despite public health and hospital-based patient safety programs. Environmental exposures such as carbon monoxide and abuse of both older (eg, ethanol) and newer (eg, "ecstasy") drugs continue to account for many deaths that are never even reported to poison control centers. Increased availability of herbal supplements without oversight by the US Food and Drug Administration has resulted in increased toxicities and drug interactions. Criminal poisonings associated with sexual assaults have increased in recent years. Finally, there is greater concern than ever before about attacks involving deadly chemicals by terrorists. The medical specialty that serves as "first-responder" to any of these exposures and scenarios is emergency medicine. Our society has never relied more heavily on physicians in our specialty to be experts in medical toxicology.

In this issue of the *Emergency Medicine Clinics of North America*, Guest Editors Holstege and Kirk have assembled an outstanding group of authors to educate us on this vital aspect of our specialty. The first articles discuss a general approach to patients with overdose as well as some special concerns in pediatric patients; later articles delve into greater depth with regard to specific toxins. The discussion is not just limited to common medications but also deals with plants, herbal substances, caustics, and criminal poisonings. The authors conclude with discussions pertaining to mass chemical

0733-8627/07/$ - see front matter © 2007 Elsevier Inc. All rights reserved.
doi:10.1016/j.emc.2007.04.001   *emed.theclinics.com*

exposures and potential agents of terrorism. These vital topics are not only relevant to individual emergency physicians but also to emergency medical systems.

This issue represents an important addition to the emergency medicine literature. Experienced emergency physicians as well as emergency medicine trainees will benefit tremendously from the expertise provided in the pages that follow. The Guest Editors and authors are to be commended for providing a single resource that covers a broad spectrum of toxicologic emergencies in a succinct, clinically relevant, and cutting-edge manner.

Amal Mattu, MD
Department of Emergency Medicine
University of Maryland School of Medicine
110 S. Paca Street, 6th Floor, Suite 100
Baltimore, MD 21201, USA

E-mail address: amattu@smail.umaryland.edu

Reference

[1] McLaughlin SA. Toxicologic emergencies. In: Mahadevan SV, Garmel GM, editors. An introduction to clinical emergency medicine. New York: Cambridge University Press; 2005.

ELSEVIER
SAUNDERS

EMERGENCY
MEDICINE
CLINICS OF
NORTH AMERICA

Emerg Med Clin N Am 25 (2007) xvii–xviii

Preface

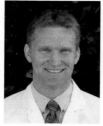 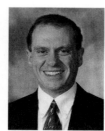

Christopher P. Holstege, MD   Mark A. Kirk, MD
Guest Editors

Innumerable potential toxins can inflict harm on humans, and they include pharmaceuticals, herbals, household products, environmental agents, occupational chemicals, drugs of abuse, and chemical terrorism threats. Each year, millions of human exposure cases are reported to the American Association of Poison Control Centers Toxic Exposure Surveillance System. The Center for Disease Control reported that poisoning (both intentional and unintentional) was one of the top 10 causes of injury related death in the United States in all adult age groups. From the beginning of written history, poisons and their effects have been well described. Paracelsus (1493–1541) correctly noted that "All substances are poisons; there is none which is not a poison. The right dose differentiates a poison...." As life in the modern era has become more complex, so has the study of poisons and their treatments.

This issue of *Emergency Medicine Clinics of North American* is dedicated to the topic of Medical Toxicology. Medical Toxicology is a subspecialty recognized by the American Board of Medical Specialties. Physicians who have trained in this area focus their practice on the prevention, diagnosis, and management of poisoning. Over the past decade, the field of Medical Toxicology has grown in conjunction with the emergence of new pharmaceuticals, abused drugs, chemicals within the work place, and agents of terrorism. As the guest editors, we considered numerous topics for inclusion in this issue. We decided upon the topics we thought represented some of the more common, controversial, or emerging areas in our field. It is our hope

doi:10.1016/j.emc.2007.04.002

that this issue will provide insight to emergency medicine personnel caring for potentially poisoned patients.

Christopher P. Holstege, MD
Director
Division of Medical Toxicology
Department of Emergency Medicine
University of Virginia
and
Blue Ridge Poison Center
University of Virginia Health System
P.O. Box 800744
1222 Jefferson Park Avenue, 4th Floor
Charlottesville, VA 22908-0774

E-mail address: ch2xf@virginia.edu

Mark A. Kirk, MD
Director
Medical Toxicology Fellowship
Blue Ridge Poison Center
Division of Medical Toxicology
Department of Emergency Medicine
University of Virginia
P.O. Box 800744
Charlottesville, VA 22908-0774

E-mail address: mak4z@virginia.edu

EMERGENCY
MEDICINE
CLINICS OF
NORTH AMERICA

ELSEVIER
SAUNDERS

Emerg Med Clin N Am 25 (2007) 249–281

The Approach to the Patient with an Unknown Overdose

Timothy B. Erickson, MD,
FACEP, FACMT, FAACT*,
Trevonne M. Thompson, MD, Jenny J. Lu, MD

*Department of Emergency Medicine, Division of Clinical Toxicology,
University of Illinois at Chicago, Toxikon Consortium, Room 471 (M/C 724),
808 South Wood Street, Chicago, IL 60612, USA*

Toxic overdose can present with various clinical symptoms, including abdominal pain, vomiting, tremor, altered mental status, seizures, cardiac dysrhythmias, and respiratory depression. These may be the only clues to diagnosis when the cause of toxicity is unknown at the time of initial assessment and management. The diagnosis may be complicated by the possibility of a multiple-drug ingestion.

The prognosis and clinical course of recovery of a patient poisoned by a specific agent depends largely on the quality of care delivered within the first few hours in the emergency setting. Fortunately, in most instances, the drug or toxin can be quickly identified by a careful history, a directed physical examination, and commonly available laboratory tests. Attempts to identify the poison should never delay life-saving supportive care, however. Once the patient has been stabilized, the physician needs to consider how to minimize the bioavailability of toxin not yet absorbed, which antidotes (if any) to administer, and if other measures to enhance elimination are necessary [1].

Clinical guidelines

Although several published position statements [2–6] and practice guidelines or consensus statements [7] exist regarding clinical toxicology diagnosis and management, most of the literature is based on retrospective case series

* Corresponding author.
E-mail address: toxboy@uic.edu (T.B. Erickson).

0733-8627/07/$ - see front matter © 2007 Elsevier Inc. All rights reserved.
doi:10.1016/j.emc.2007.02.004

analysis or isolated case reports with isolated animal or laboratory research. Well-controlled, randomized, human trials with adequate sample sizes are infrequent and difficult to perform.

Regional Poison Control Center data exist and are updated on an annual basis to document changing trends in poisoning epidemiology. This national database is predominantly presented in a retrospective fashion [8]. It is important to note, however, that most severe cases resulting in death never arrive to hospitals (ie, medical examiner cases). Published studies based on poison center data therefore are skewed toward mild to moderate poisonings and may underrepresent a small but important segment of toxic agents [9]. Unfortunately, well-designed forensic toxicology data are limited in the literature. Recently, the poison exposure data of the National Health Interview Survey and the Toxic Exposure Surveillance System have been compared to identify age-adjusted poisoning episode rates to provide a broader perspective [10].

Epidemiology

In the year 2004, more than 2.4 million human exposures to toxins were reported to the American Association of Poison Control Centers [8]. More than 75% were reported from the home and 15% from a health care facility. Two thirds of the reported exposures involved pediatric patients less than 20 years of age. The leading agents were cleaning substances, followed by analgesics and cosmetics/personal care products [8]. There were 1183 reported poisoning fatalities with children less than 6 years of age representing only 2% of these deaths. The leading fatal agents were analgesics, antidepressants, cardiovascular drugs, stimulants, and street drugs [8].

Toxicokinetics

What is it that is not a poison? All things are poison and nothing is without poison. Solely, the dose determines that a thing is not a poison.
—Paracelsus (1493–1541), the Renaissance Father of Toxicology, in his *Third Defense* [11]

As described by the Renaissance toxicologist Paracelsus, any substance should be considered a potential poison depending on the dose and duration of exposure. The pharmacokinetic movement of a xenobiotic through the human body can be described in terms of pharmacokinetics—absorption, distribution, and elimination. Toxicokinetics describes the absorption, distribution, and elimination of xenobiotics at doses capable of producing clinical toxicity. In the overdosed patient, toxicokinetic concepts are most often used in the interpretation of drug concentrations in plasma or urine. Toxicokinetics may also be used to predict the onset of symptoms and duration of toxicity [12].

Differential diagnosis of the poisoned patient

Any symptomatic patient can be a potential drug overdose. Altered mental status, gastrointestinal complaints, cardiovascular compromise, seizures, and temperature-related disorders can all be toxin-related. Some are subtle, such as the flulike symptoms seen with carbon monoxide poisoning, whereas cardiotoxins, such as digitalis, may mimic intrinsic heart disease. In the differential diagnosis, the clinician should also consider similar agents. For example, the following should be considered together as possible culprits: acetaminophen and salicylates, methanol and ethylene glycol, digitalis and beta-blockers and calcium channel antagonists.

Prehospital care

Apart from basic stabilization measures (such as oxygen administration, cardiac monitoring, and venous access establishment), emergency medical system (EMS) personnel need to do little in the field with the overdosed patient, especially when the transport time to the nearest hospital is short. EMS personnel should avoid giving ipecac because of the possibility of delaying definitive therapy and the potential for aspiration in the comatose or combative patient. Some clinical trials have studied the efficacy of prehospital charcoal administration documenting some clinical efficacy [13–15]. There is still a lack of definitive evidence to advocate the administration of charcoal in the prehospital setting, however. In the patient who has a depressed mental status EMS personnel should check a rapid serum glucose and administer intravenous dextrose when necessary. Small doses of naloxone may be required if opioids are highly suspected and the patient is hypoxic or suffering airway compromise. Benzodiazepines can be given for toxin-induced seizures. Prehospital intravenous sodium bicarbonate administration for known overdoses of cardiac sodium channel blocking agents (ie, cyclic antidepressants, propoxyphene, and cocaine) demonstrating a widened QRS complex on the cardiac monitor may also be considered.

The general approach

The general approach to the diagnosis and management of the poisoned patient can be described using a two-pronged model as seen in Fig. 1. In practice, the two prongs occur simultaneously. The left-sided prong begins with basic emergency medical care—the ABCs (airway, breathing, circulation). The mnemonic *DONT* stands for dextrose, oxygen, naloxone, thiamine. In most potentially poisoned patients, a rapid blood glucose measurement should be obtained and any derangements corrected. Supplemental oxygen, naloxone, and thiamine should be considered in the appropriate cases and situations. The various methods of decontamination should

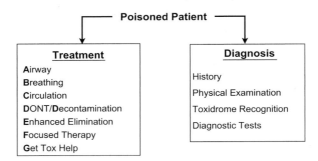

Fig. 1. The two-pronged approach to the poisoned patient.

be considered in any poisoned patient. The exact method used should be based on each individual clinical situation. Once a poisoning has been identified, methods of enhanced elimination should be considered. Focused therapy involves antidote administration when appropriate or aggressive supportive care tailored to the poison in question. Finally, when treating any poisoned patient it is prudent to consider early consultation with a toxicology service or regional poison center for further guidance.

The right-sided prong on the diagram focuses on obtaining the poisoning and other patient history, performing a focused physical examination with attention to toxidrome recognition, and deciding on the appropriate diagnostic tests to be performed. The two prongs often occur simultaneously and are integral to the diagnosis and management of the poisoned patient.

History

Historical facts should include the type of toxin or toxins, time of exposure (acute versus chronic), amount taken, and route of administration (ie, ingestion, intravenous, inhalation). It is also important to understand why the exposure occurred (accidental, suicide attempt, euphoria, therapeutic misadventure) and whether there is history of psychiatric illness or previous suicide attempts. Furthermore, it is important to inquire about all drugs taken, including prescription, over-the-counter medications, vitamins, and herbal preparations. Patients may incorrectly name the drugs they have ingested; for example, they may refer to ibuprofen as acetaminophen or vice versa. Poisoned patients can be unreliable historians, particularly if suicidal, psychotic, presenting with altered mental status, or under the influence of recreational drugs [16–18]. If unavailable from the patient, information solicited from family and friends may also prove helpful. Although issues of confidentiality may arise, it is advisable to err on the side of acting in the patient's best interest. Paramedics or emergency medical technicians are also good sources of information because they may be able to furnish details, such as the presence of empty pill bottles or drug paraphernalia that were at the scene (see Box 1 for common drugs of abuse and their respective

Box 1. Drugs of abuse and street names

Marijuana
Acapulco gold
Bhang
Doobie
Ganja
Grass
Joint
Mary Jane
Pot
Rope
Reefer

Amphetamines
Black beauties
Crank
Crystals
Cat (Methcathinone)
Ice
Ecstasy
Meth
Pep pills
Smart drug (Ritalin)
Speed
Uppers

Ecstasy
Adam
E
Lollies
Love Drug
Smarties
Vitamin E
XTC

Heroin
Boy
China white
Dust
Harry
Horse
Junk

Monkey
Smack
Speed ball (with cocaine)
Atom bomb (with marijuana)

PCP
Angel dust
Goon
Horse tranquilizer
Hog
Sherman
Tank
Wickie stick (with marijuana)

γ-hydroxybutyrate (GHB)
Bioski
Georgia home boy
Grievous bodily harm
Liquid G
Liquid ecstasy
Somatomax
Cow growth hormone

Cocaine
All American drug
Coke
Crack
Girl
Mother of pearl
Nose candy
Peruvian powder
Snow
Toot
White lady

LSD
Acid
Blotters
Microdots
Paper acid
Pyramids
Window pane
Zen

street names). In some cases it may be worthwhile to send someone to the scene to look for clues or a suicide note. Emergency personnel should inquire about the nature and progression of signs and symptoms. Further history can be obtained by consulting the patient's other physicians or by obtaining old medical records. In the case of an occupational exposure, personnel should obtain a description of the work environment and contact people at the site for relevant information.

Information regarding specific toxins may also prove useful. For example, the following may be noted following certain ingestions:

Protracted coughing with hydrocarbon ingestions
Inability to swallow or drooling with caustic ingestions
Hematemesis with iron ingestions
Intractable seizures with isoniazid overdose
Loss of consciousness with carbon monoxide

Physical examination

In the emergency setting, performing an overly detailed physical examination is a low priority compared with patient stabilization. Even a directed examination can yield important diagnostic clues, however. Once the patient is stable, a more comprehensive physical examination can reveal additional signs suggesting a specific poison. Additionally, a dynamic change in clinical appearance over time may be a more important clue than findings on a single examination. There are classic presentations that occur with specific drug classes. Even these classic presentations may not always be seen, however, and their appearance depends on the dose that the patient has ingested, the patient's premorbid condition, other substances that may have been taken, and complications that may occur in the course of the poisoning (ie, aspiration pneumonia, rhabdomyolysis, and anoxic brain injury). Emergency physicians should be aware of the classic drug syndromes that may occur, but also realize the limitations depending on other confounding factors.

Toxic vital signs

In many cases, the clinician may be able to deduce the class of drug or toxin taken simply by addressing the patient's vital signs. Mnemonics and phrases may help narrow the differential diagnosis when the patient has signs such as tachycardia, hyperthermia, or hypotension (Box 2) [19,20].

Neurologic examination

A systematic neurologic evaluation is important, particularly with patients exhibiting altered mental status. In contrast to the patient who has structural brain injury, the patient who has a toxic-metabolic cause of coma may exhibit "patchy" neurologic impairment. Toxicologic causes of

Box 2. Diagnosing toxicity from vital signs

Bradycardia (PACED)
Propranolol (beta-blockers), poppies (opiates), propoxyphene, physostigmine
Anticholinesterase drugs, antiarrhythmics
Clonidine, calcium channel blockers
Ethanol or other alcohols
Digoxin, digitalis

Tachycardia (FAST)
Free base or other forms of cocaine, freon
Anticholinergics, antihistamines, antipsychotics, amphetamines, alcohol withdrawal
Sympathomimetics (cocaine, caffeine, amphetamines, PCP), solvent abuse, strychnine
Theophylline, TCAs, thyroid hormones

Hypothermia (COOLS)
Carbon monoxide
Opioids
Oral hypoglycemics, insulin
Liquor (alcohols)
Sedative-hypnotics

Hyperthermia (NASA)
Neuroleptic malignant syndrome, nicotine
Antihistamines, alcohol withdrawal
Salicylates, sympathomimetics, serotonin syndrome
Anticholinergics, antidepressants, antipsychotics

Hypotension (CRASH)
Clonidine, calcium channel blockers
Rodenticides (containing arsenic, cyanide)
Antidepressants, aminophylline, antihypertensives
Sedative-hypnotics
Heroin or other opiates

Hypertension (CT SCAN)
Cocaine
Thyroid supplements
Sympathomimetics
Caffeine

Anticholinergics, amphetamines
Nicotine

Rapid respiration (PANT)
PCP, paraquat, pneumonitis (chemical), phosgene
ASA and other salicylates
Noncardiogenic pulmonary edema, nerve agents
Toxin-induced metabolic acidosis

Slow respiration (SLOW)
Sedative-hypnotics (barbiturates, benzodiazepines)
Liquor (alcohols)
Opioids
Weed (marijuana)

COMA
L: Lead, lithium
E: Ethanol, ethylene glycol, ethchlorvynol
T: Tricyclic antidepressants, thallium, toluene
H: Heroin, hemlock, hepatic encephalopathy, heavy metals, hydrogen sulfide, hypoglycemics
A: Arsenic, antidepressants, anticonvulsants, antipsychotics, antihistamines
R: Rohypnol (sedative hypnotics), risperidone
G: GHB
I: Isoniazid, insulin
C: Carbon monoxide, cyanide, clonidine

coma rarely cause focal neurologic deficits. These findings, along with a prolonged comatose state, loss of midbrain papillary function, and decerebrate or decorticate posturing, should prompt the clinician to evaluate for an intracranial process [21]. The Glasgow Coma Scale (GCS), although useful in head trauma victims, has a limited role in predicting the prognosis of the poisoned patient [22,23]. One recent study investigated the use of the Alert/Verbal/Painful/Unresponsive scale (AVPU) as a simple rapid method of assessing consciousness in most poisoned patients [24]. Both the GCS and AVPU scales can be used as tools to communicate level of consciousness and for evaluating the need for intubation; however, neither is suitable as a predictor of outcome in the poisoned patient.

Seizures are a common presentation of an unknown overdose, and the list of toxins that can induce a convulsion is lengthy (Box 3). Classic pupillary findings include miosis (opioids) and mydriasis (sympathomimetic agents) (Box 4). Nystagmus suggests phenytoin or phencyclidine (PCP), along with

---

Box 3. Agents that cause seizures (OTIS CAMPBELL[a])

Organophosphates, oral hypoglycemics
Tricyclic antidepressants
Isoniazid, insulin
Sympathomimetics, strychnine, salicylates
Camphor, cocaine, carbon monoxide, cyanide, chlorinated
   hydrocarbons
Amphetamines, anticholinergics
Methylxanthines (theophylline, caffeine), methanol
Phencyclidine (PCP), propranolol
Benzodiazepine withdrawal, botanicals (water hemlock, nicotine),
   bupropion, GHB
Ethanol withdrawal, ethylene glycol
Lithium, lidocaine
Lead, lindane

---

[a] Famous television "town drunk" on the Andy Griffith Show.

---

carbamazepine, lithium, ethanol, barbiturates, and sedative hypnotics. Rotary nystagmus suggests PCP toxicity, whereas vertical nystagmus represents a brainstem lesion until proven otherwise. Thiamine depletion, found in Wernicke's disease, produces ophthalmoplegia. Optic neuritis and vision loss, although seen in multiple sclerosis, may indicate advanced methanol poisoning. Other general neurologic signs include fasciculations (ie, organophosphate poisoning), rigidity (ie, tetanus and strychnine), tremors (ie, lithium and methylxanthines), speech-mumbling (ie, anticholinergics), and dystonic posturing (ie, neuroleptic agents).

Box 4. Agents that affect pupil size

Miosis (COPS)
Cholinergics, clonidine, carbamates
Opiates, organophosphates
Phenothiazines (antipsychotics), pilocarpine, pontine
   hemorrhage
Sedative-hypnotics

Mydriasis (SAW)
Sympathomimetics
Anticholinergics
Withdrawal

Skin

A careful examination of the skin should be performed. The patient's clothing should be removed and the skin assessed for color, temperature, and the presence of dryness or diaphoresis. The absence of diaphoresis is an important clinical distinction between anticholinergic and sympathomimetic poisoning. The presence of bites or similar marks may suggest spider or snake envenomations. The presence of a rash or bullae may also help provide a diagnosis. Although uncommon, bullous lesions are typically located on dependent portions of the body, such as between the fingers, knees, axilla, and back, as a result of prolonged immobility. They may be associated with any sedative hypnotic drug-induced coma, but are classically described with barbiturate poisoning [25]. Such lesions could also be indications of rhabdomyolysis or the development of compartment syndrome. A common skin finding is the presence of track marks, suggesting intravenous or subcutaneous opiate or cocaine abuse. Blue skin indicates methemoglobinemia or hypoxia; red skin may suggest niacin or boric acid exposure (Box 5). The skin examination should also include a search for pharmaceutic patches, such as opioids like fentanyl. In cases of drug abuse, these patches may be present in unusual locations, such as the vagina and scrotum.

Odors

Some poisons produce odors characteristic enough to suggest the diagnosis, such as oil of wintergreen (methylsalicylates), or garlic (organophosphate insecticides, arsenic). Some odors may be more subtle, such as the freshly mowed hay smell of phosgene or the bitter-almond scent associated with cyanide, which 30% of the population cannot detect [26]. (It is important to note that bitter almonds, which are not readily available in the United States, have a unique musty odor like dirty tennis shoes when compared with the common, or sweet, almond.) Certain odors may be overpowering and easily noted by anyone managing the patient. For example, sulfur dioxide and hydrogen sulfide produce a noxious rotten-egg smell (Table 1).

Laboratory tests

It is commonplace for many health care providers to order excessive laboratory tests when treating a poisoned patient. This testing often occurs because the offending agent is unknown or the clinician is unfamiliar with the toxin. Consultation with the regional poison center or medical toxicologist may help to narrow the scope of testing.

Routine tests

Several simple, readily available laboratory tests may provide important diagnostic clues in the symptomatic overdosed patient. These include

---

Box 5. Agents that cause skin signs

Diaphoretic skin (SOAP)
Sympathomimetics
Organophosphates
Acetylsalicylic acid or other salicylates
Phencyclidine

Dry Skin
Antihistamines, anticholinergics

Bullae
Barbiturates and other sedative-hypnotics,
Bites: Snakes and spiders

Acneiform rash
Bromides
Chlorinated aromatic hydrocarbons (dioxin)

Flushed or red appearance
Anticholinergics, niacin
Boric acid
Carbon monoxide (rare)
Cyanide (rare)

Cyanosis
Ergotamine
Nitrates
Nitrites
Aniline dyes
Phenazopyridine
Dapsone
Any agent causing hypoxemia, hypotension, or
   methemoglobinemia.

---

measurements of electrolytes, blood urea nitrogen, creatinine, serum glucose, a measured bicarbonate level, and arterial blood gases. If the patient is a female of child-bearing age, a pregnancy test is essential because these patients often overdose for suicidal or abortifacient reasons [27].

To check for anion gap metabolic acidosis, calculate the anion gap using serum mEq/L measurements:

$$Na - (Cl + HCO_3)$$

Although 8 to 12 mEq/L is traditionally accepted as the normal range for an anion gap, the measured and calculated anion gap can vary considerably

Table 1
Odors that suggest the diagnosis

Odor	Possible source
Bitter Almonds	Cyanide
Carrots	Cicutoxin (water hemlock)
Fruity	Diabetic ketoacidosis, isopropanol
Garlic	organophosphates, arsenic, dimethyl sulfoxide (DMSO), selenium
Gasoline	Petroleum distillates
Mothballs	Naphthalene, camphor
Pears	Chloral hydrate
Pungent aromatic	Ethchlorvynol
Oil of wintergreen	Methylsalicylate
Rotten eggs	Sulfur dioxide, hydrogen sulfide
Freshly mowed hay	Phosgene

[28]. When a patient presents with an elevated anion gap, the mnemonic METAL ACID GAP assists in identifying most of the common toxic causes (Box 6). In addition, knowledge of the dynamic relationship between the increase in anion gap and the decrease in bicarbonate is also important ($\Delta AG - \Delta HCO_3$) [29]. If positive and greater than 6, a metabolic alkalosis is usually present. A difference of less than 6 suggests that a hyperchloremic acidosis is present.

When a patient presents with an unexplained metabolic acidosis, a serum osmolality should be measured and the osmolal gap calculated. When an elevated osmolal gap is accompanied by anion gap acidosis immediate consideration should be given to poisoning by methanol, ethylene glycol, and other less common toxic alcohols. The osmolal gap is the difference between

---

Box 6. Agents causing an elevated anion gap (METAL ACID GAP)

Methanol, metformin, massive overdoses
Ethylene glycol
Toluene
Alcoholic ketoacidosis
Lactic acidosis
Acetaminophen (large overdoses)
Cyanide, carbon monoxide, colchicine
Isoniazid, iron, ibuprofen
Diabetic ketoacidosis
Generalized seizure-producing toxins
Acetylsalicylic acid or other salicylates
Paraldehyde, phenformin

measured serum osmolality (most accurately determined by the freezing-point depression method) and the calculated serum osmolarity, most commonly determined by the following formula:

$$2Na + \frac{Glucose}{18} + \frac{BUN}{2.8} + \frac{ETOH}{4.6}$$

An osmolal gap of 10 has been arbitrarily defined as normal. Further investigation, however, has revealed that the range of normal is approximately −15 to +10 [30]. An increase in the osmolal gap indicates the presence of a low molecular weight, osmotically active substance in the serum. The mnemonic ME DIE describes the major toxins that produce an increased osmolal gap (Box 7). It is important to understand that with toxic alcohols, the parent compound is the osmotically active component; the metabolites are not osmotically active [31]. It is generally accepted that a markedly increased osmolal gap is suggestive of toxic alcohol intoxication. Furthermore, a normal osmolal gap does not rule out toxic alcohol intoxication for several reasons: (1) the patient's baseline osmolal gap is not known; (2) as metabolism of the parent toxic alcohol compound ensues, the osmolal gap narrows (with a concomitant increase in the anion gap); (3) the contribution of any osmotically active compound to the osmolal gap is related to the compound's molecular weight. Compounds with larger molecular weights contribute less to the osmolal gap (eg, ethylene glycol has a relatively large molecular weight and a small increase in the osmolal gap results from toxic ethylene glycol levels) [30–32].

As with the calculation of ETOH/4.6, if quantitative serum levels of the other toxic alcohols are not readily available, these levels can also be estimated by using the following denominators in the above equation: methanol, 3.2; ethylene glycol, 6.2; and isopropanol, 6.0 [33].

Toxicology screens

Although technology has provided the ability to measure many toxins, most toxicologic diagnoses and therapeutic decisions are made based on historical or clinical information. The application of laboratory measurements is limited by several practical considerations: (1) laboratory turnaround time

---

Box 7. Agents increasing the osmolar gap (ME DIE)

Methanol
Ethylene glycol
Diuretics (mannitol), Diabetic ketoacidosis (acetone)
Isopropyl alcohol
Ethanol

can often be longer than the critical intervention time course of an overdose; (2) the cost and support of maintaining the instruments, staff training, and specialized labor involved in some analyses are prohibitive; (3) for many toxins there are no established cutoff levels of toxicity, making interpretation of the results difficult [34].

Although commonly ordered in a "shotgun" fashion, toxicology screens have several limitations. Most limited immunoassay screens are capable of detecting commonly abused drugs, such as marijuana and cocaine. Many other common dangerous drugs and poisons, such as isoniazid, digitalis glycosides, calcium antagonists, beta-blockers, heavy metals, and pesticides, are not routinely included. A negative screen therefore does not rule out the possibility of poisoning. Conversely, some drugs that present in therapeutic amounts, such as opioids and benzodiazepines, may be detected by the screen even though they are causing no contributing clinical symptoms. Additionally, technical limitations of the assay can cause either false-positive or false-negative results, although improvements over the past decade have rendered the tests increasingly more sensitive and specific [34–37]. Immunoassays are most widely used for discrete analyses; gas chromatography and mass spectometry techniques are used for broad screens.

The toxicology screen may have little clinical correlation if specimens are collected too early or too late for detection. Urine drug tests often detect drug metabolites and may remain positive for several days after the exposure. Blood or serum drug tests are generally positive for much shorter time periods. A comprehensive urine toxicology screen is labor intensive and intended to detect as many drugs as possible. The compounds usually detected are the alcohols, sedative hypnotics, barbiturates, benzodiazepines, anticonvulsants, antihistamines, antidepressants, antipsychotics, stimulants, opioids, cardiovascular drugs, oral hypoglycemics, and methylxanthines (caffeine, theophylline). Although comprehensive screening is unlikely to affect emergency management, the results may assist the admitting physicians in evaluating the patient if the diagnosis remains unclear [38]. Care should be given to indiscriminate ordering of such comprehensive tests; the history, physical examination, and common laboratory tests can usually narrow the differential to a few potential culprits. Additionally, potent opioids (eg, fentanyl) or sedative hypnotic agents (eg, rohypnol) may be present, but the detection limits are set too high to produce a positive result [39].

Many clinicians reflexively order a "tox screen" on all poisoned patients. This practice should be avoided. Qualitative screening panels should be used when the results will alter patient management or disposition.

Quantitative blood tests should be ordered only for those drugs or toxins for which blood levels predict toxicity or guide specific therapy. Such drugs include acetaminophen, salicylates, theophylline, lithium, lead, iron, carbon monoxide, methemoglobin, toxic alcohols, anticonvulsants, and digoxin. For unknown ingestions, a routine quantitative serum acetaminophen level is recommended because this agent is contained in many over-the-counter preparations and in overdose may not exhibit early diagnostic clues [17]. Although some sources advocate the analysis of gastric contents, this is usually reserved for forensic cases.

Urine testing

Detailed laboratory urine analysis may reveal important diagnostic clues concerning the overdosed patient. Calcium oxalate crystals are generally present in ethylene glycol poisoning. These are usually discovered late in the clinical course, however, and may be absent early in the clinical course or not detected at all if timely therapy has been instituted [40]. The Wood's lamp has been used to detect urine fluorescence following ethylene glycol ingestion [41]. More recent studies demonstrate the lack of specificity with this, however [42–44]. Urinalysis showing occult blood, with no evidence of red blood cells, suggests myoglobinuria or hemolysis. Additionally, the urinary pH is an important measurement, especially when monitoring bicarbonate therapy for salicylate overdose.

Urine color may also provide a diagnostic clue. The following are examples:

An orange to red-orange color with phenazopyridine, rifampin, deferoxamine, mercury, or chronic lead poisoning
A pink color with ampicillin or cephalosporins
A brown color with chloroquine or carbon tetrachloride
A greenish-blue color with copper sulfate or methylene blue

Radiologic studies

Abdominal films

A plain abdominal radiograph (KUB) can reveal radiopaque pills, drug-filled packets, or other toxic material. Drugs or toxins that are likely to be visible on films can be recalled by the mnemonic COINS as demonstrated in Box 8 [45].

In some cases, the vehicle in which the drug is contained, such as an enteric coating or latex, is more radiopaque than the drug itself. For this reason, a KUB may be useful in cases of body packers (drug smugglers). On the other hand, body stuffers who quickly swallow the evidence to evade the authorities typically have abdominal films that are negative for foreign body detection [46]. For many slightly radiodense drugs, such as neuroleptics and salicylates, visibility depends on the time of ingestion. A patient presenting several hours after the ingestion rarely has a positive radiograph. In practice, the KUB is probably most useful to determine the presence of a heavy metal foreign body in the gastrointestinal tract and to monitor the progress of gastrointestinal decontamination (such as whole bowel irrigation).

Box 8. Agents potentially visible on abdominal radiographs (COINS)

Chloral hydrate, cocaine packets, calcium
Opium packets
Iron; other heavy metals, such as lead, arsenic, mercury
Neuroleptic agents
Sustained-release or enteric-coated agents

Chest films

Patients who have tachypnea, hypoxia, obtundation, or coma should have a chest radiograph performed to search for potential causes of hypoxemia: chemical or aspiration pneumonitis, cardiogenic or noncardiogenic pulmonary edema (acute lung injury), and atelectasis. Drugs that can cause noncardiogenic pulmonary edema can be remembered by the mnemonic MOPS (Box 9). Chest films are also useful for detecting occasional pneumothorax or pneumomediastinum seen in patients abusing cocaine or other sympathomimetic agents.

Toxidromes

A collection of symptoms associated with certain classes of poisons is known as a toxic syndrome, or toxidrome. In patients who have unknown overdoses, a toxidrome can assist in making a diagnosis and is also useful for anticipating other symptoms that may occur. Cholinergic, anticholinergic, sympathomimetic, and narcotic agents all have characteristic toxidromes; withdrawal from many addictive agents may also produce distinctive constellations of symptoms [19]. Box 10 lists the common toxidromes. The traditional description of the anticholinergic toxidrome, for example, is "hot as a hare, dry as a bone, red as a beet, blind as a bat, mad as a hatter." (Historically, "mad as a hatter" referred to occupational mercury poisoning in the felt hat industry). Toxidromes are most clinically useful when the patient has been exposed to a single drug. When multiple drugs have been ingested, conflicting clinical effects may be present or may negate

---

Box 9. Drugs causing pneumonitis or pulmonary edema (MOPS)

Meprobamate, methadone
Opioids
Phenobarbital, propoxyphene, paraquat, phosgene
Salicylates

Box 10. Common toxidromes

Cholinergic (Examples: organophosphates, carbamates, pilocarpine)
(DUMBELLS)
    Diarrhea, diaphoresis
    Urination
    Miosis
    Bradycardia, bronchosecretions
    Emesis
    Lacrimation
    Lethargic
    Salivation

Nicotinic (recalled by the days of the week)
    Monday: Miosis
    Tuesday: Tachycardia
    Wednesday: Weakness
    Thursday: Tremors
    Friday: Fasciculations
    Saturday: Seizures
    Sunday: Somnolent

Anticholinergic (Examples: antihistamines, cyclic antidepressants, atropine, benztropine, phenothiazines, scopolamine)
Hyperthermia (HOT as a hare)
Flushed (RED as a beet)
Dry skin (DRY as a bone)
Dilated pupils (BLIND as a bat)
Delirium, hallucinations (MAD as a hatter)
Tachycardia
Urinary urgency and retention

Sympathomimetic (Examples: cocaine, amphetamines, ephedrine, phencyclidine, pseudoephedrine)
Mydriasis
Tachycardia
Hypertension
Hyperthermia
Seizures

Opioid (Examples: heroin, morphine, codeine, methadone, fentanyl, oxycodone, hydrocodone)
Miosis

Bradycardia
Hypotension
Hypoventilation
Coma

Withdrawal
Diarrhea
Mydriasis
Goose flesh
Tachycardia
Lacrimation
Hypertension
Yawning
Cramps
Hallucinations
Seizures (with alcohol and benzodiazepine withdrawal)

each other and cloud the clinical picture. In addition, the clinical onset of a specific toxic agent may be delayed when multiple substances have been ingested concomitantly. Toxidrome recognition can improve the efficiency of drug screening when these findings are communicated to laboratory personnel [47].

Treatment

The management of any clinically significant poisoning should begin with basic supportive measures. Most poisoned patients do well with supportive care alone.

ABCs

Most poisoned patients are awake and have stable vital signs. Some patients may present with an altered state of consciousness, hemodynamic instability, or active convulsions. The first priority is to stabilize the ABCs and manage life-threatening complications. When intubation is necessary, rapid sequence induction is indicated with a preference toward using short-acting paralytic agents. The emphasis should be placed on short-acting paralytics for fear of masking toxin-induced seizures. For cases in which hyperkalemia or poisoning with cholinesterase inhibitors is suspected, non-depolarizing agents are preferred.

A patient's oxygenation status can be monitored with a bedside pulse oximeter. Certain toxins, however, may demonstrate a normal pulse oximetry reading despite severe poisoning. This observation is particularly true in carbon monoxide poisoning, in which the pulse oximeter is unreliable in detecting carboxyhemoglobin [48]. The pulse oximeter only provides information regarding oxygen saturation and does not assess acid–base status. It should not be used as a substitute for obtaining an arterial blood gas or serum bicarbonate level when such information is clinically warranted.

Intravenous access should be considered in all potentially poisoned patients. This practice should be maintained even when the patient seems stable and asymptomatic. Many toxins produce delayed effects, such as hypotension or seizures, that could make obtaining intravenous access difficult.

The poisoned patient should be kept under close observation with frequent evaluations of the level of consciousness, oxygenation status, and vital signs. This observation is important, particularly with the patient who presents in a stable condition, because continued absorption of an ingested substance may lead to delayed clinical evidence of poisoning. An electrocardiogram and continuous cardiac monitoring are indicated for any agent with potential cardiac toxicity. Examples include sympathomimetic agents, cyclic antidepressants, cardiac glycosides, beta-blockers, calcium channel antagonists, antihypertensive agents, arsenic, cyanide, carbon monoxide, antidysrhythmics, citalopram, diphenhydramine, venlafaxine, chloral hydrate, methylxanthines, propoxyphene, phenothiazines, and quinine. An electrocardiogram should also be routinely obtained in patients who have polysubstance ingestions and in cases of unknown suicidal ingestions. Unlike patients who have chronic cardiopulmonary diseases whose condition worsens progressively, the poisoned patient may unexpectedly become unstable.

The patient who has an unknown poisoning may present convulsing or with a history of seizure activity. Toxin-induced seizures tend to be global central nervous system (CNS) processes as opposed to focal processes like those seen in patients who have epilepsy or CNS structural lesions [49]. Benzodiazepines, barbiturates, and valproic acid, therefore, are considered the first- and second-line therapies for toxin-induced seizures [49]. Phenytoin is generally not effective in treating toxin-induced seizures or seizures from alcohol or sedative-hypnotic withdrawal [49].

The "coma cocktail"

The "coma cocktail" refers to the empiric administration of certain medications or delivery of interventions to patients who present with unconsciousness or coma. The most common components of the coma cocktail are dextrose, naloxone, and thiamine. Flumazenil and physostigmine are sometimes included also. The approach to the unconscious poisoned patient, however, should be deliberate; empiric therapy should be used with caution.

Many toxins can potentially cause hypoglycemia. A rapid capillary glucose measurement should be obtained in all comatose patients.

Hypoglycemia should be rapidly corrected with a dextrose bolus. In situations in which a capillary glucose measurement cannot be performed, it is reasonable to administer dextrose empirically. Although some sources caution against giving a hypertonic glucose bolus to patients who have acute cerebral ischemia, this concern is probably unwarranted [50,51].

Naloxone, an opiate antagonist, may have therapeutic and diagnostic value. Patients who have opioid overdose usually become fully awake soon after its administration. If the clinical picture is consistent with the opioid toxidrome, 0.4 to 2 mg of naloxone may be given by intravenous infusion [52]. Tolerant or chronic opioid abusers typically require smaller amounts of the antidote for effect. Patients who overdose on certain potent or resistant opioids may need larger doses of naloxone. These opioids include diphenoxylate, propoxyphene, pentazocine, codeine, and fentanyl [53–55]. Although the literature is largely anecdotal, up to 10 mg of naloxone may be required in such cases [53–55]. Naloxone can precipitate acute opiate withdrawal in the opioid-dependent patient. Caution should be exercised because acute withdrawal can be accompanied by belligerence and violence [56]. Fortunately, naloxone has a short half-life, and withdrawal symptoms wear off in 1 or 2 hours. The naloxone dose should be titrated until the desired response is achieved. With long-acting opioids, an intravenous naloxone infusion dip may be required. The hourly infusion rate is two thirds of the dose required to awaken the patient. This dose is variable depending on the time of exposure and the patient's level of tolerance. If necessary, naloxone can be given intralingually, endotracheally, or subcutaneously [57]. Recently, a fatal North American fentanyl epidemic has been described, resulting in medical centers depleting their stock of naloxone [39].

Nalmefene is a long-acting opioid antagonist with a half life of approximately 10 hours. The long-lasting effect could reduce the need for continuous monitoring and repeated dosing of naloxone in opioid-intoxicated patients. The long duration of action, however, may lead to unnecessarily extended withdrawal signs and symptoms in opioid-dependent patients [58]. For this reason, cautious and limited use of nalmefene in the emergency department is warranted.

The administration of thiamine should be reserved for alcoholic patients who are malnourished. Giving thiamine to every comatose patient in an attempt to prevent Wernicke's encephalopathy is probably unwarranted [50]. Additionally, intravenous thiamine carries a small but significant risk for anaphylactoid reactions [59].

Flumazenil, a benzodiazepine antagonist, can rapidly reverse coma in benzodiazepine overdose. The drug may also induce seizures in patients who have mixed drug overdoses, however, such as cyclic antidepressant or sympathomimetic agents; it may provoke acute withdrawal in those addicted to benzodiazepines. Flumazenil should therefore be used judiciously and not administered routinely as part of the coma cocktail [60–64].

Physostigmine should not be empirically administered as part of a coma cocktail in a comatose patient who has an unknown cause. It is indicated in the case of isolated, severe anticholinergic poisoning. It is contraindicated with tricyclic antidepressant overdoses because it may exacerbate cardiotoxicity [65]. Recently, physostigmine has been recommended in potential GHB poisoning; however, efficacy in this setting is controversial [66].

Skin and eye decontamination

Data regarding proper decontamination methods are limited, but fundamental principles can be found in military chemical battlefield and radiation accident protocols [67]. If possible, hazardous materials–type decontamination is best performed in the prehospital setting. In patients who have dermal exposures, all clothing should be removed and the skin copiously irrigated and washed with a mild soap and water. The use of hot water, strong detergents, or harsh abrasives should be avoided [67]. Decontamination should not be delayed while awaiting identification of the offending agent. Emergency care providers should wear gloves, water-resistant gowns, splash-resistant goggles, and masks to protect themselves from dermal exposure. Ocular exposures to acids and alkali can be devastating. The eye should be copiously irrigated with several liters of normal saline solution and the pH of the conjunctiva closely monitored before starting other therapeutic or diagnostic interventions [7].

Gastrointestinal decontamination

Gastrointestinal decontamination is the process of preventing or reducing absorption of a substance after it has been ingested. Controversy exists concerning the roles of induced emesis, gastric lavage, activated charcoal, and cathartics in decontaminating the gastrointestinal tract. Individual circumstances determine which technique is the most appropriate in a given clinical situation [68,69]. Several experimental and clinical trials have examined gastric emptying techniques; their overall effectiveness remains limited. Regardless of the method of gastric decontamination, a significant amount of toxin remains and is available for absorption [70].

Ipecac-induced emesis

Once a preferred technique for gastric emptying, syrup of ipecac is no longer recommended for use in the emergency department [2]. Research has demonstrated no improvement in clinical outcome with its use [2]. Furthermore, the persistent vomiting that often occurs after ingestion of syrup of ipecac may delay other modes of therapy, such as administration of activated charcoal. Currently there is no role for syrup of ipecac in the prehospital management of poisonings. In 2003, the American Academy of Pediatrics issued a statement that ipecac should no longer be used routinely as a home treatment strategy and that existing ipecac in the home should be disposed of safely [71]. On June 12, 2003, the FDA Nonprescription Drugs Advisory Committee met to discuss whether there is sufficient evidence of the benefits of ipecac syrup to outweigh the potential for misuse, abuse, and adverse effects associated with it as an over-the-counter drug. At the conclusion of the meeting, the committee recommended by a six to four vote that the FDA rescind ipecac's over-the-counter status. There is no reduction in resource use or improvement in patient outcome from the use of syrup of ipecac at home. [72] The American Heart Association First Aid Task Force has made the administration of syrup of ipecac a Class III Action (more harm than benefit).

Gastric lavage

In the early 1800's Edward Jukes, a British surgeon, performed gastric lavage on himself following an ingestion of laudanum (a tincture of opium). Aside from mild gastrointestinal upset followed by a 3-hour nap, he survived with no adverse side effects. The experiment was considered a success [73]. Gastric lavage currently involves inserting a large-bore, 36- to 40-French orogastric tube. The patient should be placed in the left lateral decubitus position with the head of the bed in the Trendelenburg position. The procedure is performed by instilling approximately 250 mL (10 mL/kg in pediatric patients) of water or saline with immediate lavage of that same quantity of fluid. The technique is repeated until the recovered solution is clear of particulate matter or pill fragments [3].

Gastric lavage is no longer indicated for most ingestions [3]. Gastric lavage may be considered if a patient has ingested a potentially life-threatening amount of a toxin and presents within 1 hour of ingestion [3,74–79]. Even in this scenario, however, there is no clear evidence that its use improves clinical outcome. Gastric lavage should not be performed when a patient has ingested a corrosive substance or a volatile hydrocarbon. It should never be used as a punitive measure in cases of nontoxic overdoses or forced on patients who are combative or otherwise uncooperative. Additionally, endotracheal intubation solely to perform gastric lavage is discouraged; the decision to intubate should be independent of the decision to perform gastric lavage. Orogastric lavage is not a benign procedure and has been associated with aspiration, esophageal perforation, epistaxis, hypothermia, and death [3].

Activated charcoal

The nineteenth-century French pharmacist P.F. Tourey demonstrated the beneficial effects of charcoal when he ingested a potentially life-threatening amount of strychnine mixed with a primitive charcoal preparation in front of the French Academy of Medicine. He survived but remained underappreciated by his peers [80]. Recent evidence suggests that activated charcoal is more effective than induced emesis or gastric lavage for gastric decontamination [4]. As a result, activated charcoal administration has become the preferred method of decontamination for most poisons and is most effective when administered early after the ingestion [4]. Its routine administration in nontoxic ingestions is not indicated.

Several activated charcoal products are commercially available. Regardless of the brand, it is important to ensure the activated charcoal is thoroughly resuspended in water to achieve a 25% concentration before use. Although commonly dosed at 1 g/kg body weight, the more appropriate dose is a 10:1 ratio of activated charcoal to toxin [70]. If this dose cannot be achieved in a single dose, then serial dosing may be required.

Although studies have demonstrated reduced drug absorption with activated charcoal use, it is important to note that there is no evidence that administration of activated charcoal improves patient outcome [4]. The use of activated charcoal is contraindicated when airway reflexes are not intact or protected [4].

Multiple dose activated charcoal (MDAC) is a potential method of enhanced elimination. Some drugs undergo enterohepatic and enteroenteric recirculation. MDAC can interrupt enterohepatic and enteroenteric recirculation when such drugs have been absorbed, acting as "gut dialysis." Box 11 provides a memory aid for the drugs that may be removed using MDAC. There is no standard dose for MDAC administration. Twenty-five grams every 2 to 4 hours is a reasonable regimen. It is important that a cathartic (such as sorbitol) is not administered with MDAC because serious electrolyte abnormalities may result.

Box 11. Agents responsive to multiple doses of activated charcoal

Substances adsorbable by activated charcoal (ABCD)
Antimalarials (quinine), aminophylline (theophylline)
Barbiturates (phenobarbital)
Carbamazepine
Dapsone

Substances not adsorbable by activated charcoal (PHAILS)
Pesticides, potassium
Hydrocarbons
Acids, alkali, alcohols
Iron, insecticides
Lithium
Solvents

The substances not well adsorbed by charcoal can be recalled by the mnemonic PHAILS as listed in Box 11. The most common side effect of activated charcoal administration is constipation [4]. When given with sorbitol, gastrointestinal upset with diarrhea may result [4]. Complications of activated charcoal administration, although uncommon, include pneumonitis if aspirated, bowel obstruction, and perforation [81,82]. The reported adverse events following single-dose activated charcoal administration are few, but as with any medical intervention, a risk-to-benefit comparison should be carefully assessed [83].

Cathartics

The efficacy of cathartic use in reducing the absorption or increasing the elimination of toxins has not been established [5]. There are no published data demonstrating an improved outcome with cathartic use alone or combined with activated charcoal [5]. Cathartics, typically sorbitol, are often used with activated charcoal to reduce the gastrointestinal transit time of the toxin–charcoal mixture; however, this has not been shown to improve decontamination efficacy. Cathartic use alone has no role in the management of the poisoned patient [5]. Sorbitol may have a role in increasing charcoal therapy compliance because the sweet taste may make the activated charcoal more palatable.

A single dose of a cathartic, such as sorbitol, is typically well-tolerated. Repetitive dosing, however, can lead to serious complications. Large doses of sorbitol, especially in the extremes of age, have been associated with electrolyte imbalance and dehydration [70]. This finding is particularly important when considering multiple-dose activated charcoal because many commercially-available charcoal products contain sorbitol, and repeated doses of sorbitol may be inadvertently administered. Magnesium-containing cathartics may cause hypermagnesemia, particularly in patients who have renal insufficiency. Cathartic use should be avoided in patients who have diarrhea, ileus, recent bowel surgery, and electrolyte imbalance. Sodium-containing cathartics should be avoided in patients who have renal disease or cardiac failure [5].

Whole bowel irrigation

Whole bowel irrigation (WBI) is the process of using a large volume of a polyethylene glycol solution to clean the gastrointestinal tract by mechanical action without affecting the fluid or electrolyte balance [6]. A similar, although less rigorous, procedure has been well established to prepare patients for surgical or endoscopic procedures. Although volunteer studies have demonstrated decreased bioavailability of certain drugs using WBI, there is currently no conclusive evidence that WBI improves clinical outcome of poisoned patients [6]. In patients who are hemodynamically stable and have normal bowel function and anatomy, it is reasonable to consider using WBI with ingestions of the following substances: heavy metals, lithium, sustained-release and enteric-coated products, and substances not adsorbed by charcoal. Whole bowel irrigation may also be considered when the patient has ingested drug-filled packets or other potentially toxic foreign bodies.

Whole bowel irrigation is performed by placing a nasogastric tube and administering 1 to 2 L/h (25–50 mL/kg/h in pediatric patients) of the polyethylene glycol solution. WBI should be continued until the rectal effluent is clear. In most patients, this usually occurs within 4 to 6 hours. This procedure is generally well tolerated by most patients and has been used safely in children [6].

Antidotal therapy

The number of effective antidotes is limited and they are not for indiscriminate use. Table 2 lists selected antidotes and the substances for which they are indicated. As Paracelsus observed, all xenobiotics are potentially toxic. This observation is true for purported antidotes also. Antidotal therapy should be used carefully and in clinical circumstances when specifically indicated. With the exception of naloxone, antidotal therapy use is limited in the patient who has an unknown poisoning [84]. The clinician should be familiar with the indications for use and the availability of antidotal therapy [84]. Although administering so-called "life-saving" antidotes is often considered to be the glamorous aspect of clinical toxicology, antidotal therapy is used in a minority of poisonings. Most poisoned patients have an uneventful recovery when routine supportive care is appropriately provided.

Table 2
Antidotes and their indications

Antidote	Indication (agent)
n-acetylcysteine	Acetaminophen
Ethanol/fomepizole (4-MP)	Methanol/ethylene glycol
Oxygen/hyperbarics	Carbon monoxide
Naloxone/nalmefene	Opioids
Physostigmine	Anticholinergics
Atropine/pralidoxime (2-PAM)	Organophosphates
Methylene blue	Methemoglobinemia
Nitrites	Cyanide
Deferoxamine	Iron
Dimercaprol (BAL)	Arsenic
Succimer (DMSA)	Lead, mercury
Fab fragments	Digoxin, colchicine, crotalids
Glucagon	Beta-blockers
Sodium bicarbonate	Tricyclic antidepressants
Calcium/insulin/dextrose	Calcium channel antagonists
Dextrose, glucagon, octreotide	Oral hypoglycemics

Enhanced elimination

Enhancing elimination is the process of removing a toxin from the body once absorption has already occurred. Methods of enhanced elimination include multiple-dose activated charcoal, urinary alkalinization, and extracorporeal elimination. The role of multiple-dose activated charcoal was discussed previously. Urinary alkalinization involved the use of an intravenous sodium bicarbonate infusion and promotes urinary elimination of substances that are weak acids. It is important to maintain a normal potassium level when performing alkalinization because appropriate alkalinization cannot be achieved when hypokalemia is present. A common use of urinary alkalinization is in the salicylate-poisoned patient. Another use may be in patients who overdose on phenobarbital, although no outcome data has demonstrated this to be beneficial in terms of survivability. As an aside, urinary acidification has been recommended in the past as a method of enhanced elimination with poisoning by weak bases, such as phencyclidine and amphetamine. This procedure is no longer recommended because of the high risk for myoglobinuria and rhabdomyolysis [85].

Extracorporeal elimination

In the unstable poisoned patient, consultation with a nephrologist may be indicated before definitive diagnostic studies or drug levels become available. This consultation is particularly important when the suspected agent is a salicylate, lithium, theophylline, or a toxic alcohol (Box 12). Hemodialysis enhances removal of substances with low protein binding, small volumes of distribution, high water solubility, and low molecular weight. Charcoal hemoperfusion, if available, may be useful for theophylline, barbiturates, and carbamazepine overdose (Box 13) [86,87].

Box 12. Toxins accessible to hemodialysis (UNSTABLE)

Uremia
No response to conventional therapy
Salicylates
Theophylline
Alcohols (isopropanol, methanol)
Boric acid, barbiturates
Lithium
Ethylene glycol

Box 13. Enhanced elimination by charcoal hemoperfusion

Theophylline
Barbiturates
Carbamazepine
Paraquat
Glutethimide

Cutting-edge toxicology

The latest toxicology antidotes include fomepizole for ethylene glycol and methanol poisoning [88–90], specific immune therapy with purified Fab fragments for rattlesnake antivenin [91–94], and high-dose insulin for calcium channel antagonist poisoning [95,96]

Current controversies include challenging the widely accepted 72-hour oral *n*-acetylcysteine (NAC) treatment course for acetaminophen toxicity. Many are now suggesting a more abbreviated regimen [97]. An intravenous form of NAC has recently been approved by the US Food and Drug Administration for use in the United States [98,99]. This is a 21-hour infusion protocol with the total administered NAC dose of 300 mg/kg.

There continues to be controversy about the use of hyperbaric oxygen therapy for carbon monoxide–poisoned patients. Two recent studies show conflicting results [100,101]. Each study used distinctly different treatment protocols, which makes comparison difficult. The current Cochrane Database concludes that existing randomized trials do not establish whether the administration of HBO to patients who have carbon monoxide poisoning reduces the incidence of adverse neurologic outcomes [102].

Emergent orthotropic liver transplantation is currently the only standard treatment of fulminant hepatic failure. There is often a prolonged wait time for transplantation. The concept of a liver support device ("liver dialysis") may in the future provide a bridge to transplantation or potential recovery without transplantation [103]. Currently there are few studies in this area, especially with application in the poisoned patient, but liver support devices may play a future role in poisoned patients. Finally, the use of intravenous fat or lipid emulsion is showing promise with lipid soluble drug toxicity to treat cardiotoxicity and hemodynamic instability. Recent efficacy has been demonstrated in an animal model and in isolated human cases [104,105].

Disposition

People who have a potentially serious overdose should be observed for several hours before discharge. If signs or symptoms of intoxication develop during that time, the patient should be admitted for further observation and treatment. Some agents may require a more prolonged observation period. Such agents include sustained-release products and agents with known delayed or prolonged onset of action: calcium channel antagonists, theophylline, lithium, methadone, Lomotil, monoamine oxidase inhibitors, and oral hypoglycemic agents. Overdose with these substances may require up to 24 hours of continuous observation [106]. Although some patients admitted require observation in an intensive care unit, others can be appropriately managed on the general medical floor or in an observation unit. Consultation with a medical toxicologist or regional poison control center can help to determine the appropriate disposition.

Because many poisoned patients require less than 24 hours of observation, unnecessary hospitalization may be avoided by the use of observation units. Such units have already been developed for asthma and chest pain patients. This model may also work well for poisoned patients.

All patients presenting with an intentional poisoning should have a psychiatric evaluation and will likely require psychiatric admission. Substance abusers should be considered for drug abuse counseling.

Summary

The management of the poisoned patient who has an unknown exposure can be diagnostically and therapeutically challenging. The history and physical examination, along with a small dose of detective work, can often provide the clues to the appropriate diagnosis. The two-pronged approach as outlined in Fig. 1 provides a framework for evaluating poisoned patients. Consultation with a regional poison center or clinical toxicologist early in the care of poisoned patient can have a profound impact on the management and disposition of such patients.

References

[1] Erickson T. Managing the patient's unknown overdose ingestion. Emerg Med 1996;28: 74–88.

[2] Position paper: ipecac syrup. J Toxicol Clin Toxicol 2004;42:133–43.

[3] Vale JA, Kulig K. Position paper: gastric lavage. J Toxicol Clin Toxicol 2004;42:933–43.

[4] Chyka PA, Seger D, Krenzelok EP, et al. Position paper: single-dose activated charcoal. Clin Toxicol (Phila) 2005;43:61–87.

[5] American Academy of Clinical Toxicology. Position paper: cathartics. J Toxicol Clin Toxicol 2004;42:243–53.

[6] American Academy of Clinical Toxicology. Position paper: whole bowel irrigation. J Toxicol Clin Toxicol 2004;42:843–54.

[7] American Academy of Clinical Toxicology. Clinical policy for the initial approach to patients presenting with acute toxic ingestion or dermal or inhalation exposure. American College of Emergency Physicians. Ann Emerg Med 1995;25:570–85.

[8] Watson WA, Litovitz TL, Rodgers GCJ, et al. 2004 Annual report of the American Association of Poison Control Centers Toxic Exposure Surveillance System. Am J Emerg Med 2005;23:589–666.

[9] Hoppe-Roberts JM, Lloyd LM, Chyka PA. Poisoning mortality in the United States: comparison of national mortality statistics and poison control center reports. Ann Emerg Med 2000;35:440–8.

[10] Polivka BJ, Elliott MB, Wolowich WR. Comparison of poison exposure data: NHIS and TESS data. J Toxicol Clin Toxicol 2002;40:839–45.

[11] Deichmann WB, Henschler D, Holmsted B, et al. What is there that is not poison? A study of the Third Defense by Paracelsus. Arch Toxicol 1986;58:207–13.

[12] Watson W, Rose R. Pharmacokinetics and toxicokinetics. In: Ford M, Delaney KA, Ling L, et al, editors. Clinical toxicology. Philadelphia: Saunders; 2001.

[13] Crockett R, Krishel SJ, Manoguerra A, et al. Prehospital use of activated charcoal: a pilot study. J Emerg Med 1996;14:335–8.

[14] Greene SL, Kerins M, O'Connor N. Prehospital activated charcoal: the way forward. Emerg Med J 2005;22:734–7.

[15] Wax PM, Cobaugh DJ. Prehospital gastrointestinal decontamination of toxic ingestions: a missed opportunity. Am J Emerg Med 1998;16:114–6.

[16] Taylor RL, Cohan SL, White JD. Comprehensive toxicology screening in the emergency department: an aid to clinical diagnosis. Am J Emerg Med 1985;3:507–11.

[17] Sporer KA, Khayam-Bashi H. Acetaminophen and salicylate serum levels in patients with suicidal ingestion or altered mental status. Am J Emerg Med 1996;14:443–6.

[18] Christmas JT, Knisely JS, Dawson KS, et al. Comparison of questionnaire screening and urine toxicology for detection of pregnancy complicated by substance use. Obstet Gynecol 1992;80:750–4.

[19] Mokhlesi B, Leiken JB, Murray P, et al. Adult toxicology in critical care: part I: general approach to the intoxicated patient. Chest 2003;123:577–92.

[20] Erickson T, Aks S, Gussow L, et al. Toxicology diagnosis and management: a rational approach to managing the poisoned patient. Emergency Medicine Practice 2001; 17:676–80.

[21] Delaney KA, Kolecki P. Approach to the poisoned patient with central nervous system depression. In: Ford M, Delaney K, Ling L, et al, editors. Clinical toxicology. Philadelphia: Saunders; 2001. p. 137–45.

[22] Erickson TB, Koenigsberg M, Bunney EB, et al. Prehospital severity scoring at major rock concert events. Prehospital Disaster Med 1997;12:195–9.

[23] Merigian KS, Hedges JR, Roberts JR, et al. Use of abbreviated mental status examination in the initial assessment of overdose patients. Arch Emerg Med 1988;5: 139–45.

[24] Kelly CA, Upex A, Bateman DN. Comparison of consciousness level assessment in the poisoned patient using the alert/verbal/painful/unresponsive scale and the Glasgow Coma Scale. Ann Emerg Med 2004;44:108–13.

[25] Beveridge GW, Lawson AA. Occurrence of bullous lesions in acute barbiturate intoxication. Br Med J 1965;1:835–7.

[26] Gonzalez ER. Cyanide evades some noses, overpowers others. JAMA 1982;248:2211.

[27] Perrone J, Hoffman RS. Toxic ingestions in pregnancy: abortifacient use in a case series of pregnant overdose patients. Acad Emerg Med 1997;4:206–9.

[28] Roberts WL, Paulson WD. Method-specific reference intervals for serum anion gap and osmolality. Clin Chem 1998;44:1582.

[29] Wrenn K. The delta (delta) gap: an approach to mixed acid-base disorders. Ann Emerg Med 1990;19:1310–3.

[30] Hoffman RS, Smilkstein MJ, Howland MA, et al. Osmol gaps revisited: normal values and limitations. J Toxicol Clin Toxicol 1993;31:81–93.

[31] Glaser DS. Utility of the serum osmol gap in the diagnosis of methanol or ethylene glycol ingestion. Ann Emerg Med 1996;27:343–6.

[32] Steinhart B. Case report: severe ethylene glycol intoxication with normal osmolal gap–"a chilling thought". J Emerg Med 1990;8:583–5.

[33] Trummel J, Ford M, Austin P. Ingestion of an unknown alcohol. Ann Emerg Med 1996;27: 368–74.
[34] Osterloh JD. Utility and reliability of emergency toxicologic testing. Emerg Med Clin North Am 1990;8:693–723.
[35] Brett AS. Implications of discordance between clinical impression and toxicology analysis in drug overdose. Arch Intern Med 1988;148:437–41.
[36] Belson MG, Simon HK. Utility of comprehensive toxicologic screens in children. Am J Emerg Med 1999;17:221–4.
[37] Kellermann AL, Fihn SD, LoGerfo JP, et al. Utilization and yield of drug screening in the emergency department. Am J Emerg Med 1988;6:14–20.
[38] Osterloh JD. Laboratory testing in emergency toxicology. In: Ford M, Delaney K, Ling L, et al, editors. Clinical toxicology. Philadelphia: Saunders; 2001. p. 51–60.
[39] Drummer OH. Recent trends in narcotic deaths. Ther Drug Monit 2005;27:738–40.
[40] Haupt MC, Zull DN, Adams SL. Massive ethylene glycol poisoning without evidence of crystalluria: a case for early intervention. J Emerg Med 1988;6:295–300.
[41] Winter ML, Ellis MD, Snodgrass WR. Urine fluorescence using a Wood's lamp to detect the antifreeze additive sodium fluorescein: a qualitative adjunctive test in suspected ethylene glycol ingestions. Ann Emerg Med 1990;19:663–7.
[42] Wallace KL, Suchard JR, Curry SC, et al. Diagnostic use of physicians' detection of urine fluorescence in a simulated ingestion of sodium fluorescein-containing antifreeze. Ann Emerg Med 2001;38:49–54.
[43] Casavant MJ, Shah MN, Battels R. Does fluorescent urine indicate antifreeze ingestion by children? Pediatrics 2001;107:113–4.
[44] Parsa T, Cunningham SJ, Wall SP, et al. The usefulness of urine fluorescence for suspected antifreeze ingestion in children. Am J Emerg Med 2005;23:787–92.
[45] Savitt DL, Hawkins HH, Roberts JR. The radiopacity of ingested medications. Ann Emerg Med 1987;16:331–9.
[46] June R, Aks SE, Keys N, et al. Medical outcome of cocaine bodystuffers. J Emerg Med 2000;18:221–4.
[47] Nice A, Leikin JB, Maturen A, et al. Toxidrome recognition to improve efficiency of emergency urine drug screens. Ann Emerg Med 1988;17:676–80.
[48] Buckley RG, Aks SE, Eshom JL, et al. The pulse oximetry gap in carbon monoxide intoxication. Ann Emerg Med 1994;24:252–5.
[49] Wills B, Erickson T. Drug- and toxin-associated seizures. Med Clin North Am 2005;89: 1297–321.
[50] Hoffman RS, Goldfrank LR. The poisoned patient with altered consciousness. Controversies in the use of a "coma cocktail." JAMA 1995;274:562–9.
[51] Browning RG, Olson DW, Stueven HA, et al. 50% dextrose: antidote or toxin? Ann Emerg Med 1990;19:683–7.
[52] Hoffman JR, Schriger DL, Luo JS. The empiric use of naloxone in patients with altered mental status: a reappraisal. Ann Emerg Med 1991;20:246–52.
[53] Sporer KA. Acute heroin overdose. Ann Intern Med 1999;130:584–90.
[54] Goldfrank L, Weisman RS, Errick JK, et al. A dosing nomogram for continuous infusion intravenous naloxone. Ann Emerg Med 1986;15:566–70.
[55] Stahl SM, Kasser IS. Pentazocine overdose. Ann Emerg Med 1983;12:28–31.
[56] Gaddis GM, Watson WA. Naloxone-associated patient violence: an overlooked toxicity? Ann Pharmacother 1992;26:196–8.
[57] Wanger K, Brough L, Macmillan I, et al. Intravenous vs subcutaneous naloxone for out-of-hospital management of presumed opioid overdose. Acad Emerg Med 1998;5:293–9.
[58] Wang DS, Sternbach G, Varon J. Nalmefene: a long-acting opioid antagonist. Clinical applications in emergency medicine. J Emerg Med 1998;16:471–5.
[59] Johri S, Shetty S, Soni A, et al. Anaphylaxis from intravenous thiamine—long forgotten? Am J Emerg Med 2000;18:642–3.

[60] Votey SR, Bosse GM, Bayer MJ, et al. Flumazenil: a new benzodiazepine antagonist. Ann Emerg Med 1991;20:181–8.

[61] Lheureux P, Vranckx M, Leduc D, et al. Flumazenil in mixed benzodiazepine/tricyclic antidepressant overdose: a placebo-controlled study in the dog. Am J Emerg Med 1992; 10:184–8.

[62] Spivey WH, Roberts JR, Derlet RW. A clinical trial of escalating doses of flumazenil for reversal of suspected benzodiazepine overdose in the emergency department. Ann Emerg Med 1993;22:1813–21.

[63] Gueye PN, Hoffman JR, Taboulet P, et al. Empiric use of flumazenil in comatose patients: limited applicability of criteria to define low risk. Ann Emerg Med 1996;27:730–5.

[64] Barnett R, Grace M, Boothe P, et al. Flumazenil in drug overdose: randomized, placebo-controlled study to assess cost effectiveness. Crit Care Med 1999;27:78–81.

[65] Pentel P, Peterson CD. Asystole complicating physostigmine treatment of tricyclic antidepressant overdose. Ann Emerg Med 1980;9:588–90.

[66] Bania TC, Chu J. Physostigmine does not effect arousal but produces toxicity in an animal model of severe gamma-hydroxybutyrate intoxication. Acad Emerg Med 2005; 12:185–9.

[67] Kirk MA. Managing patients with hazardous chemical contamination. In: Ford M, Delaney K, Ling L, et al, editors. Clinical toxicology. Philadelphia: Saunders; 2001. p. 115–26.

[68] Kulig K. Initial management of ingestions of toxic substances. N Engl J Med 1992;326: 1677–81.

[69] Erickson TB, Goldfrank LR, Kulig K. How to treat the poisoned patient. Patient Care 1997;90:90–113.

[70] Nejman G, Hoekstra J, Kelley M. Journal club: gastric emptying in the poisoned patient. Am J Emerg Med 1990;8:265–9.

[71] American Academy of Pediatrics Committee on injury, violence, and poison prevention. Poison treatment in the home. Pediatrics 2003;112:1182–5.

[72] Bond GR. Home syrup of ipecac use does not reduce emergency department use or improve outcome. Pediatrics 2003;112:1061–4.

[73] Moore SW. A case of poisoning by laudanum successfully treated by means of a Juke's syringe. New York Medical Physician Journal 1835;4:91–2.

[74] Tenenbein M, Cohen S, Sitar DS. Efficacy of ipecac-induced emesis, orogastric lavage, and activated charcoal for acute drug overdose. Ann Emerg Med 1987;16:838–41.

[75] Comstock EG, Boisaubin EV, Comstock BS, et al. Assessment of the efficacy of activated charcoal following gastric lavage in acute drug emergencies. J Toxicol Clin Toxicol 1982;19: 149–65.

[76] Bosse GM, Barefoot JA, Pfeifer MP, et al. Comparison of three methods of gut decontamination in tricyclic antidepressant overdose. J Emerg Med 1995;13:203–9.

[77] Merigian KS, Woodard M, Hedges JR, et al. Prospective evaluation of gastric emptying in the self-poisoned patient. Am J Emerg Med 1990;8:479–83.

[78] Pond SM, Lewis-Driver DJ, Williams GM, et al. Gastric emptying in acute overdose: a prospective randomised controlled trial. Med J Aust 1995;163:345–9.

[79] Kulig K, Bar-Or D, Cantrill SV, et al. Management of acutely poisoned patients without gastric emptying. Ann Emerg Med 1985;14:562–7.

[80] Holt LEJ, Holz PH. The black bottle. A consideration of the role of charcoal in the treatment of poisoning in children. J Pediatr 1963;63:306–14.

[81] Moll J, Kerns Wn, Tomaszewski C, et al. Incidence of aspiration pneumonia in intubated patients receiving activated charcoal. J Emerg Med 1999;17:279–83.

[82] Gomez HF, Brent JA, Munoz DCt, et al. Charcoal stercolith with intestinal perforation in a patient treated for amitriptyline ingestion. J Emerg Med 1994;12:57–60.

[83] Seger D. Single-dose activated charcoal-backup and reassess. J Toxicol Clin Toxicol 2004; 42:101–10.

[84] Woolf AD, Chrisanthus K. On-site availability of selected antidotes: results of a survey of Massachusetts hospitals. Am J Emerg Med 1997;15:62–6.

[85] Patel R, Connor G. A review of thirty cases of rhabdomyolysis-associated acute renal failure among phencyclidine users. J Toxicol Clin Toxicol 1985;23:547–56.

[86] Pond SM. Extracorporeal techniques in the treatment of poisoned patients. Med J Aust 1991;154:617–22.

[87] Winchester JF. Use of dialysis and hemoperfusion in the treatment of poisonings. In: Daugirdas JT, Ing IS, editors. Handbook of dialysis. Boston: Boston Little Brown; 1994.

[88] Brent J, McMartin K, Phillips S, et al. Fomepizole for the treatment of methanol poisoning. N Engl J Med 2001;344:424–9.

[89] Brent J, McMartin K, Phillips S, et al. Fomepizole for the treatment of ethylene glycol poisoning. Methylpyrazole for Toxic Alcohols Study Group. N Engl J Med 1999;340:832–8.

[90] Megarbane B, Borron SW, Baud FJ. Current recommendations for treatment of severe toxic alcohol poisonings. Intensive Care Med 2005;31:189–95.

[91] Dart RC, McNally J. Efficacy, safety, and use of snake antivenoms in the United States. Ann Emerg Med 2001;37:181–8.

[92] Offerman SR, Bush SP, Moynihan JA, et al. Crotaline Fab antivenom for the treatment of children with rattlesnake envenomation. Pediatrics 2002;110:968–71.

[93] Tanen DA, Danish DC, Clark RF. Crotalidae polyvalent immune Fab antivenom limits the decrease in perfusion pressure of the anterior leg compartment in a porcine crotaline envenomation model. Ann Emerg Med 2003;41:384–90.

[94] Lavonas EJ, Gerardo CJ, O'Malley G, et al. Initial experience with Crotalidae polyvalent immune Fab (ovine) antivenom in the treatment of copperhead snakebite. Ann Emerg Med 2004;43:200–6.

[95] Yuan TH, Kerns WPn, Tomaszewski CA, et al. Insulin-glucose as adjunctive therapy for severe calcium channel antagonist poisoning. J Toxicol Clin Toxicol 1999;37:463–74.

[96] Lheureux PE, Zahir S, Gris M, et al. Bench-to-bedside review: hyperinsulinaemia/euglycaemia therapy in the management of overdose of calcium-channel blockers. Crit Care 2006; 10:212.

[97] Woo OF, Mueller PD, Olson KR, et al. Shorter duration of oral N-acetylcysteine therapy for acute acetaminophen overdose. Ann Emerg Med 2000;35:363–8.

[98] Acetylcysteine (Acetadote) for acetaminophen overdosage. Med Lett Drugs Ther 2005;47: 70–1.

[99] Calello DP, Osterhoudt KC, Henretig FM. New and novel antidotes in pediatrics. Pediatr Emerg Care 2006;22:523–30.

[100] Scheinkestel CD, Bailey M, Myles PS, et al. Hyperbaric or normobaric oxygen for acute carbon monoxide poisoning: a randomised controlled clinical trial. Med J Aust 1999;170: 203–10.

[101] Weaver LK, Hopkins RO, Chan KJ, et al. Hyperbaric oxygen for acute carbon monoxide poisoning. N Engl J Med 2002;347:1057–67.

[102] Juurlink DN, Buckley NA, Stanbrook MB, et al. Hyperbaric oxygen for carbon monoxide poisoning. Cochrane Database Syst Rev 2005:CD002041.

[103] Millis JM, Losanoff JE. Technology insight: liver support systems. Nat Clin Pract Gastroenterol Hepatol 2005;2:398–405 [quiz: 434].

[104] Bania TC, Chu J, Perez E, et al. Hemodynamic effects of intravenous fat emulsion in an animal model of severe verapamil toxicity resuscitated with atropine, calcium, and saline. Acad Emerg Med 2007;14(2):105–11.

[105] Harvey M, Cave G. Intralipid outperforms sodium bicarbonate in a rabbit model of clomipramine toxicity. Ann Emerg Med 2007;49:178–85.

[106] Bosse GM, Matyunas NJ. Delayed toxidromes. J Emerg Med 1999;17:679–90.

EMERGENCY
MEDICINE
CLINICS OF
NORTH AMERICA

ELSEVIER
SAUNDERS

Emerg Med Clin N Am 15 (2007) 283–308

Pediatric Toxicology

David L. Eldridge, MD[a],*, Jason Van Eyk, MD[b],
Chad Kornegay, MD[b]

[a]*Department of Pediatrics, Brody School of Medicine, East Carolina University,
Greenville, NC, USA*
[b]*Internal Medicine-Pediatrics Residency Program, Brody School of Medicine,
East Carolina University, Greenville, NC, USA*

The medical cliché of children being little adults is an old aphorism and a flawed view of this patient population. In the field of medical toxicology, children potentially can present with numerous unique and complex problems to emergency personnel when compared with their adult counterparts. This article reviews some of those aspects unique to children.

Fatalities in young children following toxic ingestions are rare [1]. There are, however, specific substances that have been found to be extremely toxic to children even when only small, accidental ingestions occur. It is imperative that the astute emergency physician be aware of these substances. Several over-the-counter medications (OTC) commonly are recognized as drugs of abuse [2]. This article discusses one group of OTC drugs that is not considered as commonly in this capacity. Finally, with the sun setting on the use of syrup of ipecac for managing poisonings in the home, some have advocated activated charcoal (AC) as its successor. The available evidence on the use of AC in this setting is examined.

Toxic in small amounts for small children

Children are exposed to toxic substances more frequently than any other age group [1]. According to the 2004 annual report of the American Association of Poison Control Centers (AAPCC), there were 1,250,536 exposures in children younger than 6 years old (51.3% of the total exposures) and 938,874 exposures in children age 2 or less (38.5% of the total exposures) [1]. Fortunately, the overwhelming majority of these exposures are not lethal. Since the AAPCC began reporting data in 1983, there have been

* Corresponding author.
E-mail address: eldridged@ecu.edu (D.L. Eldridge).

0733-8627/07/$ - see front matter © 2007 Published by Elsevier Inc.
doi:10.1016/j.emc.2007.02.011
emed.theclinics.com

15,447 fatalities reported, of which 537 (3.5%) occurred in children younger than 6 years old; 397 (2.6%) occurred in children age 2 or less [1,3–23].

Most pediatric poisonings do not involve pharmaceuticals. In 2004, the products most frequently involved in pediatric exposure cases were cosmetics and personal hair products, cleaning substances, and analgesics, in descending order of frequency [1]. Pharmaceuticals, however, were responsible for the majority of recorded pediatric fatalities. Of the 27 deaths reported in 2004 in children younger than 6 years of age, 19 were caused by pharmaceuticals (analgesics were reported most commonly, particularly acetaminophen and opioids), and 14 of these cases occurred in patients 2 years of age or under [1].

Even with the rarity of pediatric poisoning fatality, certain pharmaceuticals deserve special discussion. There are some medications that are toxic to children even in small amounts (eg, one or two pills). Many authors have examined this subject [24–27]. Box 1 lists some drugs and drug classes that most agree are dangerous in small amounts. Box 2 catalogs fatalities from single-agent ingestions in children 6 years and younger as reported by the AAPCC from 1983 to 2004 [1,3–23]. Many of the agents in Box 1 also are located in Box 2, further emphasizing the toxicity of these agents. Interestingly, ingestions of iron, including prenatal vitamins, are responsible for the largest number of fatalities from ingestion of a single type of agent in this database (see Box 2). However, the last iron fatality reported to the AAPCC, when looking at the data available at the time of this writing, was in 1999 [1,3–23].

Box 1. Drugs and drug classes that are potentially lethal in small children in small amounts

Antimalarials
Antidysrhythmics
Benzocaine
β-blockers
Calcium channel blockers (CCBs)
Camphor
Clonidine (and other imidazolines)
Lomotil (diphenoxylate/atropine)
Lindane
Methyl salicylate
Opioids
Theophylline
Tricyclic antidepressants (TCAs)

Data from Refs. [24–27].

Much of the concern with the agents listed in Box 1 is based largely on case reports or case series where small amounts reportedly were ingested and severe effects occurred. The strength of this evidence is often not rigorous. These reports, however, recur consistently enough that the treating physician should be particularly cautious when dealing with these agents in regards to small children. Instilling this caution is the core objective of this section. It briefly discusses some of these medications and the available evidence of significant toxicity in children exposed only to small amounts (usually only one or two doses). Discussion of all of these agents is beyond the scope of this article. Recognition of this potential danger, and not the management, is the focus of this discussion.

Tricyclic antidepressants

TCAs are a diverse group of drugs that exert various pharmacologic and toxicology effects. In the 2004 AAPCC report, antidepressants were the third most common class of medications responsible for all fatalities (including adults) [1]. The effects of TCAs are mediated by numerous different physiologic receptors [28]. Those ingesting TCAs may present with anticholinergic effects such as dry mouth, lack of bowel sounds, urinary retention, and mydriasis [28]. Death often results from cardiotoxicity and shock resulting from severe arrhythmia and hypotension [26].

In a recent review of the English literature, Rosenbaum and Kou [29] documented several case reports in which exposure to only one or two TCA pills was sufficient to kill a toddler. Each case involved a dose exceeding 15 mg/kg, with most being over 30 mg/kg, and the authors concluded that doses as low as 15 mg/kg are potentially lethal. Additional studies have demonstrated that children exposed to 5 mg/kg or less are generally asymptomatic [30,31]. In 2004, amitriptyline was the single most common antidepressant agent responsible for poison-related deaths [1]. Available in doses of 10, 25, 50, 75, 100, and 150 mg, a toddler easily could reach a lethal dose after ingestion of only one or two pills. Thus, exposures documented to be 15 mg/kg or greater should seek immediate medical attention. Observation at home can be considered for ingestions of 5 mg/kg; however, such an approach should be done with extreme caution and only if the history is absolutely clear and certainty of the dose can be assured. Otherwise, it is always better to err on the side of caution and have the child referred for formal medical evaluation.

Antimalarials

Traditionally, chloroquine and hydroxychloroquine have been used for their antiparasitic properties in treating malaria. These agents, however, increasingly are being used as second-line anti-inflammatory agents for auto-immune conditions such as rheumatoid arthritis and systemic lupus erythematosus [32]. Toxicity results from cardiotoxic effects similar to class

Box 2. Fatalities in children younger than 6 years of age caused by single pharmaceutical agents reported to the American Association of Poison Control Centers from 1983 to 2004 (total number of fatalities reported for each agent)

Analgesics
Acetaminophen (14)
Salicylates
    Aspirin/salicylate (9)
    Oil of wintergreen/methyl salicylate (5)
Other nonsteroidal anti-inflammatory drugs:
    Ibuprofen (1)
    Naproxen (1)
    Phenylbutazone (1)
Opioids
    Codeine (1)
    Fentanyl patch (1)
    Heroin (3)
    Methadone (14)
    Morphine (2)
    Morphine, long-acting (1)
    Oxycodone (2)
    Oxycodone, long-acting (3)
    Propoxyphene (2)

Anesthetics
Dibucaine ointment (3)
Halothane (1)
Ketamine (1)
Lidocaine, viscous (1)
Lidocaine (2)

Anticoagulants
Heparin (1)

Anticonvulsants
Carbamazepine (5)
Fosphenytoin (3)
Phenytoin (4)
Valproic Acid (1)
Antidepressants
Amitriptyline (6)
Amoxapine (1)
Desipramine (10)
Doxepin (2)
Imipramine (4)

Nortriptyline (1)
Sertraline (1)
Trazodone (1)

Antihistamines
Diphenhydramine (9)

Antimicrobials
Amphotericin B (1)
Cefotaxime (1)
Chloramphenicol (2)
Isoniazid (1)
Chloroquine (2)

Antineoplastics
Vincristine (1)

Antipsychotics
Chlorpromazine (1)
Clozapine (1)

Cardiovascular medications
Amrinone (1)
Clonidine (1)
Digoxin (5)
Diltiazem, long-acting (1)
Flecainide (2)
Nifedipine (5)
Nifedipine, sustained-release (SR) (1)
Nifedipine, long-acting (2)
Nitroprusside (1)
Quinidine (1)
Verapamil (3)

Cold and cough medicines
Benzonatate (3)
Dextromethorphan (1)
Pseudoephedrine (1)

Diabetic medications
Insulin (2)

Electrolytes and mineral supplements
Iron (including those listed as iron, iron sulfate, and prenatal
  vitamins) (42)
Sodium bicarbonate (2)
Sodium chloride (1)

Gastrointestinal agents
AC (1)
Bismuth subsalicylate (1)
Ipecac (2)
Promethazine (1)
Sodium phosphate (1)
Sucralfate (1)

Methylxanthines
Caffeine (1)
Theophylline (4)
Theophylline, SR (1)
Theophylline, long-acting (1)

Sedative hypnotics
Chloral hydrate (3)
Secobarbital (1)

Stimulants
Amphetamines (1)
Cocaine (2)
Methamphetamine (1)

Others
Arginine (1)
Disodium edentate (1)
Centroides antivenom (1)
Colchicine (1)
Lomotil (2)
Merthiolate topical cream
Sodium phenylbuyrate

Data from Refs. [1,3–23].

IA antiarrhythmics. Cardiac sodium and potassium channels may be blocked, resulting in arrhythmias and subsequent intractable hypotension [32,33]. In addition, severe respiratory symptoms are reported, including: tachypnea, dyspnea, pulmonary edema, and finally respiratory failure [32,33]. Central nervous system (CNS) effects range from drowsiness and coma to agitation and refractory seizures [32,33].

Chloroquine is available as a 250 and 500mg tablets as well as a 16.67 mg/mL liquid formulation. Its therapeutic dose range for children is 5 to 10 mg/kg, but doses of 30 to 50 mg/kg may be deadly [32,33]. In a recent review, Smith and Klein-Schwartz [32] concluded that children who have chloroquine ingestions of 10 mg/kg or greater should seek medical evaluation for observation and cardiac monitoring.

There are limited data on the toxicity of hydroxychloroquine in children. Animal experiments, however, suggest that chloroquine is two to three times more toxic than hydroxychloroquine [34]. Hydroxychloroquine is available as 200 mg tablets. There are no reports of toxicity from one to two tablets of hydroxychloroquine in the literature; however, given its similarities with respect to structure and pharmacology with chloroquine, caution is warranted when evaluating a potential ingestion [32].

Calcium channel blockers

Calcium channel blockers (CCBs) are used for various medical indications, including hypertension, stable angina, migraine headaches, and glaucoma [35]. CCBs exert their therapeutic effect by antagonizing L-type voltage-sensitive calcium channels in cardiac tissue and vascular smooth muscle [36]. By hindering the movement of calcium into vascular smooth muscle cells and cardiac myocytes, CCBs cause vasodilation and depress myocardial contractility and conduction [35]. Overdose patients classically present with bradycardia, often with conduction abnormalities (eg, second- or third-degree heart block), hypotension, and hyperglycemia [26].

In a 6-year retrospective case series of 283 patients by Belson and colleagues [37] involving children age 6 or less, only 2% of patients who ingested one pill or less developed symptoms with exposure, and there were no deaths. The authors concluded that children who ingest less than 2.7 mg/kg of nifedipine SR or 12 mg/kg of verapamil SR can be monitored safely at home [37]. There has been at least one fatality reported after ingestion of a single nifedipine pill, however [38].

Camphor

Camphor originally was produced as a product from the bark of the camphor tree *Cinnamomum camphora* [39]. Today it is synthesized and is a common ingredient in many nasal decongestants and ointments, and in many topical anesthetic rubs for musculoskeletal pain [39].

Toxicity usually results from oral ingestion, although there are reports of toxicity from dermal and inhalational exposure in a toddler [39]. Signs and symptoms of camphor ingestion occur primarily as a result of its direct mucosal irritation and CNS effects [39,40]. Gastrointestinal (GI) effects include oropharyngeal irritation and burning with nausea and vomiting. Camphor's CNS effects range from coma and apnea to agitation, anxiety, hallucinations, hyper-reflexia, myoclonic jerks, and seizures [39,40]. Death results from respiratory failure or intractable seizures [26].

In a recent review of the literature, Love and colleagues [39] found several case reports of serious toxicity from exposures ranging from 700 to 1500 mg. In all such cases, seizures or other signs of CNS toxicity were evident, and there were two deaths. The authors concluded that any child who ingests more than 500 mg of camphor should be evaluated at a medical facility.

Various products differ in their content of camphor [39]. For example, Campho-Phenique liquid is 10.8% camphor [39]. To reach the concerning dose of 500 mg of camphor, only 4.6 mL would have to be ingested [39]. Given that a toddler's mouthful is approximately 9.0 mL by a recent study [41], it is possible that a single mouthful of this product may pose a serious threat.

Salicylates

Besides aspirin, there are other over-the-counter preparations that contain salicylate, such as oil of wintergreen (methyl salicylate) and Pepto-Bismol (bismuth subsalicylate) [26,27]. Signs and symptoms of salicylate poisoning include metabolic acidosis with respiratory alkalosis, nausea, vomiting, tinnitus, and mental status changes. Severe intoxication results in pulmonary edema, coma, and death [27,33].

In children, salicylate toxicity has been reported to occur at 150 mg/kg [26]. Oil of wintergreen, found in analgesic balms or liniments, is 98% methyl salicylate. It has the potential to be highly toxic, as 1 mL of this liquid contains 1400 mg of salicylate [27]. Thus, in a 10 kg child, if the minimum toxic salicylate dose is considered to be 150 mg /kg, and the average swallow for a child is 9.0 mL [41], toxicity can be achieved easily with this compound.

Opioids

In addition to their use as analgesics, opioids are used as cough suppressants, antidiarrheal medications, and as adjuncts to anesthesia [42]. Opioid toxicity classically manifests as a triad of respiratory depression, miosis, and CNS depression [42,43]. Most deaths are secondary to respiratory depression [26].

Data from the AAPCC collected from 1983 to 2000 showed codeine as the most commonly ingested opioid in children younger than 6 years of age. These same data, however, showed that, starting in 1997, oxycodone ingestions have increased, and it has become the second most ingested opioid in this age group [42].

A study from 1976 demonstrated that ingestions of less than 5 mg/kg of codeine are nontoxic [44], and the authors recommended that exposure at this dosage can be monitored safely at home. In contrast, the investigators found that respiratory depression, which at times was fatal, developed in some children with ingestions greater than 5 mg/kg, so these patients should seek medical attention.

Multiple case reports are in the literature of methadone ingestions in children who have toxicity in doses as low as 5 mg [42,43]. Methadone is commonly available as 5 or 10 mg tablets or as a liquid at a concentration of 1 mg/mL. In a typical 10 kg toddler, ingestion of 0.5 mg/kg may be life-threatening, and thus any child who has ingested methadone should be evaluated in the emergency department (ED) [42].

There is limited information on the toxic doses of other common opioids, including morphine, hydrocodone, and oxycodone. There have been multiple deaths reported to the AAPCC related to these compounds, however. Given that data are available for codeine, Sachdeva and Stadnyk [42], in their review of the medical literature of pediatric opioid poisoning, recommend attempting to make a dose comparison to codeine with these other medications. They argue that at doses comparable to 5 mg/kg of codeine or less, children may be monitored at home. Higher doses should be evaluated in the ED. The exceptions noted by them were propoxyphene, methadone, and any extended-release product. These they felt all deserved ED evaluation at a minimum [42].

Sulfonylureas

Sulfonylureas are oral hypoglycemic medications that present a special challenge. When ingested by small children, they can cause a protracted hypoglycemia that may be delayed in initial presentation [45]. Clinical findings may include behavior changes, irritability, loss of appetite, weakness, seizures, and coma [46].

Data from one earlier case series of children suggested that the delay in development of hypoglycemia after ingestion necessitated observation with frequent blood glucose checks for 24 hours after ingestion [47]. One prospective, multicenter case series by Spiller and colleagues [48] looked at 185 children ages 12 years or younger who accidentally ingested sulfonylureas. Fifty-six developed hypoglycemia (blood glucose concentration of <60 mg/dL). Of those who became hypoglycemic, 54 children (96%) did so within the first 8 hours of ingestion. Spiller and colleagues [48] felt that an absence of hypoglycemia within 8 hours of ingestion signaled a benign outcome. In response to this study, a letter by another group argued that, in their experience with 313 pediatric cases, 3.5% of these (11 total) displayed hypoglycemia after 8 hours [49]. Regarding this concern, they in turn suggested that at least a 12-hour observation period (and likely longer with chlorpropamide given its long half-life) with these drugs was warranted [49].

Little and Boniface [46] performed a recent literature review of accidental ingestion of one to two sulfonylurea pills by children younger than 6 years. They concluded that ingestion of one or two tablets could lead to dangerous hypoglycemia. It was noted that although only one death was reported, up to 36% of these patients may develop hypoglycemia. Furthermore, based on their literature review, Little and Boniface [46] also advised an 8-hour observation period in an ED with frequent blood glucose monitoring. They made a point of excluding extended-release products of glipizide from this recommendation. For these they advised a longer period of observation until more clinical experience with it in this setting is available.

Lomotil

Lomotil is an antidiarrheal medication with two components—the opioid diphenoxylate and the anticholinergic agent atropine [50]. Diphenoxylate serves to inhibit GI motility, while atropine, also capable of this action, was reportedly added to deter diphenoxylate abuse [24]. One case series by McCarron and colleagues [51], which also included a review of available cases in the literature, discussed the symptoms seen in children (n = 36) with Lomotil toxicity. Anticholinergic effects reported in children with Lomotil toxicity include: tachycardia, dry mucous membranes and skin, dry mucous membranes and skin, facial flushing, urinary retention, and hyperthermia. Interestingly, mydriasis was conspicuously absent in the review by McCarron and colleagues [51]. Opioid effects, which predominated over anticholinergic effects, included miosis and CNS and respiratory depression [51]. Classically, toxicity has been described as biphasic, with early anticholinergic effects followed by narcotic effects presenting much later [52]. In the more recent review with McCarron and colleagues [51], however, only four pediatric patients of 36 showed this pattern. Twenty-one patients had anticholinergic symptoms before, during, or after opioid symptoms, while 15 patients developed only symptoms of opioid toxicity. Importantly, eight of the patients reviewed did show recurrent CNS and respiratory depression 12 to 24 hours after ingestion. This is one of the characteristics of Lomotil ingestion that make it deceptively dangerous in children. For these ingestions, McCarron and colleagues [51] recommended admission and close monitoring for 24 hours, a recommendation made in previous studies.

A case series from England by Penfold and Volans [53] looked at Lomotil overdose in 86 cases in adults and children (n = 71). In England, three of these patients (all ≤12 years old) who had symptoms including drowsiness, tachycardia, flushing, and nausea had ingested only one to five Lomotil tablets. Additionally, they reported a 2-year-old who was in a coma for 2 days after ingestion of only three or four tablets [53]. Though there have been no deaths reported from ingestion of a single pill, Lomotil tablets have shown through previous case reports their potential for disaster.

Recognition of abuse and misuse of common over-the-counter gastrointestinal agents in children and adolescents

For many children and adolescents (and their parents), there are few symptoms as distressing as nausea, vomiting, and diarrhea. These are common presenting symptoms. Quite justifiably, an emergency medicine physician often will (and correctly) conclude these symptoms are subsequent to the bad luck of an obtained infectious process. Very few would imagine that this misery would be self-induced or caused by a parent.

Although the number of ingestions that can cause GI distress adverse effects is vast, both syrup of ipecac [54] and OTC laxatives [55] have the capacity to cause profound GI adverse effects when be abused. This abuse has been recognized in adolescents who have eating disorders [54,56] and in Munchausen's by proxy (or factitious disorder by proxy) [55], a syndrome in which illnesses are inflicted on a child by a parent or caregiver to serve some particular psychological need of the perpetrator [57]. This section discusses the clinical findings caused by the chronic abuse of syrup of ipecac and laxatives to assist the emergency medicine physician in recognizing these poisonous exposures.

Syrup of ipecac

Syrup of ipecac has been available OTC since 1965 [58]. It was seen by many at that time as a key therapeutic intervention for home management of pediatric ingestions and in 1984 was a recommended part of anticipatory guidance to be included in The Injury Prevention Program (TIPP) of the American Academy of Pediatrics (AAP) [59]. Even as some were doubting its usefulness [60], others strongly defended it [61]. The debate raged on. Then in 2003, the Committee on Injury, Violence, and Poison Prevention from the AAP issued a new policy statement, "Poison Treatment in the Home" and reversed the previous philosophy from 1984 [62]. In this new position paper, the committee called for removal of ipecac from the home and declared that it "should no longer be used routinely as a poison treatment intervention in the home." The rationales for this shift in policy were multiple and based on available clinical research. The committee's specific reasons included:

Poor proof of reliability to empty the stomach even under ideal conditions
Adverse side effects such as lethargy, which may confuse the clinical picture of a poisoned child
The occurrence of prolonged vomiting that may interfere with other oral antidotes and interventions
The frequent, inappropriate use in nontoxic ingestions

Another position paper by the American Academy of Clinical Toxicology and the European Association of Poison Centers and Clinical Toxicologists (AACT/EAPCCT) subsequently was published [63]. While not calling for its immediate removal from the home or complete cessation of its use, this paper did state that, based on the available clinical data, there was no evidence that the use of ipecac alone, even if given within the recommended 60 minutes of a toxic ingestion, improved clinical outcomes. They also believed overall, however, that there were "insufficient data to support or exclude ipecac administration soon after poison ingestion."

Playing no small role in the increased scrutiny of ipecac's OTC status has been recognition of its abuse potential [64,65]. Those patients with eating disorders, like bulimia and anorexia nervosa may self-administer ipecac repetitively in order induce vomiting in an effort to lose weight [66]. Because of the secretive nature of those with these illnesses, the true prevalence of ipecac abuse may be hard to ascertain [54]. One fairly recent study looking at 851 consecutive patients in an eating disorder clinic revealed that 7.6% of this group used ipecac at least once, with 3.1% using it chronically [67]. There are deaths reported in eating disorder patients that have been attributed to the complications of abusing ipecac [68–71]. It is suspected by some that ipecac played a part in the death of singer Karen Carpenter [72]. There are numerous case reports of ipecac being used in the setting of Munchausen's by proxy [73–80].

Commercial syrup of ipecac is derived from the plants *Cephaelis ipecacuanha* and *Cephaelis accuminata*, with its chief active ingredients being two alkaloids, emetine and cephaeline [74]. These two components cause emesis with cephaeline reportedly twice as potent as emetine in this regard [60]. Vomiting is mediated by both local irritation of the GI lining and central stimulation of the chemoreceptor trigger zone of the medulla [68]. Correct dosing will produce vomiting within 30 minutes in 95% of adults and children who consume syrup of ipecac [75].

Many of the severe clinical symptoms of long-term ipecac abuse are attributed specifically to emetine [81]. These are summarized in Box 3. Emetine has been documented to remain in body organs up to 60 days after consumption [77]. With repeated dosing, emetine builds up within the body and can reach toxic levels [82]. There are some prolonged GI effects that are attributed to emetine [81]. These include protracted nausea and vomiting, abdominal cramping, diarrhea, and GI mucosal irritation and bleeding [54,73,77,81]. A pathognomic finding with chronic ipecac abuse is a skeletal myopathy [80]. Clinically, this skeletal myopathy may present as muscle weakness with accompanying hypotonia, absent deep tendon reflexes, myalgias, and possible muscle stiffness [80,83–87]. Cardiac findings caused by chronic emetine accumulation can be dramatic. Although the mechanism of emetine-induced cardiomyopathy is unknown, it is thought to be a direct toxin to the heart [79]. This cardiac toxicity has been regarded as the final cause of death in multiple cases of intentional ipecac abuse [68–71]. Clinical signs and symptoms indicative of possible cardiac distress include: chest pain, tachycardia, bradycardia, hypotension, and even shock [70,79,81]. Other CNS symptoms that have been described include convulsions, tremor, and peripheral neuropathy [77,78,81].

There are also various laboratory and diagnostic tests that may be supportive in the effort to diagnose ipecac toxicity. Serum electrolytes disturbances may be seen, including a hypokalemic, hypochloremic metabolic alkalosis caused by chronic emesis [54]. Hyponatremia also has been reported [79,81]. Leukocytosis and elevated liver enzymes may be seen [86]. Elevations in enzymes found in muscle tissue like creatinine phosphokinase, aldolase, lactate dehydrogenase frequently are elevated [54,80]. Electromyography and muscle biopsy may be helpful in making the diagnosis if the characteristic skeletal myopathy is present [84,85]. ECG findings may be

---

Box 3. Symptoms and physical examination findings of chronic ipecac exposure

Gastrointestinal
Persistent nausea and vomiting
Diarrhea
Abdominal cramping
GI bleeding

Neuromuscular
Proximal muscle weakness
Myalgias
Muscle stiffness
Hypotonia
Absent deep tendon reflexes
Peripheral neuropathy
Tremor
Convulsions

Cardiovascular
Tachycardia
Chest pain
Hypotension
Shock

Data from Refs. [54,69,70,77,79–81,84,86].

---

numerous and include: tachycardia (including sinus, ventricular, and supraventricular), bradycardia, premature atrial complexes, ventricular fibrillation, prolonged QTc interval, prolonged PR interval, and T-wave flattening or inversion [54,69,80,86,88]. Echocardiography may demonstrate ventricular dilatation and dysfunction with decreased ejection fraction and shortening fraction [54,82,88]. Atrial enlargement also has been reported by echocardiography [79]. Urine testing for cephaeline and emetine may be most helpful in establishing the diagnosis. These have been shown to be detectable in the urine of volunteers several weeks after ipecac ingestion [89].

Treatment for ipecac toxicity consists of appropriate supportive care and cessation of the exposure to ipecac. It may take weeks for these chronic symptoms to disappear, however, because emetine may persist in body organs for up to 60 days [77]. Fortunately, it is felt that the cardiac and skeletal myopathy brought on by ipecac may be reversible with cessation of emetine exposure [79,82,85,87,88].

A high degree of clinical suspicion is required when considering ipecac poisoning as a diagnosis [54]. Its intentional abuse should be considered in adolescents with unusual weight loss, and those who have histories of eating disorders [66]. Its deliberate use as a poison should be considered in small children with persistent or recurrent diarrhea and emesis of no clear etiology [80]. If these findings are accompanied by unexplained symptoms of muscle weakness or cardiac failure, suspicion should be raised even higher [54].

Laxatives

In a similar vein to syrup of ipecac, laxatives also have abused in an attempt to lose weight. The abuse of laxatives by teenagers has been documented in some poison center data from the United States [2]. Patients who have eating disorders may use them in an effort to manage their weight [90]. In one Australian study, Turner and colleagues [56] looked at 43 adolescent patients with anorexia nervosa seen consecutively at a multidisciplinary eating disorders clinic. They assessed for laxative use in this group by self-report and urine screening for the presence of some laxatives. In this population, they found that the prevalence of laxative use was as high as 32%. They cautioned the prevalence may have been even higher, because there were discrepancies in self-reporting compared with urine screening results. They also noted that their urine screen could not check for all laxatives. Patients who have eating disorders are not the only population to misuse these medications, however. One survey of 2532 high school wrestlers revealed that 1% of this group used laxatives weekly, and 0.5% used them daily as a weight loss method [91]. In addition, cases of Munchausen's by proxy have been reported in which mysterious cases of severe diarrhea later have been discovered to be secret laxative administration by a caregiver [92–94].

There are various OTC laxatives available. Bulk laxatives (like psyllium) are thought to act by retaining water and subsequently provide more liquidity to stools, making them easier to pass [95]. Osmotic agents generally consist of poorly absorbable salts like milk of magnesia (magnesium hydroxide) that act as osmotic agents and also retain water in the lumen of the gut [96]. Lubricants, like mineral oil, also reduce water absorption and subsequently soften stools [96]. Stimulant laxatives are a broad group of agents (including castor oil, senna, bisacodyl, and docusate) [96]. These drugs exert their effect by either increasing gut motility, altering electrolyte and fluid transport, or both [55,96].

There are certain common signs and symptoms that, while not specific to laxative abuse, should prompt the consideration of this entity (Box 4). Not surprisingly, a gamut of GI symptoms is common with excessive exposure to laxatives. Children and adolescents taking large amounts of laxatives will present with frequent, watery bowel movements that may amount to tremendous volumes of diarrhea [55,97]. Some report that this may alternate

---

Box 4. Signs, symptoms, and laboratory findings of laxative abuse

Clinical symptoms
General
Weight Loss
Fatigue
Generalized Muscle Weakness
Gastrointestinal
Diarrhea (at times alternating with reported periods of constipation)
Bloating
Nausea and Vomiting
Abdominal Pain/Cramping
Rectal Pain (with defecation)
Cardiovascular
Tachycardia
Hypotension
Dizziness/syncope

Common laboratory findings
Hypokalemia
Hypochloremia
Metabolic Alkalosis

Data from Refs. [55,96–99].

---

with periods of constipation [98,99]. Abdominal pain, cramping, and rectal pain with defecation are also common, while some patients will report GI bloating, nausea, and vomiting [55,97–99]. Depending on the degree of sodium and fluid loss, tachycardia, hypotension, dizziness, or syncope may occur [97]. Over a prolonged period of time, a combination of dehydration, electrolyte loss, and malnutrition can produce other symptoms such as weight loss, fatigue, lethargy, and muscle weakness [55,97]. An unusual clinical finding that has been reported in cases of the abuse of senna laxatives is finger clubbing [100–103]. The reason for this finding is unclear.

Undisclosed abuse of laxatives by adolescents or secret overdosing imposed on small children may present as chronic diarrhea of unknown etiology [97]. Definitively proving laxative abuse is difficult and relies first on clinical suspicion. Other organic disease often must be ruled out. Some laboratory testing may be helpful. If laxative abuse is suspected, serum electrolytes should be examined [97]. Vast electrolyte disarray can be seen with chronic laxative abuse because of excessive loss of both fluid and electrolytes in stool

[55,96–99]. Generally, hypokalemia is a common finding in those who have ingested excessive amounts of laxatives [55,56,96–98]. This occurs not only from stool loss but also from renal losses triggered by dehydration that subsequently causes release of renin, and ultimately results in a secondary hyperaldosteronism [96,97]. This hypokalemia is thought to then impair gut reabsorption of chloride and promote renal reabsorption of bicarbonate, leading to another commonly reported finding of hypochloremic metabolic alkalosis [55,97]. Hyponatremia, despite large sodium loss through diarrhea, is generally a rare laboratory finding because of simultaneous loss of large amounts of water [97]. Hypocalcemia and hypomagnesemia also can be seen [97,99]. If excessive osmotic laxatives consisting of salts that include sodium, magnesium, calcium, or phosphate are ingested, however, large serum excesses of these electrolytes may be detected [96]. Overuse of osmotic laxatives also may elevate measured stool osmolality greatly [98]. Finally, urine screens for detecting some laxatives have been designed [104]. Not all laxatives can be screened for, however, and false negatives have still been reported [56].

There are also some other unusual findings that may present during the diagnostic evaluation of patients exposed to large doses of laxatives. Anthraquinone laxatives (eg, senna) are linked to a phenomenon known as melanosis coli, a brown discoloration of the colonic mucosa that develops after a few months of consistent use of these laxatives [55,97]. It can be seen on endoscopy and serve as a clue to laxative abuse [99]. Cathartic colon is a radiographic finding that has been reported in those who abuse certain laxatives, particularly with those in the stimulant category. It is characterized by a dilated colon diameter, loss of haustral markings, pseudostrictures of the colon, dilated terminal ileum, and gaping of the ileocecal valve [55,96,97]. Although some literature has linked these findings with potentially irreversible damage to the colon [97–99], others question its existence as a significant clinical entity [55,105].

Acute management of laxative abuse involves appropriate supportive care and correction of fluid and electrolyte balance disturbances when appropriate [98]. As far as stopping laxatives, some caution using withdrawal schedules to minimize psychological and medical symptoms (eg, constipation and bloating) that may occur with sudden cessation [99]. Others have argued that while tolerance to some laxatives may occur, the role of a true physiologic dependence has been overstated [106]. In those patients who have suspected eating disorders, psychiatric consultation is appropriate. If Munchausen's syndrome by proxy is suspected, proving the diagnosis is difficult, but diarrhea should cease gradually with separation from the caregiver [57,92,93].

Administration of activated charcoal in the home

As has already been stated, ingestions of toxic substances by young children are common occurrences [1]. Though serious illness and fatalities remain rare with these events, part of the traditional strategy to prevent serious harm in the past was to encourage the early administration of syrup of ipecac in the home when appropriate [59]. There was an almost 50% reduction in use of ipecac syrup in 2004 compared with 2003 [1]. One factor sited for this change was recent guidelines by the AAP recommending that ipecac should be disposed of and no longer be used routinely at home [1,62].

Some began to broach the discussion that AC, being more effective than ipecac, might prove to be an appropriate home agent for GI decontamination [107]. However, even though AC is considered by many the primary means of GI decontamination in the setting of a toxic ingestion [108,109], its efficacy is not clear [110]. The AACT/EAPCCT's position statement on the use of single-dose AC in the setting of a poisonous ingestion scrutinized the available medical literature on the use of single-dose AC in the setting of a poisonous ingestion [110]. This position statement recognized that, although there is convincing evidence that AC appears to decrease drug absorption when used appropriately, there is no existing proof that it improves clinical outcome [110]. Furthermore, any clinical utility (based on drug absorption) seems to decrease if AC is given more than 1 hour after ingestion (although it also stated benefit after this point could not be excluded) [110]. Overall, they concluded AC should be given selectively and not as part of the routine management of a poisoned patient [110]. The AAP commented on home administration of AC specifically, concluding the existing evidence made it premature to recommend giving AC in this setting and placing emphasis on consulting a local poison control center first when confronted with an ingestion at home [62].

Rather than discuss the efficacy of AC this article now discusses the separate issue of the practicality of giving AC in the home based on available evidence. There have been several studies at this point that have looked at this issue [107,111–115]. The following section examines how each has addressed key questions regarding using AC in the home.

Will children take activated charcoal at home?

Offering a small child AC by mouth can be a difficult sell. This proves to be true even in the pediatric ED. Osterhoudt and colleagues [116] looked prospectively at 275 children ($\leq$18 years old) being treated for an acute poisoning. Of these, 114 were younger than age 6 and offered oral charcoal. In this group, 36 (32%) of the children would not successfully take the dose orally. Among those in this age group, it took an average of about 21 minutes for a complete dose of AC to be taken with or without flavoring.

The success of giving oral AC at home has been varied in clinical studies. Dockstader and colleagues [111] were among the first to explore the plausibility of this concept. In their published abstract, they described a study that included 50 calls to their poison center involving children age 8 months to 5 years old with reported toxic ingestions. In these cases, it was judged that

AC was a suitable therapy, and ipecac was not immediately available. The poison center helped the caller obtain AC. The caller then attempted to give the AC orally to each child. A blinded, experienced counselor then called the family back to assess its success. Thirty-five of these patients (70%) had difficulty in administration. The full, recommended dose was given successfully to 30 children (60%). Notably, 11 children (22%) vomited within 30 minutes of ingesting AC. The authors attributed this emesis to the children drinking additional water soon after administration. Though the authors report 42 of the children (84%) passing charcoal in their stool, it is not clear how much of the AC dose was ingested by the children who did not take the full dose. One criticism of this study (and subsequent others like it) is that its data rely on parental report, and that caregivers, not wanting to seem poorly compliant, may not admit failure in giving the AC as recommended [115]. Overall, however, the authors concluded, despite any troubles the children had tolerating this therapy, AC could be given at home as long as extra water was not given soon after.

Grbcich and colleagues [112] subsequently did a small study with six children, all between the ages of 1 and 5 years, who had ingested substances bound by AC. They had not been given ipecac and did not require emergency medical evaluation. Trained observers then went to the child's home and watched as a parent attempted to give charcoal. No child took the full dose (the best success was one child who took "at least 50%"). Parent satisfaction with this intervention was poor, and the investigators concluded success with administration of AC at home might also be poor. One obvious problem with this investigation is the very small sample size. Others have criticized this study for introducing the bias of bringing an outsider (ie, the trained observer) into homes and giving AC the appearance of an experimental antidote (as opposed to ipecac, the recognized standard at the time) and possibly hurting any chance of success [107].

Lamminpaa and colleagues [113] did a larger study and found more encouraging results. In their study, they prospectively interviewed over the phone and enlisted 174 households with children (age <5 years) who had ingested poison material in which charcoal was not contraindicated, and the ingestion did not require urgent attention. Parents were advised to give AC. Administration of AC was attempted in 102 children. According to their parents, the full suggested dose was given in 81 of these children (79.4%), whereas a partial dose was taken in 16 (15.7%), and completely failed in 5 (4.9%). Again, some have questioned this success given the reliance on data from parental report alone [115].

Dilger and colleagues [114] distributed 24,000 packets of AC and instructions on their use to families in Berlin with small children. They then conducted a prospective case-controlled study consisting of 858 phone discussions with households of children who had acute accidental ingestions [114]. Home AC was recommended in only 55 cases (6.4%). Of these children, home AC was administered without difficulty in only 28 (51%) of the children involved. Of the remaining 27 (49%) children, five refused the AC, and nine took only some of the recommended dose. One child received the wrong dose because parental error, and 12 parents "did not cooperate for other reasons" [114]. It is important to note that of the 33 families that had AC in the home, only 19 of them appeared to have received the formal AC packet and instructions from the investigators (the intervention group). The rest apparently had no AC or had AC but no formal instructions (the control group). It is not clear from the available published data how many of the failed or successful attempts at dosing AC were in the intervention group versus those in the control. This accuracy of this study again relied on parental report.

Next, Spiller and Rodgers [107], after encouraging pharmacies in their region to stock AC, conducted an 18-month prospective, consecutive case series where parents were followed by telephone and instructed on AC use for children with ingestions that they thought was appropriate. AC was recommended for 138 children (age range from 1 to 14 years with a mean age of 3 years), and of these 115 (83%) received AC at home. The reasons for not giving AC at home to the remaining 23 patients included: parents preferring to take child to the ED, inability to access AC, no home phone for follow-up. When AC was given, parents in this study reported 100% success, although 25.9% reported some sort of difficulty. This study again relies on correct parental reporting for its data and may make the true rate of success questionable [115]. Also of interest, the dose of AC given was based on parental estimation using the amount of AC that remained in the container. This could have led to discrepancies in whether the appropriate dose actually was given. The authors, while recognizing this weakness, argued that the optimal dose of AC currently is not defined well [107].

Finally, Scharman and colleagues [115] conducted a single-blind study involving volunteers brought to a simulated home environment. In this study, 15 children (< 3 years of age) were placed with their mothers in a playroom with a one-way mirror. They then were observed as the mothers attempted to give AC (mixed with either regular or diet cola) to their children. Children were given 30 minutes to drink the allotted AC. Only 3 children out of 15 (20%) went on to drink the defined therapeutic dose of AC (1 g/kg). Eleven of the children (73%) drank less then half of the volume offered them, and nine (60%) drank less then one quarter of the volume. Although all four children who drank at least half the AC or better had it mixed with regular cola, three others failed. The authors concluded that there was potential for failure with home AC administration [115]. This study did seem to avoid the errors of parental self-reporting and the possibility of bias introduced by the visible presence of outside observer. One weakness was that this study was fairly small (n = 15). Another criticism offered of this study was that it used volunteers [117]. The main thrust of this criticism argued that a mother confronted with a possibly poisoned child will be more motivated to give AC then a volunteer [117].

In summary, all of these studies showed widely variable success ranging from 0% to 100%. It is interesting that those that relied on parental report for confirmation reported the highest success rates of administering AC (51% to 100%) [107,113,114]. Those studies that had some degree of third-party observation were much smaller, but showed dismal success rates (0 to 20%) [112,115]. Based on the available evidence, actual success at administering AC at home is likely to be similarly mixed and likely to depend on both the individual child and his or her caregiver.

Is activated charcoal taken more quickly at home?

Considering that the available evidence that suggests that AC is at its most effective if given within 1 hour of ingestion [110], one of the hopes of home-administered AC would be a decrease in the time lapse between ingestion and the administration of AC. Some of the studies already discussed attempted to address this issue as well.

Not surprisingly, the studies that reported the most success at administering AC at home also reported quicker administration of AC when it was already available at home [107,113,114]. The time lapse in administration varied. In the study done by Lamminpaa and colleagues [113], AC was given in an average of 24.5 minutes from the time it was recommended to give AC if it was in the home. If AC was not in the home, the average delay was 41.6 minutes from the time AC was recommended. Interestingly, even in these cases where AC was not readily available, the time lapse from ingestion until dosing of AC was still an average of 56.1 minutes (range of 47.7 to 64.6 minutes), generally within one hour. Lamminpaa and colleagues [113] excluded any children who required referral for medical evaluation, so AC dosing delay in these instances was not evaluated. Dilger and colleagues found in their study that for those in their intervention group (ie, had AC available and appropriate instruction) the mean time from ingestion to AC dosing was 14 minutes. Those in the control group (ie, had no readily available AC or had AC but no formal instruction) took an average of 48 minutes to give AC. Again, even this delay was within the desired hour. In their abstract, Dilger and colleagues [114] did not address time lapses caused by referral to the ED. Finally, Spiller and Rodgers [107] found in their study that if AC was given at home, the time from ingestion to dosing of AC was an average 38 minutes (±18.3). If the child went to the ED, this time lapse went up to 73 minutes (±18.1). It is important to note that those patients in their study who received AC in the ED were smaller (n = 23) compared with those in the home (n = 115).

In the available studies that examined this issue, having AC at home appeared to decrease time lapse to its delivery. It is important to remember that all of these studies relied on parental report to track these times. The study by Lamminpaa and colleagues [113] (from Finland) seemed to show the benefits of having AC at hand by showing quicker AC delivery than if parents had to go out and find it. Dilger and colleagues [114] (from

Germany) found that formal instruction also may shorten time to AC dosing. The importance of the differences they showed is questionable, because in both studies children on the whole received AC within an hour of ingestion [113,114]. The ready availability of OTC AC in United States, however, may be different then in both Finland and Germany, and the results of similar studies may be quite different here. Although the accuracy of their data may be limited by parental report, Spiller and Rodgers [107] provided information most relevant to practice in the United States. Not only did they find that AC was given sooner after ingestion if given at home, they also showed the delay with ED referral could exceed 1 hour.

Is it safe to give activated charcoal at home?

In the studies discussed here, only the studies by the groups led by Dockstader [111] and Lamminpaa [113] quoted any adverse symptoms with AC. As previously mentioned, Dockstader and colleagues [111] reported vomiting in 11 children (22%). Some children in the study led by Lamminpaa [113] had this and other adverse effects. In their study group, 10 children had some symptoms of GI distress, including vomiting (n = 4), diarrhea, (n = 5), and constipation (n = 1). Except for the constipation, they felt some of these ill effects may have been caused by the actual ingestion. Another seven children had symptoms they thought clearly were related to the toxic ingestion and not AC (eg, one child got sleepy after ingesting sleeping pills). The other studies discussed here either make no specific mention of complications [112] or comment that there was vomiting, aspiration, or complications [107,114,115].

The most concerning adverse event involving AC is aspiration. Although rare, significant lung disease [118,119] and even fatalities [120,121] have been reported in adult and pediatric patients. Although this has, in some cases, been caused by inadvertent placement of a nasogastric tube into the airway (a concern that would not seem part of the home charcoal debate) [118], aspiration caused by vomiting and a poorly protected airway secondary to drug effect is a bigger concern [119–121]. AC is contraindicated in patients with altered mental status who may have a compromised airway and those who have ingested certain compounds (like hydrocarbons) where the aspiration risk is already elevated [110]. Although this has not borne out in any study to date, one concern would be that families might use AC when it is contraindicated, as has been the case with ipecac in the past [62]. This could lead to a rise in adverse events, like aspiration, with AC use at home.

Summary

In conclusion, the concept of home-administered AC seems advantageous because of the intuitive reasoning of the sooner the better. The evidence is not so clear, however. Studies are mixed on whether parents can give AC successfully to children at home. Although complications from AC appear rare, they do exist and the risk-benefit ratio of every potential therapy or procedure deserves serious scrutiny. Furthermore, although some studies report shortened time from ingestion to dosing of AC, the importance of this time savings is not clear. The general consensus is that AC given within 1 hour of ingestion provides better drug absorption. There is no clear benefit from AC, however, given at home or otherwise, in terms of the most important parameter, clinical outcome [110].

References

[1] Watson WA, Litovitz TL, Rodgers GC Jr, et al. 2004 Annual report of the American Association of Poison Control Centers Toxic Exposure Surveillance System. Am J Emerg Med 2005;23(5):589–666.

[2] Crouch BI, Caravati EM, Booth J. Trends in child and teen nonprescription drug abuse reported to a regional poison control center. Am J Health Syst Pharm 2004;61(12): 1252–7.

[3] Veltri JC, Litovitz TL. 1983 annual report of the American Association of Poison Control Centers National Data Collection System. Am J Emerg Med 1984;2(5):420–43.

[4] Litovitz T, Veltri JC. 1984 annual report of the American Association of Poison Control Centers National Data Collection System. Am J Emerg Med 1985;3(5):423–50.

[5] Litovitz TL, Normann SA, Veltri JC. 1985 Annual Report of the American Association of Poison Control Centers National Data Collection System. Am J Emerg Med 1986;4(5): 427–58.

[6] Litovitz TL, Martin TG, Schmitz B. 1986 annual report of the American Association of Poison Control Centers National Data Collection System. Am J Emerg Med 1987;5(5): 405–45.

[7] Litovitz TL, Schmitz BF, Matyunas N, et al. 1987 annual report of the American Association of Poison Control Centers National Data Collection System. Am J Emerg Med 1988; 6(5):479–515.

[8] Litovitz TL, Schmitz BF, Holm KC. 1988 annual report of the American Association of Poison Control Centers National Data Collection System. Am J Emerg Med 1989;7(5): 495–545.

[9] Litovitz TL, Schmitz BF, Bailey KM. 1989 annual report of the American Association of Poison Control Centers National Data Collection System. Am J Emerg Med 1990;8(5): 394–442.

[10] Litovitz TL, Bailey KM, Schmitz BF, et al. 1990 annual report of the American Association of Poison Control Centers National Data Collection System. Am J Emerg Med 1991;9(5): 461–509.

[11] Litovitz TL, Holm KC, Bailey KM, et al. 1991 annual report of the American Association of Poison Control Centers National Data Collection System. Am J Emerg Med 1992;10(5): 452–505.

[12] Litovitz TL, Holm KC, Clancy C, et al. 1992 annual report of the American Association of Poison Control Centers Toxic Exposure Surveillance System. Am J Emerg Med 1993;11(5): 494–555.

[13] Litovitz TL, Clark LR, Soloway RA. 1993 annual report of the American Association of Poison Control Centers Toxic Exposure Surveillance System. Am J Emerg Med 1994; 12(5):546–84.

[14] Litovitz TL, Felberg L, Soloway RA, et al. 1994 annual report of the American Association of Poison Control Centers Toxic Exposure Surveillance System. Am J Emerg Med 1995; 13(5):551–97.

[15] Litovitz TL, Felberg L, White S, et al. 1995 annual report of the American Association of Poison Control Centers Toxic Exposure Surveillance System. Am J Emerg Med 1996;14(5): 487–537.

[16] Litovitz TL, Smilkstein M, Felberg L, et al. 1996 annual report of the American Association of Poison Control Centers Toxic Exposure Surveillance System. Am J Emerg Med 1997; 15(5):447–500.

[17] Litovitz TL, Klein-Schwartz W, Dyer KS, et al. 1997 annual report of the American Association of Poison Control Centers Toxic Exposure Surveillance System. Am J Emerg Med 1998;16(5):443–97.

[18] Litovitz TL, Klein-Schwartz W, Caravati EM, et al. 1998 annual report of the American Association of Poison Control Centers Toxic Exposure Surveillance System. Am J Emerg Med 1999;17(5):435–87.

[19] Litovitz TL, Klein-Schwartz W, White S, et al. 1999 annual report of the American Association of Poison Control Centers Toxic Exposure Surveillance System. Am J Emerg Med 2000;18(5):517–74.

[20] Litovitz TL, Klein-Schwartz W, White S, et al. 2000 annual report of the American Association of Poison Control Centers Toxic Exposure Surveillance System. Am J Emerg Med 2001;19(5):337–95.

[21] Litovitz TL, Klein-Schwartz W, Rodgers GC Jr, et al. 2001 annual report of the American Association of Poison Control Centers Toxic Exposure Surveillance System. Am J Emerg Med 2002;20(5):391–452.

[22] Watson WA, Litovitz TL, Rodgers GC Jr, et al. 2002 annual report of the American Association of Poison Control Centers Toxic Exposure Surveillance System. Am J Emerg Med 2003;21(5):353–421.

[23] Watson WA, Litovitz TL, Klein-Schwartz W, et al. 2003 annual report of the American Association of Poison Control Centers Toxic Exposure Surveillance System. Am J Emerg Med 2004;22(5):335–404.

[24] Muller AA. Small amounts of some drugs can be toxic to young children: one pill or one swallow can require aggressive treatment. J Emerg Nurs 2003;29(3):290–3.

[25] Bar-Oz B, Levichek Z, Koren G. Medications that can be fatal for a toddler with one tablet or teaspoonful: a 2004 update. Paediatr Drugs 2004;6(2):123–6.

[26] Michael JB, Sztajnkrycer MD. Deadly pediatric poisons: nine common agents that kill at low doses. Emerg Med Clin North Am 2004;22(4):1019–50.

[27] Henry K, Harris CR. Deadly ingestions. Pediatr Clin North Am 2006;53(2):293–315.

[28] Kerr GW, McGuffie AC, Wilkie S. Tricyclic antidepressant overdose: a review. Emerg Med J 2001;18(4):236–41.

[29] Rosenbaum TG, Kou M. Are one or two dangerous? Tricyclic antidepressant exposure in toddlers. J Emerg Med 2005;28(2):169–74.

[30] McFee RB, Mofenson HC, Caraccio TR. A nationwide survey of the management of unintentional low-dose tricyclic antidepressant ingestions involving asymptomatic children: implications for the development of an evidence-based clinical guideline. J Toxicol Clin Toxicol 2000;38(1):15–9.

[31] McFee RB, Caraccio TR, Mofenson HC. Selected tricyclic antidepressant ingestions involving children 6 years old or less. Acad Emerg Med 2001;8(2):139–44.

[32] Smith ER, Klein-Schwartz W. Are 1-2 dangerous? Chloroquine and hydroxychloroquine exposure in toddlers. J Emerg Med 2005;28(4):437–43.

[33] Matteucci MJ. One pill can kill: assessing the potential for fatal poisonings in children. Pediatr Ann 2005;34(12):964–8.

[34] Jordan P, Brookes JG, Nikolic G, et al. Hydroxychloroquine overdose: toxicokinetics and management. J Toxicol Clin Toxicol 1999;37(7):861–4.

[35] DeWitt CR, Waksman JC. Pharmacology, pathophysiology and management of calcium channel blocker and beta-blocker toxicity. Toxicol Rev 2004;23(4):223–38.

[36] Vaghy PL, Williams JS, Schwartz A. Receptor pharmacology of calcium entry blocking agents. Am J Cardiol 1987;59(2):9A–17A.

[37] Belson MG, Gorman SE, Sullivan K, et al. Calcium channel blocker ingestions in children. Am J Emerg Med 2000;18(5):581–6.

[38] Lee DC, Greene T, Dougherty T, et al. Fatal nifedipine ingestions in children. J Emerg Med 2000;19(4):359–61.

[39] Love JN, Sammon M, Smereck J. Are one or two dangerous? Camphor exposure in toddlers. J Emerg Med 2004;27(1):49–54.

[40] Phelan WJ 3rd. Camphor poisoning: over-the-counter dangers. Pediatrics 1976;57(3): 428–31.

[41] Ratnapalan S, Potylitsina Y, Tan LH, et al. Measuring a toddler's mouthful: toxicologic considerations. J Pediatr 2003;142(6):729–30.

[42] Sachdeva DK, Stadnyk JM. Are one or two dangerous? Opioid exposure in toddlers. J Emerg Med 2005;29(1):77–84.

[43] Aronow R, Paul SD, Woolley PV. Childhood poisoning. An unfortunate consequence of methadone availability. JAMA 1972;219(3):321–4.

[44] von Muhlendahl KE, Scherf-Rahne B, Krienke EG, et al. Codeine intoxication in childhood. Lancet 1976;2(7980):303–5.

[45] Bosse GM, Matyunas NJ. Delayed toxidromes. J Emerg Med 1999;17(4):679–90.

[46] Little GL, Boniface KS. Are one or two dangerous? Sulfonylurea exposure in toddlers. J Emerg Med 2005;28(3):305–10.

[47] Quadrani DA, Spiller HA, Widder P. Five-year retrospective evaluation of sulfonylurea ingestion in children. J Toxicol Clin Toxicol 1996;34(3):267–70.

[48] Spiller HA, Villalobos D, Krenzelok EP, et al. Prospective multicenter study of sulfonylurea ingestion in children. J Pediatr 1997;131(1 Pt 1):141–6.

[49] Borowski H, Caraccio T, Mofenson H. Sulfonylurea ingestion in children: is an 8-hour observation period sufficient? J Pediatr 1998;133(4):584–5.

[50] Rumack BH, Temple AR. Lomotil poisoning. Pediatrics 1974;53(4):495–500.

[51] McCarron MM, Challoner KR, Thompson GA. Diphenoxylate-atropine (Lomotil) overdose in children: an update (report of eight cases and review of the literature). Pediatrics 1991;87(5):694–700.

[52] Wasserman GS, Green VA, Wise GW. Lomotil ingestions in children. Am Fam Physician 1975;11(6):93–7.

[53] Penfold D, Volans GN. Overdose from Lomotil. Br Med J 1977;2(6099):1401–2.

[54] Silber TJ. Ipecac syrup abuse, morbidity, and mortality: isn't it time to repeal its over-the-counter status? J Adolesc Health 2005;37(3):256–60.

[55] Wald A. Is chronic use of stimulant laxatives harmful to the colon? J Clin Gastroenterol 2003;36(5):386–9.

[56] Turner J, Batik M, Palmer LJ, et al. Detection and importance of laxative use in adolescents with anorexia nervosa. J Am Acad Child Adolesc Psychiatry 2000;39(3):378–85.

[57] Schreier H. Munchausen by proxy defined. Pediatrics 2002;110(5):985–8.

[58] Shannon M. The demise of ipecac. Pediatrics 2003;112(5):1180–1.

[59] Krassner L. TIPP usage. Pediatrics 1984;74(5 Pt 2):976–80.

[60] Vale JA, Meredith TJ, Proudfoot AT. Syrup of ipecacuanha: is it really useful? Br Med J (Clin Res Ed) 1986;293(6558):1321–2.

[61] Litovitz T. In defense of retaining ipecac syrup as an over-the-counter drug. Pediatrics 1988; 82(3 Pt 2):514–6.

[62] Poison treatment in the home. American Academy of Pediatrics Committee on Injury, Violence, and Poison Prevention. Pediatrics 2003;112(5):1182–5.

[63] Position paper: ipecac syrup. J Toxicol Clin Toxicol 2004;42(2):133–43.

[64] Ente G, Penzer PH. New abuse of ipecac. Pediatrics 1986;77(1):134–5.

[65] Cooper C, Kilham H, Ryan M. Ipecac—a substance of abuse. Med J Aust 1998;168(2):94–5.

[66] Vanin JR. Ipecac abuse—danger. J Am Coll Health 1992;40(5):237–8.

[67] Greenfeld D, Mickley D, Quinlan DM, et al. Ipecac abuse in a sample of eating disordered outpatients. Int J Eat Disord 1993;13(4):411–4.

[68] Dawson JA, Yager J. A case of abuse of syrup of ipecac resulting in death. J Am Coll Health 1986;34(6):280–2.

[69] Schiff RJ, Wurzel CL, Brunson SC, et al. Death due to chronic syrup of ipecac use in a patient with bulimia. Pediatrics 1986;78(3):412–6.

[70] Adler AG, Walinsky P, Krall RA, et al. Death resulting from ipecac syrup poisoning. JAMA 1980;243(19):1927–8.

[71] Friedman EJ. Death from ipecac intoxication in a patient with anorexia nervosa. Am J Psychiatry 1984;141(5):702–3.

[72] Pope HG Jr, Hudson JI, Nixon RA, et al. The epidemiology of ipecac abuse. N Engl J Med 1986;314(4):245–6.

[73] Andersen JM, Keljo DJ, Argyle JC. Secretory diarrhea caused by ipecac poisoning. J Pediatr Gastroenterol Nutr 1997;24(5):612–5.

[74] Bader AA, Kerzner B. Ipecac toxicity in Munchausen syndrome by proxy. Ther Drug Monit 1999;21(2):259–60.

[75] Cooper CP, Kamath KR. A toddler with persistent vomiting and diarrhoea. Eur J Pediatr 1998;157(9):775–6.

[76] Goebel J, Gremse DA, Artman M. Cardiomyopathy from ipecac administration in Munchausen syndrome by proxy. Pediatrics 1993;92(4):601–3.

[77] McClung HJ, Murray R, Braden NJ, et al. Intentional ipecac poisoning in children. Am J Dis Child 1988;142(6):637–9.

[78] Santangelo WC, Richey JE, Rivera L, et al. Surreptitious ipecac administration simulating intestinal pseudo-obstruction. Ann Intern Med 1989;110(12):1031–2.

[79] Schneider DJ, Perez A, Knilamus TE, et al. Clinical and pathologic aspects of cardiomyopathy from ipecac administration in Munchausen's syndrome by proxy. Pediatrics 1996; 97(6 Pt 1):902–6.

[80] Sutphen JL, Saulsbury FT. Intentional ipecac poisoning: Munchausen syndrome by proxy. Pediatrics 1988;82(3 Pt 2):453–6.

[81] Manno BR, Manno JE. Toxicology of ipecac: a review. Clin Toxicol 1977;10(2): 221–42.

[82] Dresser LP, Massey EW, Johnson EE, et al. Ipecac myopathy and cardiomyopathy. J Neurol Neurosurg Psychiatry 1993;56(5):560–2.

[83] Carraccio C, Blotny K, Ringel R. Sudden onset of profound weakness in a toddler. J Pediatr 1993;122(4):663–7.

[84] Halbig L, Gutmann L, Goebel HH, et al. Ultrastructural pathology in emetine-induced myopathy. Acta Neuropathol (Berl) 1988;75(6):577–82.

[85] Mateer JE, Farrell BJ, Chou SS, et al. Reversible ipecac myopathy. Arch Neurol 1985;42(2): 188–90.

[86] Rashid N. Medically unexplained myopathy due to ipecac abuse. Psychosomatics 2006; 47(2):167–9.

[87] Palmer EP, Guay AT. Reversible myopathy secondary to abuse of ipecac in patients with major eating disorders. N Engl J Med 1985;313(23):1457–9.

[88] Ho PC, Dweik R, Cohen MC. Rapidly reversible cardiomyopathy associated with chronic ipecac ingestion. Clin Cardiol 1998;21(10):780–3.

[89] Yamashita M, Yamashita M, Azuma J. Urinary excretion of ipecac alkaloids in human volunteers. Vet Hum Toxicol 2002;44(5):257–9.

[90] Mitchell JE, Boutacoff LI, Hatsukami D, et al. Laxative abuse as a variant of bulimia. J Nerv Ment Dis 1986;174(3):174–6.

[91] Kiningham RB, Gorenflo DW. Weight loss methods of high school wrestlers. Med Sci Sports Exerc 2001;33(5):810–3.

[92] Ackerman NB Jr, Strobel CT. Polle syndrome: chronic diarrhea in Munchausen's child. Gastroenterology 1981;81(6):1140–2.

[93] Epstein MA, Markowitz RL, Gallo DM, et al. Munchausen syndrome by proxy: considerations in diagnosis and confirmation by video surveillance. Pediatrics 1987;80(2):220–4.

[94] Volk D. Factitious diarrhea in two children. Am J Dis Child 1982;136(11):10127–8.

[95] Thompson WG. Laxatives: clinical pharmacology and rational use. Drugs 1980;19(1):49–58.

[96] Xing JH, Soffer EE. Adverse effects of laxatives. Dis Colon Rectum 2001;44(8):1201–9.

[97] Baker EH, Sandle GI. Complications of laxative abuse. Annu Rev Med 1996;47:127–34.

[98] Oster JR, Materson BJ, Rogers AI. Laxative abuse syndrome. Am J Gastroenterol 1980; 74(5):451–8.

[99] Vanin JR, Saylor KE. Laxative abuse: a hazardous habit for weight control. J Am Coll Health 1989;37(5):227–30.

[100] Malmquist J, Ericsson B, Hulten-Nosslin MB, et al. Finger clubbing and aspartylglucos-amine excretion in a laxative-abusing patient. Postgrad Med J 1980;56(662):862–4.

[101] Pines A, Olchovsky D, Bregman J, et al. Finger clubbing associated with laxative abuse. South Med J 1983;76(8):1071–2.

[102] Prior J, White I. Tetany and clubbing in patient who ingested large quantities of senna. Lancet 1978;2(8096):947.

[103] Silk DB, Gibson JA, Murray CR. Reversible finger clubbing in a case of purgative abuse. Gastroenterology 1975;68(4 Pt 1):790–4.

[104] Stolk LM, Hoogtanders K. Detection of laxative abuse by urine analysis with HPLC and diode array detection. Pharm World Sci 1999;21(1):40–3.

[105] Muller-Lissner S. What has happened to the cathartic colon? Gut 1996;39(3):486–8.

[106] Wald A. Constipation in the primary care setting: current concepts and misconceptions. Am J Med 2006;119(9):736–9.

[107] Spiller HA, Rodgers GC Jr. Evaluation of administration of activated charcoal in the home. Pediatrics 2001;108(6):E100.

[108] Burns MM. Activated charcoal as the sole intervention for treatment after childhood poisoning. Curr Opin Pediatr 2000;12(2):166–71.

[109] Tenenbein M. Gastrointestinal decontamination of the overdose patient in the year 2000. Clinical Pediatric Emergency Medicine 2000;1(3):195–9.

[110] Chyka PA, Seger D, Krenzelok EP, et al. Position paper: single-dose activated charcoal. Clin Toxicol (Phila) 2005;43(2):61–87.

[111] Dockstader LL, Lawrence RA, Bresnick HL. Home administration of activated charcoal: feasibility and acceptance. Vet Hum Toxicol 1986;28(5):471.

[112] Grbcich PA, Lacouture PG, Woolf A. Administration of charcoal in the home. Vet Hum Toxicol 1987;29(6):458.

[113] Lamminpaa A, Vilska J, Hoppu K. Medical charcoal for a child's poisoning at home: availability and success of administration in Finland. Hum Exp Toxicol 1993;12(1):29–32.

[114] Dilger I, Brockstedt M, Oberdisse U, et al. Activated charcoal is needed rarely in children but can be administered safely by the lay public. J Toxicol Clin Toxicol 1999;37:402–3.

[115] Scharman EJ, Cloonan HA, Durback-Morris LF. Home administration of charcoal: can mothers administer a therapeutic dose? J Emerg Med 2001;21(4):357–61.

[116] Osterhoudt KC, Alpern ER, Durbin D, et al. Activated charcoal administration in a pediatric emergency department. Pediatr Emerg Care 2004;20(8):493–8.

[117] Spiller HA. Home administration of charcoal. J Emerg Med 2003;25(1):106–7 [author reply: 107].

[118] Graff GR, Stark J, Berkenbosch JW, et al. Chronic lung disease after activated charcoal aspiration. Pediatrics 2002;109(5):959–61.

[119] Justiniani FR, Hippalgaonkar R, Martinez LO. Charcoal-containing empyema complicating treatment for overdose. Chest 1985;87(3):404–5.

[120] Elliott CG, Colby TV, Kelly TM, et al. Charcoal lung. Bronchiolitis obliterans after aspiration of activated charcoal. Chest 1989;96(3):672–4.

[121] Menzies DG, Busuttil A, Prescott LF. Fatal pulmonary aspiration of oral activated charcoal. BMJ 1988;297(6646):459–60.

ELSEVIER
SAUNDERS

EMERGENCY
MEDICINE
CLINICS OF
NORTH AMERICA

Emerg Med Clin N Am 25 (2007) 309–331

Management of β-Adrenergic Blocker and Calcium Channel Antagonist Toxicity

William Kerns II, MD, FACEP, FACMT

*Division of Toxicology, Department of Emergency Medicine, Carolinas Medical Center,
Medical Education Building, 3rd floor, 1000 Blythe Boulevard, Charlotte, NC 28203, USA*

This review intends to update the management portion of a comprehensive description of β-adrenergic blocker (BB) and calcium channel antagonist (CCA) toxicity that appeared in the 1994 *Emergency Medicine Clinics of North America* [1]. Over the last 13 years, these two classes of drugs remain invaluable treatments for various cardiovascular and other medical conditions. Unfortunately, they also remain common causes of cardiovascular collapse following accidental or intentional overdose. Toxicity is associated with significant mortality. According to American Association of Poison Control Centers Toxic Exposure Surveillance System (AAPCC TESS) data, deaths amongst cardiovascular agents like BBs and CCAs are only exceeded by abused sympathomimetics such as cocaine (Fig. 1) [2–6].

The most significant changes with BB and CCA toxicity occurring in the last 13 years deal with the search for improved treatment. New therapies have evolved and continue to evolve. Once a novel therapy, investigation with insulin-euglycemia yielded insight into metabolic abnormalities that occur with drug-induced shock and now provides a valuable treatment. There are new formulations of standard antidotes such as recombinant glucagon. There is additional experience with efficacy and safety of calcium supplements. Emphasis on early and aggressive goal-directed therapy of shock has brought more critical care skills into the emergency department, including more rapid diagnosis of cardiogenic shock with the advent of emergency department ultrasound [7,8].

A review of the mechanism of BB- and CCA-induced toxicity will facilitate understanding various antidotal strategies. Calcium is critical for physiologic signaling. Calcium enters cells by way of specific channels and once

---

E-mail address: rkerns@carolinashealthcare.org

0733-8627/07/$ - see front matter © 2007 Elsevier Inc. All rights reserved.
doi:10.1016/j.emc.2007.02.001
emed.theclinics.com

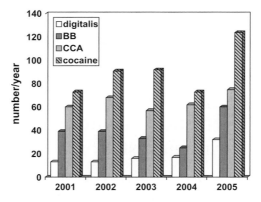

Fig. 1. Cardiovascular drug annual mortality from AAPCC TESS Data. (*Data from* Refs. [2–6].)

in the cell, participates in multiple processes. In myocardial cells, calcium entry by way of L-type or voltage-gated calcium channels initiates calcium release from intracellular storage organelles that is necessary to affect excitation–contraction coupling [9]. It is also critical for action potential generation in sinoatrial tissue [9]. In vascular smooth muscle, calcium influx maintains tone [9]. Adrenergic stimulation can modulate the effects of calcium. For example, β_1-adrenergic receptor stimulation facilitates calcium entry into cardiac myocytes by increasing the number of open calcium channels. β-adrenergic–facilitated calcium entry involves activation of adenyl cyclase, a membrane-bound enzyme that catalyzes cyclic adenosine monophosphate (cAMP) formation. Formation of cAMP leads to phosphorylation of the L-type channel with subsequent opening and calcium influx [10]. Although they act through differing mechanisms, both BBs and CCAs inhibit calcium entry. β-adrenergic–blocking drugs inhibit facilitated L-type calcium channel opening, and CCAs maintain the channel in the closed state [11]. Excessive inhibition of calcium entry results in hallmark toxicity of bradycardia, conduction abnormalities, hypotension, and, if severe, hypodynamic shock [1,12].

Calcium signaling is critical to other processes that are affected by cardiac drug toxicity including carbohydrate metabolism. During drug-induced shock due to either BBs or CCAs, the heart switches its preferred source of energy substrate from free fatty acids to carbohydrates [13,14]. In response, the liver increases glucose availability by way of glycogenolysis. Even though circulating glucose is sufficient enough to support the heart during stress, CCAs block calcium-mediated insulin release by pancreatic β-islet cells that is necessary for myocardial cells to use the additional glucose [15]. The resulting metabolic manifestations resemble diabetic ketoacidosis with insulin deficiency, hyperglycemia, and acidemia [16].

Beyond general supportive care, the goals for both new and established therapies for management of BB and CCA drug toxicity are to achieve improved perfusion by increasing blood pressure and reversing myocardial dysfunction.

Supportive care

Initial resuscitation

Attention to airway, breathing, and circulation is paramount in improving patient survival following BB and CCA overdose. Although some patients maintain surprising alertness despite significant cardiovascular compromise, many will have abrupt central nervous system depression with loss of airway protective reflexes and require intubation and mechanical ventilation. For patients that present with hallmark bradycardia and hypotension, atropine and normal saline fluid bolus are reasonable initial therapies. In cases of mild toxicity, these measures may suffice. However, atropine and fluid bolus more often fail to improve heart rate and blood pressure in significant overdose, and the health care provider should anticipate quickly moving on to other resuscitation measures [17,18].

Critically ill patients who have shock require prompt evaluation of the source(s) of hypotension to guide therapy. Emergency department bedside cardiac ultrasound is increasingly available and serves as a rapid, noninvasive screening tool to assess myocardial function [8]. If ultrasound identifies a hypodynamic myocardium, then pharmacologic therapy can focus on cardiotonic drugs to improve contractility and output (see later discussion). Emergent formal echocardiography is useful if screening ultrasonography is not readily available. If ultrasonography demonstrates adequate contractility, then placement of a more invasive device such as an arterial blood pressure monitor and/or pulmonary artery catheter may be necessary. If lowered peripheral resistance is identified, then pharmacologic therapy can be directed to vasoactive agents such as norepinephrine to improve blood pressure. If the patient requires more resuscitation than a simple fluid bolus, then a Foley catheter is indicated to monitor urine output.

Determination of acid-base status is important because acidemia can worsen myocardial dysfunction due to CCAs. The mechanism of enhanced myocardial depression with acidosis is not fully elucidated but may be due to increased drug-binding at the calcium channel [19]. Acidemia can be treated by using appropriate ventilator settings or administering bicarbonate with a target of maintaining blood pH of at least 7.4. Bicarbonate therapy can improve hemodynamics. Bicarbonate administration increased mean arterial pressure and cardiac output in a toxic verapamil model [20].

Continuous cardiac monitoring and a 12-lead electrocardiogram are essential to identify cardiac conduction abnormalities. Because several BBs and CCAs can antagonize myocardial fast sodium channel function similar to that of tricyclic antidepressants, the 12-lead electrocardiogram will also assess QRS duration and act as a treatment indicator [21,22]. Consider 1 to 2 mEq/kg sodium bicarbonate bolus for QRS duration greater than 120 milliseconds.

Diagnostic studies

In addition to bedside cardiac ultrasound, invasive monitors, electrocardiogram, and arterial blood gas analysis, other important studies specific to BB and CCA toxicity include analysis of blood lactate, glucose, and renal function as well as chest radiography.

Assessment of glucose and lactate is necessary because significant CCA overdose can induce a diabetogenic state with hyperglycemia and lactate accumulation [23–25]. This is due to altered glucose metabolism, insulin deficiency, and insulin resistance [16]. The extent of hyperglycemia and lactic acidosis serves as a marker of the degree of calcium channel poisoning [16].

Hypoglycemia has often been associated with BB overdose, but it is actually extremely rare [1,12]. Like serious CCA toxicity, BB overdose can occasionally present with hyperglycemia [26–28]. Insulin is indicated for hyperglycemia and hyperlactatemia (see later discussion).

A plain chest radiograph serves as an adjunct to the physical examination looking for pulmonary edema that may limit fluid and solute administration during resuscitation [29,30].

Specific serum BB and CCA drug levels may be obtained for later confirmation of exposure, but will not be available in a timely fashion to guide therapy.

Gastrointestinal decontamination

When considering the cumulative poisoning literature, there is insufficient evidence that gastrointestinal decontamination improves overall outcome. For this reason, airway, ventilation, and cardiovascular resuscitation take precedence over gastrointestinal decontamination following overdose. However, if the patient is stable and there is a suspicion of BB and CCA overdose, decontamination may be appropriate because of the potential mortality from these cardiovascular drugs.

Gastric lavage is not routinely indicated but may be useful if the patient presents within 1 to 2 hours of a "life-threatening ingestion" according to consensus review by toxicologists [31]. What constitutes a life-threatening ingestion can be determined on a case-by-case basis, weighing potential morbidity and mortality due to cardiac drug overdose versus risks of the lavage procedure itself.

It is reasonable to administer 1 gm/kg activated charcoal within 1 to 2 hours of ingestion to decrease systemic drug absorption [32]. The first 2 hours postingestion are considered the greatest window of opportunity to decrease drug absorption. However, many BBs and CCAs are available as sustained release preparations with delayed systemic absorption leading to onset of toxicity greater than 12 hours [18,33]. Thus, there is additional time to institute effective gastrointestinal decontamination compared with regular release formulations. For example, charcoal given 4 hours after sustained release verapamil reduced bioavailability by nearly one third in a controlled volunteer study [34]. Whole bowel irrigation is a plausible adjunct to activated charcoal in the case of sustained release drug ingestion [35]. Whole bowel irrigation has been used in several cases of CCA ingestion [36,37]. A cooperative patient who does not have evidence of gut dysfunction is prerequisite for whole bowel irrigation.

Specific pharmacologic therapy

Calcium

Calcium is a logical therapy for CCA toxicity. In theory, augmentation of extracellular calcium may overcome competitive antagonism of the calcium channel or maximize calcium entry through unblocked channels. From animal investigations, calcium is expected to increase inotropy and improve blood pressure, but have little effect on conduction blocks and heart rate [38–40]. Calcium affords some survival effect in these studies [14,40].

Clinical experience is mixed. Calcium infusion alone has improved blood pressure in some instances [33,37,41]. In a large series of CCA overdoses (n = 139), 23 patients were treated with calcium. Blood pressure increased in 16 (70%) of these patients [18]. However, calcium failed in many cases [25,42–45].

Calcium has been used to treat BB toxicity as well, but evidence to support its use is less substantial than for CCA toxicity. In rodent and canine models, calcium reversed negative inotropy induced by various betablockers, but did not reverse bradycardia or conduction abnormalities [46–48]. These studies did not test for survival. Inotropic benefit without chronotropic effect has been observed in limited human application, although no case report used calcium alone to treat BB toxicity [49–52]. In one unusual case, a patient demonstrated dramatic restoration of pulse and conduction in addition to blood pressure in temporal relationship to calcium boluses when other agents failed [53]. Calcium often failed to improve hemodynamics [51].

There are no clear guidelines as to what form or dose of calcium to use. Animal models of CCA toxicity demonstrate that large doses are needed. A twofold to threefold increase in serum calcium was associated with improved inotropy in two models [14,38]. Little can be inferred from human case reports regarding the necessary dose because most refer to the total dose in terms of grams rather than milliequivalents. The largest case series of CCA toxicity reported doses ranging from 4.5 to 95 mEq [18].

Calcium is available in two forms: chloride and gluconate. Calcium chloride contains more calcium in terms of milliequivalents than calcium gluconate. A 10 mL vial of 10% calcium chloride solution contains 13.5 mEq of calcium, whereas a similar volume and concentration of calcium gluconate provides 4.5 mEq. However, when given as equivalent doses, the chloride and gluconate form provide similar increases in ionized calcium [54,55].

Most patients tolerate the necessary large doses of calcium without problems, including one patient whose total serum calcium peaked at 23.8 mg/dL (5.9 mmol/L) following 30 gm of calcium [56]. However, calcium administration has potential adverse cardiac effects (albeit rare) including hypotension, conduction blockade, bradycardia, and, asystole if given too rapidly [57]. There is also the theoretic risk of inadvertently giving calcium to a digitalis-intoxicated patient who has resultant excessive cardiac myocyte calcium overload and asystole. Tissue injury due to extravasation of calcium preparations is more of a concern, especially due to the chloride form. Thus, central intravenous administration is recommended when using calcium chloride. Given the greater risk of tissue injury with calcium chloride and similar ability of the various forms to raise calcium levels, it seems prudent to use the gluconate form during cardiac drug resuscitation.

A reasonable approach to calcium therapy is to give a 0.6-mL/kg bolus of 10% calcium gluconate (0.2 mL/kg 10% calcium chloride) over 5 to 10 minutes. After the bolus, initiate a continuous calcium gluconate infusion at 0.6 to 1.5 mL/kg/hour (0.2–0.5 mL/kg/hour 10% calcium chloride), because bolus administration only briefly increases ionized calcium (5–10 minutes) [54,55]. Titrate the infusion to affect either improved blood pressure or contractility. Follow serial ionized calcium levels every 30 minutes initially and then every 2 hours with a goal of maintaining ionized calcium at approximately twice normal.

In summary, although calcium is a logical agent to resuscitate cardiac drug toxicity, clinical experience is mixed and disappointing at times. When beneficial, it appears to provide primarily inotropic effect. The calcium gluconate form is the safest of the available preparations to use.

Glucagon

Glucagon is produced in pancreatic α-cells from cleavage of proglucagon. It is a regulatory hormone that opposes the hypoglycemic action of insulin, hence its first clinical application for treatment of hypoglycemia. During stress states, including shock, glucagon stimulates hepatic glycogenolysis resulting in increased circulating glucose. Glucagon also has direct myocardial action and has been investigated as an inotrope in both ischemic and nonischemic heart failure [58]. Thus, it is an attractive antidote for drug-induced myocardial failure.

Since 1998, pharmaceutic glucagon has been produced by way of recombinant technology. Before that time, glucagon consisted of a purified bovine or porcine pancreatic extract. This is important to understand because virtually all research and published clinical experience regarding antidotal glucagon use used the older bovine or porcine-derived form. The animal-derived glucagon product also contains insulin [14]. Because pure glucagon has not been used in cardiac drug toxicity models until recently [59], it is unclear what contribution the insulin contaminant plays in the apparent efficacy of glucagon. Lastly, unlike bovine and porcine glucagon, recombinant glucagon does not contain phenol, so concerns with secondary toxicity due to excessive administration of this preservative are no longer necessary.

Glucagon pharmacokinetics are well characterized. The onset of action is rapid and the duration of effect is short. Increased cardiodynamic changes occur in 1 to 3 minutes in nonpoisoned individuals, peak at 5 to 7 minutes, and persist for 10 to 15 minutes [58]. The hyperglycemic effect peaks at 20 to 30 minutes after administration [60].

Glucagon exerts positive inotropic and chronotropic effects on the myocardium by stimulating adenyl cyclase similar to catecholamines, but through a separate receptor [61,62]. This property makes glucagon particularly attractive as an antidote for BB toxicity by providing cAMP necessary for myocardial cell performance in the face of β-adrenergic receptor blockade. Glucagon's positive chronotropic and inotropic effects are demonstrated in several animal models of β-blockade, including isolated, perfused myocardial tissue and intact canine models [63,64].

Several canine studies directly compare glucagon with other purported BB antidotes. Glucagon was superior to isoproterenol in reversing β-blockade with 2 mg/kg propranolol [65]. Another investigation compared glucagon with amrinone, a phosphodiesterase inhibitor. Although both agents reversed depressed myocardial contractility induced by 10 mg/kg propranolol, glucagon was superior in reversing bradycardia [66]. In a study that compared survival after propranolol intoxication, glucagon was superior to epinephrine but inferior to insulin-euglycemia [67]. In a rodent model of beta-blocker toxicity, glucagon alone did not alter survival but worsened survival when used in combination with dopamine [68].

The first published human case of BB overdose treated with glucagon appeared in 1973 [65]. The patient developed coma, bradycardia, and hypotension following an overdose of propranolol, imipramine, and valium. After 90 minutes of failed isoproterenol infusion, 10 mg glucagon increased heart rate from 52 to 70 beats per minute (bpm) and blood pressure from 60 to 95 mm Hg. Unfortunately, the patient later died from urosepsis. From this modest start, antidotal glucagon use increased, and many subsequent reports described good clinical response often after conventional therapy failed [17,28,69–77]. Despite the abundance of cases promoting glucagon's efficacy, there are only a few reports whereby glucagon was the sole pharmacologic agent used to treat BB poisoning [76–78]. Glucagon failed in several other instances [27,79–82]. There are no human controlled trials of glucagon for BB toxicity.

Laboratory and clinical experience also support the use of glucagon for CCA toxicity. In isolated heart preparations, glucagon reversed bradycardia and hypotension induced by diltiazem, nifedipine, and verapamil [83]. In intact rat and canine studies, glucagon consistently increased heart rate and contractility following verapamil infusion [77,84–87]. In addition to cardiodynamic effects, glucagon reversed conduction blocks due to diltiazem and verapamil [87–89]. Only one animal study directly compared glucagon with other standard antidotes for survival effect following severe verapamil toxicity [87]. In this study, glucagon provided similar survival compared with epinephrine but was inferior to insulin-euglycemia.

As in the case of glucagon use in human BB toxicity, there are no clinical trials to assess efficacy in CCA overdose. There are published cases demonstrating glucagon's efficacy [25,77,90–94]. Glucagon failed to improve heart rate and blood pressure in several cases as well [18,25,95].

The recommended initial dose of glucagon is 50 to 150 µg/kg, roughly 3 to 10 mg in a 70-kg patient. Smaller initial doses frequently fail to produce adequate cardiodynamic responses [72,75]. Glucagon works rapidly. Responses in heart rate and blood pressure often occur within minutes [65,75,76]. Bolus therapy may be repeated again in 3 to 5 minutes. There is no established ceiling dose to bolus therapy with up to 30 mg cumulative dose in one case [71]. Rather than give repeated bolus doses, it makes more kinetic sense to initiate a glucagon infusion following the initial bolus because of the short duration of cardiac effects [58]. A reasonable guideline for determining the infusion dose is to give the effective bolus dose each hour. For example, if heart rate increased after two successive 5-mg boluses, then administer 10 mg/hour. The infusion rate can then be titrated to the desired effect. There is no established maximum dose for continuous infusion. One patient required 411 mg given over 41 hours following propranolol overdose [75].

The adverse effects of glucagon are well described. Nausea and vomiting are common and the occurrence is dose related [58,60,72,96,97]. Emesis may pose a substantial problem in the patient who has depressed mentation and tenuous airway status. Transient hyperglycemia may also occur [58,60]. Hyperglycemia is expected based on glucagon's stimulation of glycogenolysis and typically does not require intervention. Hypoglycemia is infrequently reported during glucagon therapy for noncardiac drug–related conditions, possibly because of pre-existing poor hepatic glycogen stores [98]. Relevance during resuscitation of cardiac drug toxicity is unknown. In experimental verapamil poisoning, glucagon-treated animals develop hypoglycemia following initial hyperglycemia [14,87]. However, to the author's best knowledge, there are no human reports of hypoglycemia following antidotal glucagon use in the setting of cardiac drug toxicity. Lastly, glucagon availability is a common shortcoming because many hospitals do not have sufficient pharmacy stock to provide adequate resuscitation [76,99,100].

All in all, the available animal data, human clinical experience, and minimal adverse effect profile support the use of glucagon early in the course of both BB and CCA toxicity. It seems to be most effective in increasing heart rate.

Adrenergic receptor agonists—catecholamines

Adrenergic receptor agonists are a rational therapeutic choice in drug-induced shock for their cardiotonic and vasoactive effects. All of the available catecholamines, including dopamine, dobutamine, epinephrine, isoproterenol, and norepinephrine, have been used to resuscitate BB and CCA toxicity [17,18,22,101,102]. In general, there is no single agent that is predictably successful for all cases. In theory, the choice of adrenergic agonist could be based upon the pharmacologic activity of the offending agent. For example, in the case of β-receptor blockade with hemodynamically significant bradycardia, predominant β-stimulation with isoproterenol is reasonable. However, this has not borne out in clinical application. In one series of 39 BB overdoses, isoproterenol faired poorly compared with other catecholamines, raising heart rate in only 11% and blood pressure in 22% of cases compared with epinephrine (67% and 50%) or dopamine (25% each) [17]. A better approach is to select an agent based upon specific hemodynamic and cardiodynamic monitoring. For example, the patient who has depressed contractility and decreased peripheral resistance may benefit from norepinephrine or epinephrine, because these drugs possess both β- and α-agonist properties.

One aspect of treating with a catecholamine that is clear from experimental models and clinical reports of severe cardiac drug toxicity is that large doses may be necessary for successful resuscitation. The doses of isoproterenol and dopamine had to be increased 15 fold and 5 fold, respectively, to reverse propranolol-induced hemodynamic changes in canines [103]. After labetolol infusion in volunteers, isoproterenol at 26 times the control dose was needed to restore blood pressure [104]. Following combined diltiazem and metoprolol overdose, epinephrine at 30 to 100 μg/minute raised blood pressure [105]. Epinephrine at 0.8 μg/kg/minute raised blood pressure following verapamil overdose [42]. Even with extraordinary doses and combining multiple catecholamines, this class of agents often fails to restore adequate perfusion [27,86,106].

Adverse effects of catecholamine administration include tissue injury, hypotension, and detrimental metabolic consequences. Extravasation of potent α-agonists from peripheral intravenous sites may lead to skin and local tissue necrosis. Thus, central intravenous administration is preferable to peripheral administration whenever possible. Catecholamines, such as isoproterenol and dobutamine, that possess predominant β-receptor activity and little α-agonist activity may decrease peripheral resistance and worsen hypotension [107]. Lastly, adrenergic agonists enhance free fatty acid use by the heart, and this may be detrimental during shock (see insulin-euglycemia discussion) [14].

A reasonable approach to catecholamine use is based on cardiodynamic and hemodynamic monitoring, using norepinephrine as a first line agent for hypotension due to low systemic resistance. Because of potential detrimental metabolic effects on the heart from catecholamines and marginal efficacy in animal studies, other cardiotonic agents are better initial choices for improving depressed myocardial function.

In summary, there is no one catecholamine that is superior for cardiovascular drug toxicity. Large doses of multiple adrenergic agents may be required.

Insulin-euglycemia

Insulin is a pancreatic polypeptide that plays an essential role in glucose homeostasis. It is secreted by β-islet cells primarily in response to elevated circulating glucose. Insulin promotes glucose use and storage and inhibits glucose release, gluconeogenesis, and lipolysis. Insulin is necessary for glucose uptake by most tissues, including the heart. Insulin also possesses inotropic properties, improving myocardial function in depressed hearts due to ischemic and nonischemic causes [108–112]. Interest in insulin as a treatment for cardiovascular drug overdose arose from insulin's inotropic property. The beneficial effect in drug-induced shock may be due to its role in carbohydrate metabolism.

Insulin was first used specifically for cardiac drug toxicity in an anesthetized canine model of verapamil poisoning in 1993 [87]. In this model, 4 IU/minute insulin infused with dextrose to maintain euglycemia (HIE) improved contractility and coronary blood flow compared with calcium, epinephrine, and glucagon. Most importantly, HIE provided superior survival compared with standard treatments; all HIE animals survived. Similar findings were observed in a subsequent study using nonanesthetized, verapamil-toxic animals [113]. HIE treatment was also tested in a model of propranolol toxicity [67]. As in the verapamil investigations, HIE reversed myocardial failure, increased coronary blood flow, and improved survival compared with standard antidotes.

The mechanism of insulin's beneficial effect is not fully understood. Initially the inotropic effect was thought due to catecholamine release [109]. This is unlikely because β-receptor blockade does not impair the increased inotropy afforded by insulin [110]. Additionally, catecholamine levels did not increase after insulin administration in the verapamil canine study [16]. The best explanation lies in metabolic rescue.

The metabolic consequences of drug-induced shock provide a milieu that is ideal for insulin treatment—namely hyperglycemia and insulin deficiency. During nonstress conditions, the heart prefers free fatty acid as its primary substrate from which to generate energy molecules. During drug-induced shock, the preferred myocardial energy substrate shifts from free fatty acids to carbohydrates [13,14,110]. Glucose release occurs by way of hepatic glycogenolysis to meet increased carbohydrate demand. Both animal models and human cases of CCAs, especially verapamil, show marked hyperglycemia [16,23,114]. Although not as common, hyperglycemia can be seen during severe BB toxicity as well [26–28,115]. As an added insult, CCA toxicity is associated with insulin deficiency. Insulin release by the pancreatic β-islet cells is calcium channel–mediated and CCAs inhibit insulin release [15,16].

Cellular glucose uptake becomes concentration-dependent rather than insulin-mediated [116]. Critical tissues such as the myocardium may not efficiently or adequately use needed glucose during shock. Impaired substrate use—metabolic starvation—worsens depressed contractility already present from direct myocardial calcium channel antagonism.

Supplemental insulin provides metabolic support to the heart during shock by promoting carbohydrate metabolism. Following beta-blockade, insulin increased myocardial glucose uptake and improved function [110]. In severe CCA toxicity, insulin increased both glucose and lactate uptake [14]. Further evaluation of metabolic changes during verapamil toxicity showed that HIE increased lactate extraction to a greater extent than glucose extraction [116]. Improved function following insulin treatment occurs without an increase in myocardial work [14,110]. In contrast, treatment with calcium, glucagon, or epinephrine promotes free fatty acid use with subsequent increased myocardial work [14]. This metabolic difference may explain why standard treatments often fail to resuscitate severe drug-induced myocardial depression.

Clinical experience with insulin is favorable. Insulin was first used to treat hyperglycemia associated with CCA toxicity with good outcome [23]. HIE was specifically used for its inotropic properties to resuscitate five patients who had hypodynamic shock due to cardiac drug overdose in 1999 [25]. Since the initial 1999 case series, HIE has been used at the author's institution for five additional patients who had improved cardiovascular performance and all survived. Fifty-eight additional cases have been reported in the literature [117–128].

These 68 patients ingested CCAs [63], combined CCA–BB [4], and BB [1]. HIE was typically used as a rescue therapy after patients received varying doses of multiple pharmacologic antidotes. There are no cases whereby cardiotoxic drug overdose was managed with HIE alone. Given this framework for making clinical conclusions, most authors report good cardiodynamic and hemodynamic response to HIE, often when other therapies failed. Blood pressure and contractility typically increased within 15 to 60 minutes after initiating HIE [25]. This time course is similar to animal investigations [67,87]. Heart rate response is less dramatic and consistent with a lack of chronotropic effect in animal models [67,87]. In two cases managed at the author's institution, patients converted from third degree heart block to normal sinus rhythm in temporal relationship to HIE, but restoration of normal conduction was not reported in other published cases. Three reports (5 total patients) found HIE unhelpful in managing hypotension, although the insulin dose may have been suboptimal in one case [125], was unreported in a second [120], and may have been started too late in 2 patients [121]. Overall survival in the 68 patients was 85%. However, no randomized clinical trial has formally studied mortality nor adverse events with HIE versus other antidotes.

The insulin regimens used to treat these 68 patients varied, and details were often incomplete. The maximum insulin infusion ranged from 0.1 to

2.5 IU/kg/hour with 0.5 IU/kg/hour (39/55 patients) as the most common dose and 1.0 IU/kg/hour as the next most used dose (15/55). Fifteen patients received an insulin bolus (range 10–90 IU) before continuous infusion. Three patients were managed with a single bolus only, including a patient that inadvertently received 1000 IU with good cardiovascular response and no adverse events [117]. The duration of insulin infusion varied widely as well with a mean of 31 hours and ranged from .75 to 96 hours (n = 20 patients). Euglycemia was maintained by way of exogenous dextrose. The average maximum dextrose requirement was 24 gm/hour, but ranged from 0.5 to 75 gm/hour (n = 14 patients). The mean duration of dextrose infusion was 47 hours and ranged from 9 to 100 hours (n = 10 patients). Dextrose was required after cessation of insulin in 7 of these 10 patients.

Adverse events with HIE were predictable and infrequent. Numeric hypoglycemia (blood glucose < 60 mg/dL or 3.3 mmol/L) was reported in 9 of 55 patients. In most cases, additional dextrose was administered and HIE was continued without further hypoglycemia. However, in one series totaling 37 patients, 5 patients developed hypoglycemia that led to early cessation of insulin infusion [127]. These 5 patients had less hypotension on presentation than the remaining patients and thus may have been more insulin sensitive (communication with coauthor of Ref. [127]). HIE treatment lowers serum potassium. In the initial case series, serum potassium fell as low as 2.2 mEq/L (2.2 mmol/L) without sequelae [25]. Keep in mind that HIE does not deplete potassium; it simply shifts potassium from the extracellular to intracellular compartment. Potassium administration in these cases can theoretically result in potassium excess. Other asymptomatic electrolyte findings include hypophosphatemia and hypomagnesemia [25]. It is not clear if changes in magnesium and phosphate are due to the cardiac drug insult, general critical illness, or HIE. Similar changes are observed following insulin therapy for diabetic ketoacidosis [129,130].

Based on the animal data and clinical experience to date, a reasonable HIE regimen consists of the following: 1 IU/kg regular insulin bolus to maximally saturate receptors followed by a regular insulin infusion starting at 0.5 IU/kg/hour. The infusion can be titrated upward every 30 minutes to achieve the desired effect on contractility or blood pressure. (Bedside echocardiography is an ideal, rapid, and noninvasive technique for measuring myocardial response.) Euglycemia is defined as blood glucose between 100 and 250 mg/dL (5.5–14 mmol/L) and is maintained by administering intravenous dextrose. Unless the patient is markedly hyperglycemic (> 400 mg/dL or 22 mmol/L), a 25-gm dextrose bolus is given with the initial insulin bolus and is followed by dextrose infusion at 0.5 gm/kg/hour. Because this amount of dextrose is associated with a large volume of solute (25 gm/hour = 250 mL/hr of a 10% solution), establish central intravenous access so that smaller volume, more concentrated solutions can be given. The glucose infusion is titrated based on frequent bedside glucose monitoring—every 20 to 30 minutes until blood glucose is stable—and then at least every 1 to 2 hours. Potassium can be measured, but does not need to be replaced unless it falls below 2.5 mEq/dL (2.5 mmol/L) and there is a source of potassium loss.

In summary, HIE is a safe and effective therapy for significant CCA or BB toxicity. Animal and clinical data suggest that the best indication is when there is evidence of a hypodynamic myocardium. Additionally, the response to HIE is not immediate, so early detection of depressed contractility and early initiation of HIE therapy will increase the chance of benefit.

Sodium bicarbonate therapy

Sodium bicarbonate is used to treat acidemia and sodium channel blockade.

As discussed under supportive therapy, acidemia worsens CCA toxicity [19], and sodium bicarbonate treatment improves hemodynamics [20].

Both BB and CCA drugs appear to antagonize myocardial sodium channels. β-blockers with the so-called "membrane stabilizing effect" include acebutolol, betoxalol, carvedilol, metoprolol, oxprenolol, and propranolol [131]. Thus, toxicity from these drugs may include widened QRS in addition to bradycardia [53,132,133]. At high doses, CCAs impair myocardial sodium channels, although experimental evidence is mixed [134–137]. Patients who have wide complex QRS abnormalities are reported following CCA overdose [21,22].

Sodium bicarbonate is the traditional treatment for wide complex QRS conduction abnormalities due to sodium channel antagonism. Bicarbonate has been evaluated in animal studies of BB and CCA toxicity and has been used anecdotally in human poisoning. Bicarbonate therapy alone did not alter QRS duration or hemodynamics in a canine model of mild BB toxicity [138]. However, it reversed QRS widening following acebutolol overdose in one case report [100]. Diltiazem and verapamil overdoses resulted in QRS prolongation responsive to bicarbonate boluses [21].

Despite limited evidence to fully support bicarbonate use for BB and CCA toxicity, it may be a useful adjunct to other resuscitation measures in cases of either BB or CCA toxicity with QRS prolongation greater than 120 milliseconds.

Nonpharmacologic modalities

Hemodialysis

Extracorporeal drug removal has limited usefulness following BB and CCA overdose. All three classes of CCAs are lipophilic, highly protein bound, and primarily undergo hepatic metabolism [1,12]. Thus, one would predict little drug removal with dialysis. The same is true for most BBs, with a few exceptions. Atenolol, nadolol, and sotalol have properties that render them amenable to hemodialysis including: protein binding less than 25%, volume of distribution less than 2 L/kg, and renal elimination [139]. Dialysis was used in three confirmed cases of atenolol toxicity [26,140,141].

Cardiac pacing

Transvenous or transthoracic electrical pacing may be required to maintain heart rate [17,18,22,142]. However, pacing often fails to achieve electrical capture, and if electrical capture occurs, blood pressure is not always restored [17,18,73]. The disconnect between electrical capture and lack of improved contractility or increased blood pressure lies in the lack of intracellular calcium necessary for contraction. This is especially true for CCAs whereby there is increased time required for calcium to enter myocytes during diastole [143]. For this reason, the optimal pacing rate is probably 50 to 60 bpm—lower than the target rate suggested to treat other causes of hemodynamically significant bradycardia. Attempts to pace at higher rates may not provide sufficient time for the myocardium to attain a forceful contraction.

Extraordinary measures

Extracorporeal circulatory support, aortic balloon pump, and prolonged cardiopulmonary resuscitation (CPR) have been employed in severe toxicity when standard pharmacologic measures failed. Following a massive propranolol overdose that resulted in a witnessed cardiac arrest and 4 hours of CPR, 6 hours of extracorporeal support resulted in full neurologic recovery [73]. Cardiopulmonary bypass has also been used for verapamil toxicity. Bypass was started after 2.5 hours of CPR and failed pharmacologic therapy. Return of spontaneous circulation occurred during bypass; the patient survived and fully recovered [144]. In another report, bypass failed to resuscitate a toddler after accidental verapamil ingestion [145]. Resuscitation of an atenolol overdose included extracorporeal membrane oxygenation before hemodialysis [26]. Placement of an intra-aortic balloon pump after 2.75 hours of CPR and pharmacologic resuscitation sustained a propranolol overdose through cardiogenic shock [146]. The patient survived without neurologic sequelae. Aortic balloon pump was used with multiple drugs to stabilize a combined atenolol and verapamil overdose [147]. In addition to demonstrating the utility of unusual resuscitation techniques, these cases also demonstrate that patients who have cardiac drug toxicity may survive prolonged cardiac arrest (2.5–4 hr) with good neurologic outcome.

Continued research

There are several recent investigations of novel therapies for BBs and CCAs. Immunotherapy has been explored for CCA toxicity. In a model using rat ventricular tissue, verapamil-specific IgG attenuated decreases in

Table 1
Treatment options for BB and CCA toxicity

Indication	Treatment	Dose	Comments
↓ Contractility	Insulin-euglycemia (HIE)	1 IU/kg regular insulin + 0.5 gm/kg dextrose IV bolus, then 0.5–1 IU/kg/hr regular insulin + 0.5 gm/kg/hr dextrose continuous IV infusion	1) Initiate HIE simultaneously with either calcium, glucagon, or norepinephrine 2) If blood glucose is >400 mg/dL (22 mmol/L), omit dextrose bolus 3) Titrate dextrose infusion to maintain blood glucose 100–250 mg/dL (5.5–14 mmol/L) 4) Monitor blood glucose q 20–30 min until stable, then q 1–2 hr 5) K+ replacement not needed unless <2.5 mEq/L
	10% Calcium gluconate	0.6 mL/kg IV bolus, then 0.6–1.5 mL/kg/hr IV continuous infusion	1) Calcium chloride can be substituted but requires central IV access 2) Used primarily for CCA toxicity but can be considered for BB toxicity
	Glucagon	50–150 mcg/kg (3–10 mg) IV bolus, then 50–150 mcg/kg/hr continuous IV infusion	Used primarily for BB toxicity, but can also be used for CCA toxicity
↓ Peripheral resistance	Norepinephrine	Titrate to age-appropriate systolic blood pressure	Administered via central IV access
	Norepinephrine	Titrate to age-appropriate systolic blood pressure	Administered via central IV access
Heart rate <50 bpm	Glucagon	50–150 mcg/kg (3–10 mg) IV bolus, then 50–150 mcg/kg/hr continuous IV infusion	Used primarily for BB toxicity, but can also be used for CCA toxicity
	Norepinephrine	Titrate to age-appropriate systolic blood pressure	Administered via central IV access
	Cardiac pacing		Target heart rate is 60 bpm
QRS>120 ms	Sodium bicarbonate	1–2 mEq/kg IV bolus	Can repeat for recurrent QRS widening

Abbreviation: IV, intravenous.

myocardial contractility [148]. Intralipid has also been evaluated for CCAs. In theory, administration of an exogenous lipid compound provides an additional pharmacologic compartment in which highly lipid-soluble drugs can partition, thus reducing drug burden at target tissues. In verapamil toxic rats, intralipid infusion attenuated bradycardia, doubled survival time, and increased the lethal dose [149]. Vasopressin has been studied for both β-adrenergic blockade and calcium channel antagonism. It is a hypothalamic hormone released in response to lowered blood pressure. It stimulates smooth muscle V_1-receptors that increase vascular tone. Vasopressin is attractive for use in cardiac drug overdose, especially because it may increase the response to catecholamines [150]. It has been anecdotally used for caffeine, amitriptyline, milrinone, and amlodipine overdose [125,151–153]. In the amlodipine case report, vasopressin increased blood pressure after calcium, catecholamines, insulin, and charcoal hemoperfusion failed [125]. Three animal studies have evaluated vasopressin for treatment of cardiac drug toxicity: two investigating CCAs and one BB drug toxicity [59, 152,153]. Unfortunately, these studies did not demonstrate any hemodynamic benefit, although all studies administered vasopressin as a single agent, and coadministration of a catecholamine was not tested.

Therapeutic goals

The overall objective of therapy is to improve organ perfusion with subsequent increases in survival. Reasonable clinical and physiologic markers of the efficacy of therapy include improvement in myocardial ejection fraction (EF) ($\geq 50\%$ EF); increased blood pressure (≥ 90 mm Hg in adult); adequate heart rate (≥ 60 bpm); resolution of acidemia, euglycemia, adequate urine flow (1–2 mL/kg/hour); reversal of cardiac conduction abnormalities (QRS ≤ 120 milliseconds); and improved mentation. It is unlikely that any single therapeutic modality will accomplish these multisystem goals. Thus, health care providers can anticipate that successful resuscitation of BB and/or CCA toxicity will require combined use of the agents previously described. To facilitate management, treatment options, doses, and guidelines are summarized in Table 1.

References

[1] Kerns W, Kline J, Ford MD. Beta-blocker and calcium channel blocker toxicity. Emerg Med Clin North Am 1994;12:365–90.
[2] Watson WA, Litovitz TL, Rodgers GC, et al. 2002 Annual report of the American Association of Poison Control Centers Toxic Exposure Surveillance System. Am J Emerg Med 2003;21:353–421.
[3] Litovitz TL, Klein-Schwartz W, Rodgers GC, et al. 2001 Annual report of the American Association of Poison Control Centers Toxic Exposure Surveillance System. Am J Emerg Med 2002;20:391–452.

[4] Watson WA, Litovitz TL, Klein-Schwartz W, et al. 2003 Annual report of the American Association of Poison Control Centers Toxic Exposure Surveillance System. Am J Emerg Med 2004;22:335–404.

[5] Watson WA, Litovitz TL, Rodgers GC, et al. 2004 Annual report of the American Association of Poison Control Centers Toxic Exposure Surveillance System. Am J Emerg Med 2005;23:589–666.

[6] Lai MW, Klein-Schwartz W, Rodgers GC, et al. 2005 Annual report of the American Association of Poison Control Centers' National Poisoning and Exposure Database. Clin Toxicol 2006;44:803–932.

[7] Rivers E, Nguyen B, Havstad S, et al. Early goal-directed therapy in the treatment of severe sepsis and septic shock. N Engl J Med 2001;345:1368–77.

[8] Jones AE, Tayal VS, Sullivan DM, et al. Randomized, controlled trial of immediate versus delayed goal-directed ultrasound to identify the cause of nontraumatic hypotension in emergency department patients. Crit Care Med 2004;32:1703–8.

[9] Katz AM. Calcium channel diversity in the cardiovascular system. J Am Coll Cardiol 1996; 28:522–9.

[10] Sperelakis N, Wahler GM. Regulation of Ca2+ influx in myocardial cells by beta adrenergic receptors, cyclic nucleotides, and phosphorylation. Mol Cell Biochem 1988;82:19–28.

[11] Katz AM. Selectivity and toxicity of antiarrhythmic drugs: molecular interactions with ion channels. Am J Med 1998;104:179–95.

[12] DeWitt CR, Waksman JC. Pharmacology, pathophysiology, and management of calcium channel blocker and beta-blocker toxicity. Toxicol Rev 2004;23:223–38.

[13] Masters TN, Glaviano VV. Effects of d,l-propranolol on myocardial free fatty acid and carbohydrate metabolism. J Pharmacol Exp Ther 1969;167:187–93.

[14] Kline J, Leonova E, Raymond RM. Beneficial myocardial metabolic effects of insulin during verapamil toxicity in the anesthetized canine. Crit Care Med 1995;23:1251–63.

[15] Devis G, Somers G, Obberghen E, et al. Calcium antagonists and islet function. I. Inhibition of insulin release by verapamil. Diabetes 1975;24:247–51.

[16] Kline JA, Raymond RM, Schroeder JD, et al. The diabetogenic effects of acute verapamil poisoning. Toxicol Appl Pharmacol 1997;145:357–62.

[17] Weinstein RS. Recognition and management of poisoning with beta-adrenergic blocking agents. Ann Emerg Med 1984;13:1123–31.

[18] Ramoska EA, Spiller HA, Winter M, et al. A one-year evaluation of calcium channel blocker overdoses: toxicity and treatment. Ann Emerg Med 1993;22:196–200.

[19] Smith HJ, Briscoe MG. The relative sensitization by acidosis of five calcium blockers in cat papillary muscles. J Mol Cell Cardiol 1985;17:1709–16.

[20] Tanen DA, Ruha AM, Curry SC, et al. Hypertonic sodium bicarbonate is effective in the acute management of verapamil toxicity in a swine model. Ann Emerg Med 2000;36: 547–53.

[21] Holstege CP, Kirk MA, Furbee RB, et al. Wide complex dysrhythmia in calcium channel blocker overdose responsive to sodium bicarbonate therapy [abstract]. J Toxicol Clin Toxicol 1998;36:509.

[22] Watling SM, Crain JL, Edwards TD, et al. Verapamil overdose: case report and review of the literature. Ann Pharmacother 1992;26:1373–8.

[23] Enyeart JJ, Price WA, Hoffman DA, et al. Profound hyperglycemia and metabolic acidosis after verapamil overdose. J Am Coll Cardiol 1983;2:1228–31.

[24] Roth A, Miller HI, Belhassen B, et al. Slow-release verapamil and hyperglycemic metabolic acidosis. Ann Intern Med 1989;110:171–2.

[25] Yuan TH, Kerns WP, Tomaszewski CA, et al. Insulin-glucose as adjunctive therapy for severe calcium channel antagonist poisoning. J Toxicol Clin Toxicol 1999;37:463–7.

[26] Rooney M, Massey KL, Jamali F, et al. Acebutolol overdose treated with hemodialysis and extracorporeal membrane oxygenation. J Clin Pharmacol 1996;36:760–3.

[27] Shore ET, Cepin D, Davidson MJ. Metoprolol overdose. Ann Emerg Med 1981;10:524–7.

326   KERNS

[28] Buiumsohn A, Eisenberg ES, Jacob H, et al. Seizures and intraventricular conduction defect in propranolol poisoning. A report of two cases. Ann Intern Med 1979;91:860–2.

[29] Herrington DM, Insley BM, Weinmann GG. Nifedipine overdose. Am J Med 1986;81: 344–6.

[30] Humbert VH, Munn NJ, Hawkins RF. Noncardiogenic pulmonary edema complicating massive diltiazem overdose. Chest 1991;99:258–60.

[31] American Academy of Clinical Toxicology. European Association of Poison Centres and Clinical Toxicologists. Position paper: gastric lavage. J Toxicol Clin Toxicol 2004;42: 933–43.

[32] American Academy of Clinical Toxicology. European Association of Poison Centres and Clinical Toxicologists. Position statement: single-dose activated charcoal. J Toxicol Clin Toxicol 1997;35:721–41.

[33] Spiller HA, Meyers A, Ziemba T, et al. Delayed onset of cardiac arrhythmias from sustained-release verapamil. Ann Emerg Med 1991;20:201–3.

[34] Laine K, Kivisto KT, Neuvonen PJ. Effect of delayed administration of activated charcoal on the absorption of conventional and slow-release verapamil. J Toxicol Clin Toxicol 1997; 35:263–8.

[35] American Academy of Clinical Toxicology. European Association of Poison Centres and Clinical Toxicologists. Position paper: whole bowel irrigation. J Toxicol Clin Toxicol 2004;42:843–54.

[36] Buckley N, Dawson AH, Howarth D, et al. Slow-release verapamil poisoning: use of polyethylene glycol whole bowel irrigation and high-dose calcium. Med J Aust 1993;158:202–4.

[37] Haddad LM. Resuscitation after nifedipine overdose exclusively with intravenous calcium. Am J Emerg Med 1996;14:602–3.

[38] Hariman RJ, Mangiardi LM, McAllister RG, et al. Reversal of the cardiovascular effects of verapamil by calcium and sodium: differences between electrophysiologic and hemodynamic responses. Circulation 1979;59:797–804.

[39] Gay R, Algeo S, Lee R, et al. Treatment of verapamil toxicity in intact dogs. J Clin Invest 1986;77:1805–11.

[40] Strubelt O, Diederich K-W. Experimental investigations of the antidotal treatment of nifedipine overdosage. Clin Toxicol 1986;24:135–49.

[41] Perkins CM. Serious verapamil poisoning: treatment with intravenous calcium gluconate. Br Med J 1978;2:1127.

[42] Chimienti M, Previtali M, Medici A, et al. Acute verapamil poisoning: successful treatment with epinephrine. Clin Cardiol 1982;5:219–22.

[43] Crump BJ, Holt DW, Vale JA. Lack of response to intravenous calcium in severe verapamil poisoning. Lancet 1982;2:939–40.

[44] Horowitz BZ, Rhee KJ. Massive verapamil ingestion: a report of two cases and a review of the literature. Am J Emerg Med 1989;7:624–31.

[45] Li Saw Hee FL, Lip GYH. Case report: fatal verapamil overdosage despite intensive therapy and use of high dose intravenous calcium. J Hum Hypertens 1996;10:495–6.

[46] Strubelt O. Evaluation of antidotes against the acute cardiovascular toxicity of propranolol. Toxicology 2006;31:261–70.

[47] Langemeijer J, de Wildt D, de Groot G, et al. Calcium interferes with the cardiodepressive effects of beta-blocker overdose in isolated rat hearts. J Toxicol Clin Toxicol 1986;24: 111–33.

[48] Love JN, Hanfling D, Howell JM. Hemodynamic effects of calcium chloride in a canine model of acute propranolol intoxication. Ann Emerg Med 1996;28:1–6.

[49] Jones JL. Metoprolol overdose. Ann Emerg Med 1982;11:114–5.

[50] Sangster B, de Wildt D, van Dijk A, et al. A case of acebutolol intoxication. J Toxicol Clin Toxicol 1983;20:69–77.

[51] Tai YT, Lo CW, Chow WH, et al. Successful resuscitation and survival following massive overdose of metoprolol. Br J Clin Pract 1990;44:746–7.

[52] Pertoldi F, D'Olando L, Mercante WP. Electromechanical dissociation 48 hours after atenolol overdose: usefulness of calcium chloride. Ann Emerg Med 1998;31:777–81.
[53] Brimacombe JR, Scully M, Swainston R. Propranolol overdose–a dramatic response to calcium chloride. Med J Aust 1991;155:267–8.
[54] Cote CJ, Drop LJ, Daniels AL, et al. Calcium chloride versus calcium gluconate: comparison of ionization and cardiovascular effects in children and dogs. Anesthesiology 1987;66: 465–70.
[55] Martin TJ, Kang Y, Robertson KM, et al. Ionization and hemodynamic effects of calcium chloride and calcium gluconate in the absence of hepatic function. Anesthesiology 1990;73: 62–5.
[56] Buckley N, Whyte IM, Dawson AH. Overdose with calcium channel blockers. Br Med J 1994;308:1639.
[57] Carlon GC, Howland WS, Goldiner PL, et al. Adverse effects of calcium administration. Report of two cases. Arch Surg 1978;113:882–5.
[58] Parmley WW. The role of glucagon in cardiac therapy. N Engl J Med 1971;285:801–2.
[59] Holger JS, Engebretsen KM, Obetz CL, et al. A comparison of vasopressin and glucagon in beta-blocker induced toxicity. Clin Toxicol 2006;44:45–51.
[60] Chernish SM, Maglinte DDT, Brunelle RL. The laboratory response to glucagon: dosages used in gastrointestinal examinations. Invest Radiol 1988;23:847–52.
[61] Murad F, Vaughn M. Effect of glucagon on rat heart adenyl cyclase. Biochem Pharmacol 1969;18:1053–9.
[62] Levey GS, Fletcher MA, Klein I, et al. The characterization of I125-glucagon binding in a solubilized preparation of cat myocardial adenylate cyclase. J Biol Chem 1974;249:2665–73.
[63] Glick G, Parmley WW, Wechsler AS, et al. Glucagon: its enhancement of cardiac performance in the cat and dog and persistence of its inotropic action despite beta-receptor blockade with propranolol. Circ Res 1968;22:789–99.
[64] Lucchesi BR. Cardiac actions of glucagon. Circ Res 1968;22:777–87.
[65] Kosinski EJ, Malindzak GS. Glucagon and isoproterenol in reversing propranolol toxicity. Arch Intern Med 1973;132:840–3.
[66] Love JN, Leasure JA, Mundt DJ, et al. A comparison of amrinone and glucagon therapy for cardiovascular depression associated with propranolol toxicity in a canine model. J Toxicol Clin Toxicol 1992;30:399–412.
[67] Kerns W, Schroeder JD, Williams C, et al. Insulin improves survival in a canine model of acute beta-blocker toxicity. Ann Emerg Med 1997;29:748–57.
[68] Toet AE, Wemer J, Vleeming W, et al. Experimental study of the detrimental effect of dopamine/glucagon combination in d,l-propranolol intoxication. Hum Exp Toxicol 1996;15:411–21.
[69] Adlerfliegel F, Leeman M, Demaeyer P, et al. Sotalol poisoning associated with asystole. Intensive Care Med 1993;19:57–8.
[70] Ehgartner GR, Zelinka MA. Hemodynamic instability following intentional nadolol overdose. Arch Intern Med 1988;148:801–2.
[71] Lewis M, Kallenbach J, Germond C, et al. Survival following massive overdose of adrenergic blocking agents (acebutolol and labetalol). Eur Heart J 1983;4:328–32.
[72] Illingworth RN. Glucagon for beta-blocker poisoning. Practitioner 1978;223:683–5.
[73] McVey FK, Corke CF. Extracorporeal circulation in the management of massive propranolol overdose. Anaesthesia 1991;46:744–6.
[74] O'Mahony D, O'Leary P, Molloy MG. Severe oxprenolol poisoning: the importance of glucagon infusion. Hum Exp Toxicol 1990;9:101–3.
[75] Peterson CD, Leeder JS, Sterner S. Glucagon therapy for beta-blocker overdose. Drug Intell Clin Pharm 1984;18:394–8.
[76] Smith RC, Wilkinson J, Hull RL. Glucagon for propranolol overdose. J Am Med Assoc 1985;254:2412.

[77] Love JN, Sachdeva DK, Bessman ES, et al. A potential role for glucagon in the treatment of drug-induced symptomatic bradycardia. Chest 1998;114:323–6.

[78] Wilkinson J. Beta blocker overdoses. Ann Emerg Med 1986;15:982.

[79] Freestone S, Thomas HM, Bhamra HK, et al. Severe atenolol poisoning: treatment with prenalterol. Hum Toxicol 1986;5:343–5.

[80] Gerkin R, Curry SC. Significant bradycardia following acute self-poisoning with atenolol [abstract]. Vet Hum Toxicol 1987;29:479.

[81] Hurwitz MD, Kallenbach J, Pincus JS. Massive propranolol overdose. Am J Med 1986;81: 1118.

[82] Perrot D, Bui-Xuan B, Bouffard Y, et al. A case of sotalol poisoning with fatal outcome. J Toxicol Clin Toxicol 1988;26:389–96.

[83] Zaritsky AL, Horowitz M, Chernow B. Glucagon antagonism of calcium channel blocker-induced myocardial dysfunction. Crit Care Med 1988;16:246–51.

[84] Stone CK, May WA, Carroll R. Glucagon and phenylephrine combination vs glucagon alone in experimental verapamil overdose. Ann Emerg Med 1995;25:369–74.

[85] Stone CK, Thomas SH, Koury SI, et al. Glucagon and phenylephrine combination vs glucagon alone in experimental verapamil overdose. Acad Emerg Med 1996;3:120–5.

[86] Tuncok Y, Apaydin S, Kalkan S, et al. The effects of amrinone and glucagon on verapamil-induced cardiovascular toxicity in anaesthetized rats. International Journal of Investigative Pathology 1996;77:207–12.

[87] Kline JA, Tomaszewski CA, Schroeder JD, et al. Insulin is a superior antidote for cardio-vascular toxicity induced by verapamil in the anesthetized canine. J Pharmacol Exp Ther 1993;267:744–50.

[88] Jolly SR, Kipnis JN, Lucchesi BR. Cardiovascular depression by verapamil: reversal by glucagon and interactions with propranolol. Pharmacology 1987;35:249–55.

[89] Sabatier J, Pouyet T, Shelvey G, et al. Antagonistic effects of epinephrine, glucagon and methylatropine but not calcium chloride against atrio-ventricular conduction disturbances produced by high doses of diltiazem, in conscious dogs. Fundam Clin Pharmacol 1991;5: 93–106.

[90] Doyon S, Roberts JR. The use of glucagon in a case of calcium channel blocker overdose. Ann Emerg Med 1993;22:1229–33.

[91] Pollack CV. Utility of glucagon in the emergency department. J Emerg Med 1993;11: 195–205.

[92] Quezado Z, Lippmann M, Wertheimer J. Severe cardiac, respiratory, and metabolic complications of massive verapamil overdose. Crit Care Med 1991;19:436–8.

[93] Walter FG, Frye G, Mullen JT, et al. Amelioration of nifedipine poisoning associated with glucagon therapy. Ann Emerg Med 1993;22:1234–7.

[94] Wolf LR, Spadafora MP, Otten EJ. Use of amrinone and glucagon in a case of calcium channel blocker overdose. Ann Emerg Med 1993;22:1225–8.

[95] Erickson FC, Ling LJ, Grande GA, et al. Diltiazem overdose: case report and review. J Emerg Med 1991;9:357–66.

[96] Williams JF, Childress RH, Chip JN, et al. Hemodynamic effects of glucagon in patients with heart disease. Circulation 1969;39:38–47.

[97] vander Ark CR, Reynolds EW. Clinical evaluation of glucagon by continuous infusion in the treatment of low cardiac output states. Am Heart J 1970;79:481–7.

[98] Hall-Boyer K, Zaloga GP, Chernow B. Glucagon: hormone or therapeutic agent? Crit Care Med 1984;12:584–9.

[99] Love JN, Tandy TK. Beta-adrenoceptor antagonist toxicity: a survey of glucagon availability. Ann Emerg Med 1993;22:267–8.

[100] Donovan KD, Gerace RV, Dreyer JF. Acebutolol-induced ventricular tachycardia reversed with sodium bicarbonate. J Toxicol Clin Toxicol 1999;37:481–4.

[101] Lindvall K, Sojgren A. High-dose prenalterol in beta-blockade intoxication. Acta Med Scand 1985;218:525–8.

[102] Goenen M, Col J, Compere A, et al. Treatment of severe verapamil poisoning with combined amrinone-isoproterenol therapy. Am J Cardiol 1986;58:1142–3.

[103] Avery GJ, Spotnitz HM, Rose EA, et al. Pharmacologic antagonism of beta-adrenergic blockade in dogs. I. Hemodynamic effects of isoproterenol, dopamine, and epinephrine in acute propranolol administration. J Thorac Cardiovasc Surg 1979;77:267–76.

[104] Richards DA, Prichard BN, Boakes AJ, et al. Pharmacological basis for antihypertensive effects of intravenous labetalol. Br Heart J 1977;39:99–106.

[105] Anthony T, Jastremski M, Elliott W, et al. Charcoal hemoperfusion for the treatment of a combined diltiazem and metoprolol overdose. Ann Emerg Med 1986;15:1344–8.

[106] Koch AR, Vogelaers GP, Decruyenaere JM, et al. Fatal intoxication with amlodipine. J Toxicol Clin Toxicol 1995;33:253–6.

[107] Hoffman BB, Lefkowitz RJ. Catecholamines, sympathomimetic drugs, and adrenergic receptor antagonists. In: Hardman JG, Limbird LE, Molinoff PB, et al, editors. Goodman and Gilman's the pharmacological basis of therapeutics. New York: McGraw-Hill; 1996. p. 199–248.

[108] Weissler AM, Altschuld RA, Gibb LE, et al. Effect of insulin on the performance and metabolism of the anoxic isolated perfused rat heart. Circ Res 1973;32:108–16.

[109] Farah AE, Alousi AA. The actions of insulin on cardiac contractility. Life Sci 1981;29: 975–1000.

[110] Reikeras O, Gunnes P, Sorlie D, et al. Metabolic effects of high doses of insulin during acute left ventricular failure in dogs. Eur Heart J 1985;6:451–7.

[111] Law WR, McLane MP, Raymond RM. Effect of insulin on myocardial contractility during canine endotoxin shock. Cardiovasc Res 1988;22:777–85.

[112] Raymond RM, McLane MP, Law WR, et al. Myocardial insulin resistance during acute endotoxin shock in dogs. Diabetes 1988;37:1684–8.

[113] Kline JA, Raymond RM, Leonova E, et al. Insulin improves heart function and metabolism during non-ischemic cardiogenic shock in awake canines. Cardiovasc Res 1997;34: 289–98.

[114] Spurlock BW, Virani NA, Henry CA. Verapamil overdose. West J Med 1991;154:208–11.

[115] Howard DC. Glucagon for reaction to combined calcium channel blocker and beta-blocker use. J Emerg Nurs 1996;22:173–5.

[116] Kline JA, Leonova E, Williams TC, et al. Myocardial metabolism during graded intraportal verapamil infusion in awake dogs. J Cardiovasc Pharmacol 1996;27:719–26.

[117] Place R, Carlson A, Leiken J, et al. Hyperinsulin therapy in the treatment of verapamil overdose [abstract]. J Toxicol Clin Toxicol 2000;38:576–7.

[118] Boyer EW, Duic PA, Evans A. Hyperinsulinemia/euglycemia therapy for calcium channel blocker poisoning. Pediatr Emerg Care 2002;18:36–7.

[119] Boyer EW, Shannon M. Treatment of calcium-channel-blocker intoxication with insulin infusion. N Engl J Med 2001;344:1721–2.

[120] Herbert JX, O'Malley C, Tracey JA, et al. Verapamil overdosage unresponsive to dextrose/insulin therapy [abstract]. J Toxicol Clin Toxicol 2001;39:293–4.

[121] Cumpston K, Mycyk M, Pallasch E, et al. Failure of hyperinsulinemia/euglycemia therapy in severe diltiazem overdose [abstract]. J Toxicol Clin Toxicol 2002;40:618.

[122] Marques M, Gomes E, de Oliviera J. Treatment of calcium channel blocker intoxication with insulin infusion: case report and literature review. Resuscitation 2003;57:211–3.

[123] Rasmussen L, Husted SE, Johnsen SP. Severe intoxication after an intentional overdose of amlodipine. Acta Anaesthesiol Scand 2003;47:1038–40.

[124] Meyer M, Stremski E, Scanlon M. Verapamil-induced hypotension reversed with dextrose-insulin [abstract]. J Toxicol Clin Toxicol 2001;39:500.

[125] Marraffa JM, Stork CM, Medicis JJ, et al. Massive amlodipine overdose successfully treated using high-dose vasopressin [abstract]. J Toxicol Clin Toxicol 2004;42:732–3.

[126] Greene SL, Gawarammana IB, Dargan PI, et al. Safety of high dose insulin therapy in calcium channel antagonist overdose [abstract]. J Toxicol Clin Toxicol 2006;44:758.

[127] Miller AD, Maloney GE, Kanter MZ, et al. Hypoglycemia in patients treated with high-dose insulin for calcium channel blocker poisoning [abstract]. J Toxicol Clin Toxicol 2006;44:782–3.

[128] Harris NS. Case records of the Massachusetts General Hospital. Case 24-2006. A 40-year-old woman with hypotension after an overdose of amlodipine. N Engl J Med 2006;355: 602–11.

[129] Kebler R, McDonald FD, Cadnapaphornchai P. Dynamic changes in serum phosphorus levels in diabetic ketoacidosis. Am J Med 1985;79:571–6.

[130] Ionescu-Tirgoviste C, Bruckner I, Mihalache N, et al. Plasma phosphorus and magnesium values during treatment of severe diabetic ketoacidosis. Med Interne 1981;19:66–8.

[131] Frishman WH. Beta-adrenergic blockers. Med Clin North Am 1988;72:37–81.

[132] Nicolas F, Villers D, Rozo L, et al. Severe self-poisoning with acebutolol in association with alcohol. Crit Care Med 1987;15:173–4.

[133] Offenstadt G, Hericord P, Amstutz P. Intoxication volontaire par le pindolol [Intentional overdose of pindolol]. Nouv Presse Med 1976;5:1539.

[134] Rosen MR, Ilvento JP, Gelband H, et al. Effects of verapamil on electrophysiologic properties of canine cardiac Purkinje fibers. J Pharmacol Exp Ther 1974;189:414–22.

[135] Henry PD. Comparative pharmacology of calcium antagonists: nifedipine, verapamil, and diltiazem. Am J Cardiol 1980;46:1047–58.

[136] Yatani A, Brown AM. The calcium channel blocker nitrendipine blocks sodium channels in neonatal rat cardiac myocytes. Circ Res 1985;57:868–75.

[137] Prakash P, Tripathi O. Verapamil and TTX inhibit +Vmax but differentially alter the duration of action potential of adult chicken ventricular myocardium. Indian J Biochem Biophys 1998;35:123–30.

[138] Love JN, Howell JM, Newsome JT, et al. The effect of sodium bicarbonate on propranolol-induced cardiovascular toxicity in a canine model. J Toxicol Clin Toxicol 2000;38: 421–8.

[139] Brubacher JR. Beta-adrenergic antagonists. In: Goldfrank LR, Flomenbaum NE, Lewin NA, et al, editors. Goldfrank's toxicologic emergencies. New York: McGraw-Hill; 2002. p. 741–61.

[140] Saitz R, Williams BW, Farber HW. Atenolol-induced cardiovascular collapse treated with hemodialysis. Crit Care Med 1991;19:116–8.

[141] Salhanick SD, Wax PM. Treatment of atenolol overdose in a patient with renal failure using serial hemodialysis and hemoperfusion and associated echocardiographic findings. Vet Hum Toxicol 2000;42:224–5.

[142] Kenyon CJ, Aldinger GE, Joshipura P, et al. Successful resuscitation using external cardiac pacing in beta adrenergic antagonist-induced bradyasystolic arrest. Ann Emerg Med 1988; 17:711–3.

[143] Ehara T, Daufmann R. The voltage- and time-dependent effects of (-)-verapamil on the slow inward current in isolated cat ventricular myocardium. J Pharmacol Exp Ther 1978; 207:49–55.

[144] Holzer M, Sterz F, Schoerkhuber W, et al. Successful resuscitation of a verapamil-intoxicated patient with percutaneous cardiopulmonary bypass. Crit Care Med 1999;27:2818–23.

[145] Hendren WG, Schieber RS, Garrettson LK. Extracorporeal bypass for the treatment of verapamil poisoning. Ann Emerg Med 1989;18:984–7.

[146] Lane AS, Woodward AC, Goldman MR. Massive propranolol overdose poorly responsive to pharmacologic therapy: use of the intra-aortic balloon pump. Ann Emerg Med 1987;16: 1381–3.

[147] Frierson J, Bailly D, Shultz T, et al. Refractory cardiogenic shock and complete heart block after unsuspected verapamil-SR and atenolol overdose. Clin Cardiol 1991;14:933–5.

[148] Hill RE, Heard K, Bogdan GM, et al. Attenuation of verapamil-induced myocardial toxicity in an ex-vivo rat model using a verapamil-specific ovine immunoglobin. Acad Emerg Med 2001;8:950–5.

[149] Tebbutt S, Harvey M, Nicholson T, et al. Intralipid prolongs survival in a rat model of verapamil toxicity. Acad Emerg Med 2006;13:134–9.

[150] Noguera I, Medina P, Segarra G, et al. Potentiation by vasopressin of adrenergic vasoconstriction in the rat isolated mesenteric artery. Br J Pharmacol 1997;122:1315–20.

[151] Holstege CP, Hunter Y, Baer AB, et al. Massive caffeine overdose requiring vasopressin infusion and hemodialysis. J Toxicol Clin Toxicol 2003;41:1003–8.

[152] Sztajnkrycer MD, Bond GR, Johnson SB, et al. Use of vasopressin in a canine model of severe verapamil poisoning: a preliminary descriptive study. Acad Emerg Med 2004;11: 1253–61.

[153] Barry JD, Durkovich DW, Richardson W, et al. Vasopressin treatment of verapamil toxicity in the porcine model. J Med Toxicol 2005;1:3–10.

ELSEVIER
SAUNDERS

EMERGENCY
MEDICINE
CLINICS OF
NORTH AMERICA

Emerg Med Clin N Am 25 (2007) 333–346

Emergency Department Management of the Salicylate-Poisoned Patient

Gerald F. O'Malley, DO[a,b,c,d,*]

[a]Division of Toxicology, Albert Einstein Medical Center, 5501 Old York Road,
Philadelphia, PA 19141, USA
[b]Thomas Jefferson University Hospital, Philadelphia, PA 19141, USA
[c]Children's Hospital of Philadelphia, Philadelphia, PA 19141, USA
[d]Philadelphia Poison Control Center, Philadelphia, PA 19141, USA

The term salicylate refers to any of a group of chemicals that are derived from salicylic acid. The best known is acetylsalicylic acid (aspirin). Acetylsalicylic acid is metabolized to salicylic acid (salicylate) after ingestion. The salicylates originally were derived from salicin, the active ingredient in willow bark, which Hippocrates used 2500 years ago for treating pain and fever [1,2]. Salicylates also occur naturally in many plants such as strawberries, almonds, and tomatoes [3].

Poisoning by aspirin is common and is under-represented in poison center data, because it is often not recognized [4–6]. The in-hospital mortality for unrecognized chronic aspirin poisoning is reportedly three times higher than if the diagnosis is made in the emergency department [7]. Familiarity with the clinical presentation during the various stages of acute and chronic aspirin poisoning is important for the practice of emergency medicine. The most challenging aspect of the clinical evaluation and management of the aspirin-poisoned patient may be recognition of the subtle signs and symptoms of chronic, nonintentional aspirin overdose (Box 1).

Epidemiology

Salicylate poisoning continues to be an important overdose that frequently presents to emergency departments [8–10]. There were over 21,000

* Department of Emergency Medicine, Albert Einstein Medical Center, 5501 Old York Road, Philadelphia, PA 19141.
E-mail address: omalleyg@einstein.edu

0733-8627/07/$ - see front matter © 2007 Elsevier Inc. All rights reserved.
doi:10.1016/j.emc.2007.02.012

Box 1. Pitfalls in the emergency department management of salicylate–poisoned patients

Failure to recognize the presence of salicylate toxicity

Failure to appreciate the presence of continued absorption of salicylate

Misinterpreting clinical significance of serum salicylate levels, because units of measure were unclear

Reliance on one or two serum levels of salicylate that may not describe a trend of decreasing total body burden of aspirin clearly

Misinterpretation of low serum salicylate levels as nontoxic and failure to comprehend the changing acid–base status of the patient

Waiting until serum salicylate levels are determined before beginning urinary alkalinization

Accidentally adding bicarbonate to isotonic saline (creating a hypertonic solution) rather than intravenous dextrose/water solutions to alkalinize the urine

Forgetting to add potassium to the urinary alkalinization infusion

Failure to recognize the emergent need for definitive therapy (hemodialysis) on the basis of impending end organ injury (Box 2).

Inappropriately or prematurely initiating intubation and mechanical ventilation without hyperventilation and without simultaneous hemodialysis

Prematurely discharging patients without demonstrating metabolic stability, declining salicylate levels, and the absence of an aspirin bezoar

---

aspirin and nonaspirin salicylate exposures reported to the United States poison centers in 2004, with 43 deaths and 12,968 patients requiring hospital treatment [11]. Because poison center data are collected passively, that statistic is certainly an underestimate of the true incidence of salicylate poisoning occur in the United States. One half of the reported exposures (10,786) were categorized as intentional overdoses. The incidence of chronic aspirin poisoning is not known, but it is misdiagnosed frequently [12].

In recent years, packaging strategies such as child-resistant packaging and reducing the amount of medication in each package of over-the-counter analgesics have impacted the incidence of poisoning. It is estimated that the use of child-resistant packaging for salicylate-containing medications has resulted in a 34% reduction in the salicylate-related child mortality rate [13]. In England, Australia, and Ireland, analgesics are packaged and sold in small amounts (ie, 4 g of acetaminophen). This has resulted in a 30% decrease in the number of patients requiring liver transplantation for acetaminophen-induced hepatic failure and a 22% reduction in suicidal deaths from acetaminophen and salicylate [14]. Large aspirin overdoses were reduced by 39% on average in the countries in which the limited package formulation is required [14,15].

Pathophysiologic basis for poisoning

Salicylate is a metabolic poison. Understanding the pathophysiology of its metabolic effects can help to understand the clinical manifestations of toxicity. The metabolic derangements induced by salicylate poisoning are multifactorial, but the principal pathophysiologic mechanism in salicylate poisoning is interference with aerobic metabolism by means of uncoupling of mitochondrial oxidative phosphorylation [15a,16]. This leads to the interruption of a series of enzyme-mediated mitochondrial functions and increased anaerobic metabolism with cellular conversion of pyruvate to lactate and rapid development of lactic acidosis [17,18]. The inefficiency of anaerobic metabolism results in less energy being used to create ATP and release of the energy created during the metabolism of glucose in the electron transport chain as heat, so salicylate poisoned patients may become febrile [19]. The absence of fever, however, does not rule out salicylate poisoning.

The acidosis is caused by anaerobic metabolism and the inability to buffer hydrogen ions, which is reflected by the accumulation of lactate. The presence of acetasalicylic acid or salicylate molecules probably contributes little to the acidotic state [15a,20].

Interference with oxidative phosphorylation by salicylate also will impact glucose homeostasis negatively by causing glycogen depletion, gluconeogenesis, and catabolism of proteins and free fatty acids, the end result being low serum glucose levels and central nervous system (CNS) hypoglycemia relative to serum glucose levels [15a].

Absorption and metabolism of salicylate

The pharmacokinetic profile of aspirin is unique and explains the unique characteristics of clinical poisoning. The ionization constant (pKa) of aspirin is 3, which means that at a pH of 3, approximately half of the available chemical is in the ionized state. In an acidic environment like the stomach, more of the drug will be absorbed compared with tissues at a higher pH [21]. The absorption of aspirin from the stomach can be delayed by the presence of food in the stomach and the formulation of the aspirin, (eg, enteric coating of pills may create concretions and bezoars that limit available surface area for absorption) [22]. Aspirin is thought to cause spasm of the pyloric sphincter, increasing gastric transit time and prolonging the time that aspirin is in the acidic environment of the stomach, favoring increased absorption [21]. Salicylates also are absorbed readily in the unionized form from the small intestine [23,24].

Dermal salicylate formulations typically do not result in tissue penetration much deeper than 3 to 4 mm in animal studies [25,26] and human volunteer experiments [27]. Methyl salicylate has less dermal absorption than either camphor or menthol, with lower mean plasma levels and shorter elimination half-life than either compound in people [28]. Significant amounts of salicylate typically are not absorbed through the skin except in select patients, such as children and patients with compromised skin such as burn patients or patients who have severe psoriasis [29–31].

In therapeutic doses, the major route of salicylate biotransformation is conjugation with glycine in the liver. A small amount of aspirin is excreted unchanged in the urine [15a]. In overdose, the liver's ability to metabolize the drug is overwhelmed, and unchanged salicylate excretion through the kidney becomes a much more important elimination route.

Salicylate–induced acid-base changes

Respiratory alkalosis

Salicylate toxicity initially will create a pure respiratory alkalosis because of direct stimulatory effects on the respiratory centers of the cerebral medulla. This is characterized in the blood gas by a decrease in the partial pressure of dissolved CO_2 accompanied by an elevated pH and normal to slightly lower levels of serum HCO_3 [32]. There is some controversy as to whether pediatric aspirin poisoned patients demonstrate this phase of acid–base derangement. Pediatric patients may present later in the course of the poisoning, or the centrally mediated hyperventilatory phase of aspirin poisoning may be so subtle in children that it often is missed [33–36].

Mixed acid–base disturbances

As the poisoning progresses and more of the aspirin is absorbed into the serum and is incorporated into the mitochondria, uncoupling oxidative phosphorylation, lactic acid accumulates in the serum, and metabolic compensatory mechanisms are initiated [16]. Hyperventilation becomes a true compensatory mechanism in addition to the byproduct of central medullary stimulation [20]. This phase is characterized metabolically by a continued decrease in the pCO_2, marked decline in measured HCO_3 and possibly a decrease in serum pH, depending on the ability of the patient to maintain the respiratory demands of the developing acidosis and to retain bicarbonate in the kidney [37]. A common error at this stage of the poisoning is to acknowledge that the serum pH is close to 7.4 or slightly higher than 7.4, and assume that the patient is compensating adequately for the acidosis.

Metabolic acidosis

As the ability to compensate for the acidosis is overwhelmed, pH drops; lactic acid accumulates, and serum bicarbonate is consumed. Patients who reach the stage of aspirin poisoning where pH is less than 7.4 with decreased pCO2 and low serum bicarbonate are dangerously unstable, likely to decompensate hemodynamically and will begin to demonstrate other symptoms of end-organ injury [37].

Clinical presentation

Classic salicylism

The triad of salicylate poisoning consists of hyperventilation, tinnitus, and gastrointestinal (GI) irritation [38,39]. Physicians should remain aware that patients may hyperventilate with a normal respiratory rate by increasing tidal volume (hyperpnea) and should make it a habit to observe respiratory patterns carefully. Ototoxicity is a well-described phenomenon with salicylism, and it is thought to be secondary to interference with chloride channels in the cochlear hair cells that transmit sound waves [40,41]. The ototoxicity is most noticeable in the range of serum salicylate from 20 to 40 mg/dL [40,42]. Aspirin, especially enteric-coated formulations, are known to develop concretions and bezoars in the stomach and act as a direct GI irritant leading to nausea, vomiting, and abdominal pain [22,43,44].

Early presentation

Patients who present early in the course of salicylate poisoning may have modest symptoms, and the hyperventilation may be mistaken for emotional excitation or anxiety. GI irritation may or may not be present, and tinnitus or other symptoms of ototoxicity may be overlooked unless the physician specifically tests for them with direct questioning or confrontational hearing testing. Vital signs may reflect emotional agitation and CNS stimulation with tachycardia, increased work of breathing (increased minute ventilation), and overall autonomic up-regulation. Early in the course of acute poisoning, fever generally will be absent [39]. Clinical symptoms will be variable if the patient ingested more than one drug, or the ingested aspirin formulation contained a CNS depressant, which might blunt the expected hyperventilation and respiratory alkalosis [45].

Laboratory values early in the course of aspirin poisoning will be largely normal or will reflect the direct stimulatory effect of salicylate on the cerebral respiratory center. Serum aspirin levels may be elevated modestly (20 to 40 mg/dL), and blood gas analysis may demonstrate pure respiratory alkalosis with elevated pH and low pCO_2 with normal or near-normal HCO_3 [39]. The decision to determine serum salicylate concentrations is not difficult. Although serum salicylate levels may not be required to screen every asymptomatic overdose, liberal use of the laboratory to make the diagnosis and follow resuscitative efforts is advisable [46–48].

Late presentation

As salicylate enters the mitochondria, dramatic changes in vital signs and clinical stability occur. Serum salicylate levels alone are not adequate to accurately assess and follow seriously poisoned patients [49]. Serum salicylate levels do not reflect the total body burden of salicylate, and so to evaluate the rapidly changing acid base status of an aspirin poisoned patient, serial salicylate levels should be accompanied by serial blood gas analysis [5]. Patients who present in the late phases of salicylate toxicity often are misdiagnosed as sepsis [50], myocardial infarction [51], or as agitated or otherwise psychiatrically disturbed [43,52,53].

Death from salicylism

The progression to death from salicylate poisoning is particularly tumultuous. The toxic effects of the salicylate molecule on mitochondrial function and subsequent basement membrane leakage overwhelm the compensatory capacity of the organism. This leads to marked metabolic acidosis with development of pulmonary and cerebral edema. Myocardial depression and hypotension secondary to the acidosis and volume deficit occur, and CNS depression with seizures secondary to hypoxia, hypoglycemia, and direct CNS toxicity often precedes cardiopulmonary arrest [54].

In one study, nearly half (45%) of the patients who died from salicylate poisoning arrived at the emergency department alert and deteriorated while there [55]. In another study, 39% of the patients who had severe salicylate poisoning requiring ICU management arrived alert with minimal symptoms [56]. Mean postmortem salicylate serum levels on 16 patients who presented dead on arrival after aspirin overdose were 51 mg/dL (range 17 to 101 mg/dL) [55]. Postmortem examination of salicylate-poisoned patients demonstrated several unique findings including myocardial necrosis suggestive of toxic myocarditis [57], pulmonary congestion, hemorrhagic gastritis with unabsorbed salicylate and GI ulceration, cerebral edema, and paratonia (extreme muscle rigidity) [55,56].

Emergency department evaluation of the salicylate-poisoned patient

Done nomogram

The aspirin nomogram, commonly referred to as the Done nomogram, after its creator Done [58,59], was first published in 1960. Data from pediatric patients who ingested a one-time dose of aspirin were plotted over time to create an instrument to predict toxicity. Several important limitations exist with regards to the development of the Done nomogram that limit its generalizability, including the fact that patients who had polydrug ingestion were included in the analysis, making the clinical correlation difficult to interpret. In addition, the nomogram assumed an elimination half-life of 20 hours in all patients and did not allow for the change from first-order to zero-order elimination kinetics that occurs when serum levels exceed the elimination enzyme systems [60]. Although innovative and often accurate for the intended (pediatric) population, the Done nomogram has been demonstrated to have very limited applicability and usefulness for most aspirin-poisoned patients, and its routine use is discouraged [49].

Laboratory evaluation

Physicians should make liberal use of blood tests in the evaluation of potentially aspirin-poisoned patients. Different clinical laboratories may report salicylate levels in different units of measure (mg/dL versus mmol/L). Clinicians should maintain consistent use of the respective units of measure to avoid confusion. Seriously aspirin-poisoned patients may display symptoms that allow an astute practitioner to perform comparative serial examinations and assess developing toxicity. Accurate recognition of worsening signs of toxicity, however, is an inexact science with uncertain sensitivity and specificity, especially in the event of polypharmaceutical ingestion or pediatric patients [45,61–63]. Serum salicylate levels frequently do not reflect the severity of the poisoning. Depending on the time since ingestion, presence of food in the stomach, coingestants, and presence of concretions, among other variables, symptoms may or may not correlate with serum salicylate levels. Symptomatic patients suspected of aspirin ingestion or salicylate poisoning should have serial aspirin levels and blood gas analysis performed until a clear trend toward decreasing (not plateau or modestly increasing) levels and metabolic stability as described by the blood gas is present.

Radiographic evaluation of the aspirin poisoned patient is rarely helpful, except for seriously ill patients who may have pulmonary edema or patients who have altered mental status that might require CT scanning of the head to eliminate the possibility of an alternative cause for a changed level of consciousness. Large bezoars of ingested enteric-coated aspirin tablets may or may not be visible on a radiograph, and the absence of opacity on an abdominal radiograph is not adequate to rule out the presence of a large amount of salicylate in the gut [64].

Treatment of the salicylate-poisoned patient

Resuscitation

Depending on the acuity of the poisoning and the presence of end-organ injury and hemodynamic instability, patients may require early, aggressive resuscitation and treatment. Most patients who have consequential aspirin overdose will be somewhat volume deficient because of fluid losses caused by increased respiration, fever, and metabolic activity [15a]. Volume resuscitation with alkalinized intravenous fluids is reasonable and advisable and should be initiated early in the course of the patient's treatment so that valuable time is not lost waiting for laboratory confirmation of elevated salicylate levels [65]. Begin by placing a sufficient volume of sodium bicarbonate (three ampules $NaHCO_3$ with 44 mEq $Na+$/ampule) into a liter of a glucose-containing hypotonic solution, such as 5% dextrose and water and infusing at 2 to 3 mL/kg per hour to promote brisk urine output. A total of 40 mEq of KCl per liter should be added to prevent hypokalemia.

Salicylate-poisoned patients who require advanced airway management are particularly challenging. Salicylate-intoxicated patients who have depressed mental status from the salicylate-induced cerebral hypoglycemia or acidosis or coingestants who require endotracheal intubation and mechanical ventilation pose a clinical no-win situation for emergency physicians, because positive pressure ventilation simply cannot maintain the respiratory rate and metabolic demands of seriously salicylate-poisoned patients. Hemodynamic instability and worsening of acid–base status will almost definitely be the consequence [66]. Patients who require endotracheal intubation for airway protection and maintenance almost always should be hemodialyzed simultaneously to remove salicylate and the accumulated organic acids. Careful attention to maintaining a favorable acid–base status through the judicious manipulation of ventilator settings should occur so as not to allow hypoventilation and the accumulation of CO_2.

Gastric decontamination

The unique characteristics of aspirin in the stomach make gastric decontamination particularly problematic. Gastric irritation, induction of nausea, and decreased mental alertness all combine to put the salicylate-poisoned patient at substantial risk for vomiting and aspiration from any attempt at GI decontamination. Clinicians must weigh the very real risk of aspiration versus the possible benefits from any method of gastric decontamination.

Activated charcoal has been demonstrated to be effective in decreasing the area under the curve for absorbed aspirin, and it is the most widely used method of gastric decontamination for salicylate-poisoned patients [67,68]. Multidose activated charcoal similarly has been shown to reduce absorption of aspirin and results in decreased serum levels, but this has not translated into an improved morbidity or mortality rate [69]. Given that multiple doses of activated charcoal are quite safe and generally well tolerated and seem to result in lower total body burden of aspirin, it is reasonable to recommend 25 g of activated charcoal without sorbitol given orally every 3 hours while the patient is being monitored with serial aspirin and blood gas measurements. Before each 25 g dose of activated charcoal, bowel sounds should be checked, and if absent, the activated charcoal should not be withheld.

Whole-bowel irrigation is not recommended in aspirin-poisoned patients, because there are very little data to support its use in salicylate poisoning.

What data do exist do not demonstrate an improved outcome [70,71]. Whole-bowel irrigation with balanced electrolyte solutions decreases gut transit time but may increase total surface area available for absorption and possibly lead to increased serum levels of aspirin. It is universally poorly tolerated and difficult to perform [70,71].

Gastric lavage largely has been abandoned in the management of poisoned patients with the possible exception of overdose with a life-threatening drug and early presentation of the patient in the course of the poisoning [72–74]. Serious aspirin poisoning is certainly a life threat and given the unique potential of enteric-coated aspirin to form concretions and remain in the stomach due to pylorospasm [22], it is reasonable to consider gastric lavage with a large-bore endogastric tube (36 French or larger) if substantial salicylate poisoning is suspected, and there is no likelihood of airway compromise [74–76].

Enhanced elimination

Restoring intravascular volume and alkalinization of the serum and urine is an important first-line treatment for acetasalicylic acid toxicity. Bicarbonate diuresis is the mainstay and first-line treatment for aspirin toxicity, and it should be initiated early in every case of moderate salicylate poisoning [65]. The (pKa) is a logarithmic function, so a small change in urine pH will have a disproportionately larger effect on salicylate clearance, so theoretically elimination of salicylic acid is increased substantially in alkaline urine [77]. The most practical method of creating an isotonic alkaline solution in the emergency department is to add sodium bicarbonate to 5% dextrose in water. In general, one 50 mL ampule of 40% sodium bicarbonate should contain 43 mEq of sodium. By putting three ampules (150 mL total volume) of sodium bicarbonate into one liter of D5W, the resulting solution should have 132 mEq of sodium, which is essentially 0.9% (normal) saline [15a]. A total of 40 mEq of KCl per liter should be added to prevent hypokalemia. This solution should be infused rapidly at a rate of at least 2 to 3 mL/kg/hour to maintain a brisk urine output of 1 to 2 mL/kg/hr. The enhanced excretion of salicylate requires not just raising the pH of the urine, but also increasing the glomerular filtration rate [65].

The development of cerebral or pulmonary edema following salicylate poisoning is an important consideration, but a concern for possibly causing these complications should not lead to inadequate or inefficient urinary alkalinization or intravascular volume restoration. Patients who develop worsening respiratory function with increased work of breathing and hypoxia consistent with pulmonary edema or who develop altered or decreased mental status consistent with cerebral edema should have their hydration and urinary alkalinization interrupted and be evaluated immediately for definitive treatment (hemodialysis).

Box 2. Indications for hemodialysis in salicylate—poisoned patients

Severe acidosis or hypotension refractory to optimal supportive
    care (regardless of absolute serum aspirin concentration)
Evidence of end-organ injury (ie, seizures, rhabdomyolysis,
    pulmonary edema)
Renal failure
High serum aspirin concentration (>100 mg/dL) despite relatively
    stable metabolic picture
Consider for patients who require endotracheal intubation unless
    that indication for mechanical ventilation is respiratory
    depression secondary to a coingestant.

Potassium replacement long has been an important aspect of urinary alkalinization despite a paucity of clinical evidence to support the routine practice [15a]. Chronic potassium depletion causes increased reabsorption of bicarbonate in the proximal renal tubules and difficulty achieving an alkaline urine. The effects of acute potassium depletion on urinary excretion of bicarbonate are uncertain [78]. It seems reasonable to infuse potassium and NaHCO3 simultaneously, especially in patients who are already hypokalemic. Urinary alkalinization should be delayed while attempts are made to replace the serum potassium [15a].

Hemodialysis is the definitive treatment to prevent and treat salicylate-induced end-organ injury [79]. Indications for dialysis are listed in Box 2. Hemodialysis will remove aspirin in the serum and lactate efficiently [80]. Patients may have metabolized their aspirin and have a low measured serum concentration of salicylate, but they still may benefit from hemodialysis to remove the byproducts of mitochondrial poisoning. Charcoal hemoperfusion is not practical in most circumstances [81], and hemodialysis has become the preferred method of enhanced elimination of excess serum salicylate.

Summary

Aspirin carries both significant adverse effects in therapeutic doses and a substantial risk in overdose, for which there is no antidote. Its risk-benefit profile is probably the poorest of all analgesics currently available over the counter; this is reflected in current trends in analgesic use and overdose figures [8] Emergency physicians must have a healthy respect for the erratic and unpredictable absorption and elimination kinetics of aspirin, the devastating physiologic effects of aspirin overdose and the subtle manifestations, presentation, and increased mortality of chronic aspirin toxicity. Consultation with the regional poison control center is advised to assist with the management and follow-up of all poisoned patients.

References

[1] Hedner T, Everts B. The early clinical history of salicylates in rheumatology and pain. Clin Rheumatol 1998;17(1):17–25.

[2] Mueller RL, Scheidt S. History of drugs for thrombotic disease. Discovery, development, and directions for the future. Circulation 1994;89(1):432–49.

[3] Hare LG, Woodside JV, Young IS. Dietary salicylates. Journal of Clinical Pathology 2003; 56:649–50.

[4] Fink CW. Acute versus chronic salicylate poisoning. Pediatrics 1983;71(5):862–3.

[5] Flomenbaum N. Salicylates. In: Goldfrank LR, Flomenbaum N, Lewin N, editors. Goldfrank's toxicologic emergencies. 7th edition. New York: McGraw-Hill Medical Publishing Division; 2003. p. 513.

[6] Vivian AS, Goldberg IB. Recognizing chronic salicylate intoxication in the elderly. Geriatrics 1982;37(11):91–7.

[7] Anderson RJ, Potts DE, Gabow PA, et al. Unrecognized adult salicylate intoxication. Ann Intern Med 1976;85(6):745–8.

[8] Jones A. Over-the-counter analgesics: a toxicologic perspective. Am J Ther 2002;9(3): 245–57.

[9] Pirmohamed M, James S, Meakin S, et al. Adverse drug reactions as cause of admission to hospital: prospective analysis of 18,820 patients. BMJ 2004;329(7456):15–9.

[10] Wazaify M, Kennedy S, Hughes CM, et al. Prevalence of over-the-counter drug-related overdoses at accident and emergency departments in Northern Ireland—a retrospective evaluation. J Clin Pharm Ther 2005;30(1):39–44.

[11] Watson WA, Litovitz TL, Rodgers GC Jr, et al. 2004 Annual report of the American Association of Poison Control Centers Toxic Exposure Surveillance System. Am J Emerg Med 2005;23(5):589–666.

[12] Gittelman DK. Chronic salicylate intoxication. South Med J 1993;86(6):683–5.

[13] Rodgers GB. The effectiveness of child-resistant packaging for aspirin. Arch Pediatr Adolesc Med 2002;156(9):929–33.

[14] Hawton K, Simkins S, Decks J, et al. UK legislation on analgesic packs: before-and-after study of long-term effect on poisonings. BMJ 2004;329(7474):1076.

[15] Sheen CL, Dillon JF, Bateman DN, et al. Paracetamol pack size restriction: the impact on paracetamol poisoning and the over-the-counter supply of paracetamol, aspirin, and ibuprofen. Pharmacoepidemiol Drug Saf 2002;11(4):329–31.

[15a] Yip L, Dart RC, Gabrow PA. Concepts and controversies in salicylate toxicity. Emerg Med Clin N Am 1994;12(2):351–64.

[16] Petrescu I, Tarba C. Uncoupling effects of diclofenac and aspirin in the perfused liver and isolated hepatic mitochondria of rat. Biochim Biophys Acta 1997;1318(3):385–94.

[17] Krause DS, Wolf BA, Shaw LM. Acute aspirin overdose: mechanisms of toxicity. Ther Drug Monit 1992;14(6):441–51.

[18] Temple AR. Pathophysiology of aspirin overdosage toxicity, with implications for management [review]. Pediatrics 1978;62(5 Pt 2 Suppl):873–6.

[19] Leatherman JW, Schmitz PG. Fever, hyperdynamic shock, and multiple-system organ failure. A pseudo-sepsis syndrome associated with chronic salicylate intoxication. Chest 1991; 100(5):1391–6.

[20] Schwartz R, Landy G. Organic acid excretion in salicylate intoxication. J Pediatr 1965;66: 658–66.

[21] Hill JB. Salicylate intoxication. N Engl J Med 1973;288:1110–3.

[22] Rivera W, Kleinschmidt KC, Velez LI, et al. Delayed salicylate toxicity at 35 hours without early manifestations following a single salicylate ingestion. Ann Pharmacother 2004;38(7–8): 1186–8.

[23] Myers B, Evans DN, Rhodes J, et al. Metabolism and urinary excretion of 5-amino salicylic acid in healthy volunteers when given intravenously or released for absorption at different sites in the gastrointestinal tract. Gut 1987;28:196–200.

[24] Schanker LS, Tocco DJ, Brodie BB, et al. Absorption of drugs from the rat small intestine. J Pharmacol Exp Ther 1958;123(1):81–8.

[25] Singh P, Roberts MS. Dermal and underlying tissue pharmacokinetics of salicylic acid after topical application. J Pharmacokinet Biopharm 1993;21(4):368–70.

[26] Singh P, Roberts MS. Skin permeability and local tissue concentrations of nonsteroidal anti-inflammatory drugs after topical application. J Pharmacol Exp Ther 1994;268(1):144–51.

[27] Cross SE, Anderson C, Roberts MS. Topical penetration of commercial salicylate esters and salts using human isolated skin and clinical microdialysis studies. Br J Clin Pharmacol 1998; 46(1):29–35.

[28] Martin D, Valdez J, Boren J, et al. Dermal absorption of camphor, menthol, and methyl salicylate in humans. J Clin Pharmacol 2004;44:1151–7.

[29] Bell AJ, Duggin G. Acute methyl salicylate toxicity complicating herbal skin treatment for psoriasis. Emerg Med (Fremantle) 2002;14(2):188–90.

[30] Lebwohl M. The role of salicylic acid in the treatment of psoriasis. Int J Dermatol 1999;38(1): 20–2.

[31] Taylor JR, Halprin KM. Percutaneous absorption of salicylic acid. Arch Dermatol 1975; 111(6):740–3.

[32] Martin L. All you really need to interpret arterial blood gases. 2nd edition. Philadelphia: Lippincott, Williams and Wilkins; 1999.

[33] Chrichton JU, Elliott GB. Salicylate—a dangerous drug in infancy and childhood. Can Med Assoc J 1960;83:1144.

[34] Done AK. Treatment of salicylate poisoning: review of personal and published experiences. Clin Toxicol 1968;1:451.

[35] Gaudreault P, Temple AR, Lovejoy FH. The relative severity of acute versus chronic salicylate poisoning in children: a clinical comparison. Pediatrics 1982;70:567–8.

[36] Jepsen F, Ryan M. Poisoning in children. Current Paediatrics 2005;15(7):563–8.

[37] Wrathall G, Sinclair R, Moore A, et al. Three case reports of the use of haemodiafiltration in the treatment of salicylate overdose. Hum Exp Toxicol 2001;20(9):491–5.

[38] Grabe DW, Manley HJ, Kim JS, et al. Respiratory distress caused by salicylism confirmed by lung biopsy. Clin Drug Investig 1999;17(1):79–81.

[39] Proudfoot AT. Toxicity of salicylates. Am J Med 1983;75(Suppl):100–2.

[40] Cazals Y. Auditory sensori-neural alterations induced by salicylate. Prog Neurobiol 2000; 62(6):583–631.

[41] Wecker H, Laubert A. Reversible hearing loss in acute salicylate intoxication. HNO 2004; 52(4):347–51.

[42] Mongan E, Kelly P, Nies K, et al. Tinnitus as an indication of therapeutic serum salicylate levels. JAMA 1973;226(2):142–5.

[43] Taylor JR, Streetman, DS, Castle SS. Medication bezoars: a literature review and report of a case. Ann Pharmacother 1998;32(9):940–6.

[44] Stack PE, Thomas E. Pharmacobezoar: an evolving new entity. Dig Dis 1995;13(6):356–64.

[45] Gabow PA, Anderson RJ, Potts DE, et al. Acid–base disturbances in the salicylate-intoxicated adult. Arch Intern Med 1978;138:1482–3.

[46] Dale C, Aulaqi AA, Baker A, et al. Assessment of a point-of-care test for paracetamol and salicylate in blood. QJM 2005;98(2):113–8.

[47] Graham CA, Irons AJ, Munro PT. Paracetamol and salicylate testing: routinely required for all overdose patients? Eur J Emerg Med 2006;13(1):26–8.

[48] Wood DM, Dargan PI, Jones AL. Measuring plasma salicylate concentrations in all patients with drug overdose or altered consciousness: is it necessary? Emerg Med J 2005;22(6):401–3.

[49] Dugandzic RM, Tierney MG, Dickinson GE, et al. Evaluation of the validity of the Done nomogram in the management of acute salicylate intoxication. Ann Emerg Med 1989;18: 1186–90.

[50] Chalasani N, Roman J, Jurado RL. Systemic inflammatory response syndrome caused by chronic salicylate intoxication. South Med J 1996;89(5):479–82.

[51] Paul BN. Salicylate poisoning in the elderly: diagnostic pitfalls. J Am Geriatr Soc 1972;20: 388–9.

[52] Bailey RB, Jones SR. Chronic salicylate intoxication: a common cause of morbidity in the elderly. J Am Geriatr Soc 1989;37:556.

[53] Steele TE, Morton WA. Salicylate-induced delirium. Psychosomatics 1986;27:455–6.

[54] Dargan PI, Wallace CI, Jones AL. An evidence-based flowchart to guide the management of acute salicylate (aspirin) overdose. Emerg Med J 2002;19:206–9.

[55] McGuigan MA. A two-year review of salicylate deaths in Ontario. Arch Intern Med 1987; 147:510–2.

[56] Thisted B, Krantz T, Stroom J. Acute salicylate self-poisoning in 177 consecutive patients treated in ICU. Acta Anaesthesiol Scand 1987;31(4):312–6.

[57] Pena-Alonso YR, Montoya-Cabrera MA, Bustos-Cordoba E. Aspirin intoxication in a child associated with myocardial necrosis: Is this a drug-related lesion? Pediatr Dev Pathol 2003;3: 342–7.

[58] Done AK. Salicylate intoxication: significance of measurements of salicylate in blood in cases of acute ingestion. Pediatrics 1960;26:805–6.

[59] Done AK. Aspirin overdosage: incidence, diagnosis, and management. Pediatrics 1978; 62(Suppl):890–7.

[60] Kulig K. Salicylate intoxication: is the Done nomogram reliable? [Comment in AACT] Clinical Toxicology UPDATE 1990;3(2):2–3.

[61] Chabali R. Diagnostic use of anion and osmolal gaps in pediatric emergency medicine. Pediatr Emerg Care 1997;13(3):204–10.

[62] Litovitz T, Manoguerra A. Comparison of pediatric poisoning hazards: an analysis of 3.8 million exposure incidents. A report from the American Association of Poison Control Centers. Pediatrics 1992;89(6 Pt 1):999–1006.

[63] Mitchell AA, Lovejoy FH Jr, Slone D, et al. Acetaminophen and aspirin. Prescription, use, and accidental ingestion among children. Am J Dis Child 1982;136(11):976–9.

[64] Erzurumlu K, Malagirt Z, Bektas A, et al. Gastrointestinal bezoars: a retrospective analysis of 34 cases. World J Gastroenterol 2005;11(12):1813–7.

[65] Proudfoot AT, Krenzelok EP, Vale JA. Position paper on urine alkalinization. J Toxicol Clin Toxicol 2004;42(1):1–26.

[66] Greenberg MI, Hendrickson RG, Hofman M. Deleterious effects of endotracheal intubation in salicylate poisoning. Ann Emerg Med 2003;41(4):583–4.

[67] Kirshenbaum LA, Mathews SC, Sitar DS, et al. Does multiple-dose charcoal therapy enhance salicylate excretion? Arch Intern Med 1990;150(6):1281–3.

[68] Park GD, Spector R, Goldberg MJ, et al. Expanded role of charcoal therapy in the poisoned and overdosed patient. Arch Intern Med 1986;146(5):969–73.

[69] Vale JA, Krenzolak E, Barceloux GD. Position statement and practice guidelines on the use of multidose activated charcoal in the treatment of acute poisoning. American Academy of Clinical Toxicology; European Association of Poisons Centres and Clinical Toxicologists. J Toxicol Clin Toxicol 1999;37(6):731–51.

[70] Lheureux P, Tenenbein M. Position paper: whole bowel irrigation. J Toxicol Clin Toxicol 2004;42(6):843–54.

[71] Tenenbein M. Position statement: whole bowel irrigation. American Academy of Clinical Toxicology; European Association of Poisons Centres and Clinical Toxicologists. J Toxicol Clin Toxicol 1997;35(7):753–62.

[72] Daly FF, Little M, Murray L. A risk assessment-based approach to the management of acute poisoning. Emerg Med J 2006;23(5):396–9.
[73] Heard K. The changing indications of gastrointestinal decontamination in poisonings. Clin Lab Med 2006;26(1):1–12, vii.
[74] Worthley LI. Clinical toxicology: part I. Diagnosis and management of common drug overdosage. Crit Care Resusc 2002;4(3):192–215.
[75] Heard K. Gastrointestinal decontamination. Med Clin North Am 2005;89(6):1067–78.
[76] Osterhoudt KC, Durbin D, Alpern ER, et al. Risk factors for emesis after therapeutic use of activated charcoal in acutely poisoned children. Pediatrics 2004;113(4):806–10.
[77] Proudfoot AT, Krenzelok EP, Brent J, et al. Does urinary alkalinization increase salicylate elimination? If so, why? Toxicol Rev 2003;22(3):129–36.
[78] Chang YL, Biagi B, Giebish G. Control mechanism for bicarbonate transport across the rat proximal convoluted tubule. Am J Physiol 1982;242:532–43.
[79] Lund B, Seifert SA, Mayersohn M. Efficacy of sustained low-efficiency dialysis in the treatment of salicylate toxicity. Nephrol Dial Transplant 2005;20(7):1483–4.
[80] Higgins RM, Connolly JO, Hendry BM. Alkalinization and hemodialysis in severe salicylate poisoning: comparison of elimination techniques in the same patient. Clin Nephrol 1998; 50(3):178–83.
[81] Shalkham AS, Kirrane BM, Hoffman RS, et al. The availability and use of charcoal hemoperfusion in the treatment of poisoned patients. Am J Kidney Dis 2006;48(2):239–41.

ELSEVIER
SAUNDERS

EMERGENCY
MEDICINE
CLINICS OF
NORTH AMERICA

Emerg Med Clin N Am 25 (2007) 347–356

Emergency Management of Oral Hypoglycemic Drug Toxicity

Adam K. Rowden, DO[a,*], Charles J. Fasano, DO[a,b]

[a]Department of Emergency Medicine, Albert Einstein Medical Center,
5501 Old York Road, Philadelphia, PA 19141, USA
[b]Department of Emergency Medicine, Thomas Jefferson University,
Philadelphia, PA 19107-5587, USA

Exposure to oral hypoglycemic agents is a common problem confronting the emergency physician. In 2004, there were more than 10,000 exposures to these medications reported to the American Association of Poison Control Centers (AAPCC). Of these exposures, 40% involved sulfonylureas, 40% involved metformin, and the remaining 20% involved other or unknown oral hypoglycemic agents [1]. Because of the large array of oral diabetic agents available, their diverse mechanisms of action, and large variations in the potential for adverse outcomes, the emergency physician must have knowledge of the available agents and the potential for toxicity.

Oral hypoglycemic agents likely to cause hypoglycemia

Sulfonylureas

This class of drugs is a mainstay of treatment of type II diabetes. The sulfonylureas are separated into first- and second-generation drugs. The primary difference in this classification is that the second-generation agents have a shorter elimination half-life ($t_{1/2}$) than the first-generation agents. These agents stimulate insulin secretion from pancreatic beta cells [2–4]. Most of the sulfonylureas are metabolized through the liver and excreted by the kidney. Many of the metabolites are themselves active, although to a lesser degree than the parent compound. These active metabolites likely account for the long duration of action that may be seen following overdose [3]. The extremely long $t_{1/2}$ and duration of action of these medications is beneficial for glucose control and medication compliance, but can be problematic when toxicity is encountered.

---

* Corresponding author.
E-mail address: rowdena@einstein.edu (A.K. Rowden).

0733-8627/07/$ - see front matter © 2007 Elsevier Inc. All rights reserved.
doi:10.1016/j.emc.2007.02.010

The toxicity of sulfonylureas in overdose is an extension of their therapeutic mechanism. With toxicity, the pancreas secretes excessive insulin with a resultant decrease in blood sugar [2–4]. Because of the long duration of action, those patients who have sulfonylurea-induced hypoglycemia can have repeated episodes of hypoglycemia that can be refractory to treatment [5]. Typically, patients require glucose monitoring for 24 hours, but in rare cases hypoglycemic episodes continue as many as 27 days after the initial ingestion [6]. The management of sulfonylurea toxicity is simply repeat assessment of blood glucose levels and correction of hypoglycemia if it develops. Patients who have intentional overdoses of these agents may require more aggressive management and prolonged monitoring for hypoglycemia.

Diabetic patients who take their therapeutic sulfonylurea dose and then experience hypoglycemia present a unique challenge to the emergency physician. After correction of the hypoglycemia, a search for the underlying cause of the hypoglycemia must be completed. Some common causes include drug–drug interactions, decreased drug metabolism, or decreased drug excretion [7]. The complicated nature of these problems coupled with the extended $t_{1/2}$ and active metabolites of the sulfonylureas makes a compelling argument for prolonged observation or inpatient admission of these patients [3,4,8].

A child exposed, or potentially exposed, to a sulfonylurea is commonly encountered in emergency medicine. In 2004, 1400 exposures to sulfonylureas in children less than 6 years of age were reported to the AAPCC [1]. Even one pill is enough to cause clinically significant hypoglycemia in toddlers [9–11]. The onset of hypoglycemia can also be delayed with rare case reports suggesting a delay of 11 to 21 hours for specific agents [10–13]. In a large, prospective, observational series, Spiller found that no child had an onset of hypoglycemic symptoms more than 8 hours after exposure [11]. Extrapolating these data, 8 hours of euglycemia is the minimum time period that a child should be watched to predict a benign outcome. If hypoglycemia develops during that time period, however, the patient should then be admitted and observed [12,14].

Multiple cases of surreptitious or accidental poisoning by sulfonylureas are reported in the literature. Intentional surreptitious ingestion [15], pharmacy dispensing errors, [16,17] contaminated herbal products [18], and cases of Munchausen by proxy in pediatric, adult, and geriatric patients [19–22] have been described. In such cases the C-peptide test, used to differentiate endogenous from exogenous insulin, is elevated because sulfonylurea exposure results in secretion of endogenous insulin from the pancreas [15]. Assays are available to screen for sulfonylureas [23], but because of the multitude of products available, false negatives have been encountered [24,25] making more specific testing necessary in some clinical scenarios.

Meglitinides

Repaglinide and nateglinide are the two meglitinides available in the United States and are novel agents for type II diabetes. They have a mechanism similar to the sulfonylureas but with a faster onset and shorter duration of action [3]. Limited experience in overdose suggests that hypoglycemia is possible but may not be as long lasting as that caused by sulfonylureas [26,27]. In a case reported by Hirsberg [26], a patient experienced repeated episodes of hypoglycemia and was subsequently evaluated for the possibility of an insulinoma. It was later discovered that he was intentionally overdosing on repaglinide. Likewise, Nakayama [27] reported a case of hypoglycemia in a patient after intentional overdose of nateglinide. In both cases, hypoglycemia was easily treated with dextrose solutions and the duration of action was short. Hypoglycemia also has been reported following therapeutic dosing of these agents [28]. Nagai [28] reported a woman who was started on nateglinide and experienced repeated episodes of hypoglycemia during therapeutic dosing even after her initial dose was halved. The patient's decreased creatinine clearance was speculated to be the cause along with the nateglinide. In a controlled volunteer study, Fonseca and colleagues [29] found that patients who had diabetes who were mildly hyperglycemic and were given therapeutic doses of repaglinide were more likely to experience hypoglycemia than controls. Until further data are available, treating physicians should err on the side of caution in regard to the treatment and disposition of meglitinide exposures and approach them in similar manner as the sulfonylureas.

Treatment of oral hypoglycemic-induced hypoglycemia

As with any poisoned patient, the initial assessment is focused on addressing airway, breathing, and circulation. After the primary survey, any patient who has altered mental status should have his or her blood glucose evaluated. After initial stabilization, preventing absorption and enhancing elimination of the causative agent and possible antidotal therapy can be considered.

There is controversy regarding the effectiveness of activated charcoal in the setting of sulfonylurea overdose. With the exception of tolbutamide, the first-generation agents do not seem to be effectively bound by activated charcoal [30]. The second-generation agents seem to have higher affinity for charcoal [31]. As with any overdose, when considering gastrointestinal decontamination the risk for aspiration should be weighed against any potential benefit. Hemodialysis and charcoal hemoperfusion [32] have been attempted for sulfonylurea toxicity in case reports, but are not routinely recommended.

Hypoglycemia is a common presentation to the emergency department [33]. Regardless of the cause, the emergency management of hypoglycemia includes early recognition and administration of rapidly metabolized carbohydrates in the form of oral glucose or intravenous (IV) dextrose.

In patients who have altered mental status, hypoglycemia is treated with a rapid bolus of IV 50% dextrose and dextrose-containing IV fluids [34]. The initial dose of dextrose is a 50 mL bolus of 50% dextrose IV, which provides 25 g of glucose. This dose may be repeated as needed for persistent episodes of hypoglycemia. In children, the initial recommended dose of dextrose for the treatment of hypoglycemia is a 2 mL/kg bolus of 25% dextrose in water IV, and in infants the dose is 2 to 4 mL/kg of 10% dextrose in water IV. When the patient's mental status is normalized after initial treatment, long-acting oral carbohydrates or a continuous intravenous infusion of dextrose may need to be administered to prevent subsequent episodes.

The hypoglycemic patient who does not have IV access presents a challenge to the treating physician. These patients are often confused and combative making the placement of IV catheters difficult. Sublingual administration of dextrose has been shown to be effective in children who have hypoglycemia [35]. Glucagon is an FDA-approved agent for the treatment of hypoglycemia and should be administered if attempts at IV access are unsuccessful [36].

The treatment of sulfonylurea-induced hypoglycemia is much more complex than insulin-induced hypoglycemia. Poisoning may be refractory to the routine treatments rendered for hypoglycemia and often requires repeated supplemental glucose administration, higher concentrations of glucose, and antidotal therapy.

Octreotide

Octreotide is a somatostatin analog that is known to suppress insulin secretion [37]. Several case reports and one prospective study in healthy volunteers have demonstrated the safety and efficacy of octreotide administration for the treatment of sulfonylurea-induced hypoglycemia [38–41]. McLaughlin and colleagues [40] published a retrospective case series of nine patients and concluded that octreotide is safe and effective in preventing rebound hypoglycemia after sulfonylurea ingestion. Boyle and colleagues [38] showed that octreotide was superior to glucose and diazoxide in preventing recurrent hypoglycemia in eight glipizide-poisoned volunteers. Octreotide has been shown to be effective in massive sulfonylurea overdose. Case reports have demonstrated the efficacy of octreotide in intentional glyburide overdose in adults [42,43] and in accidental overdose in children [44].

The indications and dosage intervals of octreotide have not been clearly defined. Some authors recommend a single 50 to100 µg subcutaneous injection after a single hypoglycemia episode [40], whereas others recommend serial subcutaneous injections every 6 to 8 hours or constant intravenous infusion after a second hypoglycemic episode [4,42,45–47].

A recently published prospective pilot study enrolled patients who presented to the emergency department with a single sulfonylurea-induced hypoglycemic episode and randomized them to receive either standard therapy consisting of 50% dextrose IV and oral carbohydrates or standard therapy plus 50 µg subcutaneous octreotide. Preliminary data demonstrated a trend toward a decrease in frequency of hypoglycemic episodes and an increase in mean glucose at specified intervals in those patients receiving octreotide compared with placebo [48]. Future protocols need to be developed to further confirm the above-mentioned efficacy of octreotide and define the ideal dosage and interval [40,48,49].

Glucagon

Glucagon is a polypeptide hormone approved for the treatment of hypoglycemia. Glucagon is of particular interest to emergency personnel because it is efficacious for the treatment of hypoglycemia when given subcutaneously or intramuscularly, thereby negating the need for an IV line. Numerous studies have shown the efficacy and safety of glucagon for the treatment of hypoglycemia [50–52]. Vukmir and colleagues [52] showed an approximate 100 mg/dL increase in serum glucose in 49 of 50 prehospital hypoglycemic patients who received subcutaneous glucagon. In separate studies, Howell and Guly [51] and Carstens and Sprehn [50] concluded that subcutaneous glucagon administration is a safe and efficacious treatment of hypoglycemia, and it should be strongly considered when intravenous dextrose cannot be given because of the lack of IV access.

Ideally, intravenous dextrose should be used to treat hypoglycemia. If this is impossible, glucagon should be administered at the dose of 1 mg in adults (greater than 20 kg) and 0.5 mg in children (less then 20 kg) by way of subcutaneous or intramuscular injection. Several studies from Europe in the 1990s showed the safety and efficacy of intranasal glucagon for the treatment of hypoglycemia [53–55]. Glucagon should be used with caution in patients who have presumed sulfonylurea-induced hypoglycemia. Its mechanism of action involves inducing gluconeogenesis by recruiting hepatic glycogen stores. This increase in serum glucose in addition to the physiologic response of insulin released by glucagon in theory could exacerbate clinical hypoglycemia in a patient who is already in a toxin-induced hyperinsulinemic state [4].

Diazoxide

Diazoxide directly inhibits insulin secretion from pancreatic beta cells. It has been shown to be an effective treatment of refractory sulfonylurea-induced hypoglycemia [5]. Because of its potential for hypotension, diazoxide should be used with caution. Hypotension may be limited by slow intravenous infusion (300 mg over 30 minutes every 4 hours).

Disposition

Patients who are exposed to sulfonylureas or meglitinides and experience hypoglycemia should be admitted for serial monitoring of their blood glucose. Exposures (ie, an intentional overdose in an adult or a child who is found ingesting a pill) that present without hypoglycemia should be observed for a minimum of 8 hours. If hypoglycemia develops during that observation period, the patient should be admitted for further monitoring [8,11,47].

Oral hypoglycemic agents that do not cause hypoglycemia

Biguanides

Metformin is the only biguanide agent available in the United States. It controls type II diabetes by several mechanisms that have not been fully elucidated. Limiting gluconeogenesis in the liver seems to be its primary mechanism. It also increases insulin receptors in muscle tissue, thereby increasing glucose uptake into cells [3,4,8,56]. It has not been shown to increase insulin secretion from the pancreas or interfere with the hormonal regulation of insulin secretion [56,57]. It therefore does not result in hypoglycemia in either therapeutic or overdose situations. Reports of metformin-related hypoglycemia involve a combination of metformin and another antidiabetic agent [8,58–60].

Lactic acidosis is a rare but serious major complication of metformin use in overdose and therapeutic situations [8,57–60]. The incidence of lactic acidosis during therapeutic dosing is low and has been estimated 1 per 10,000 patient years [61]. The most important risk factor for developing lactic acidosis during therapeutic dosing is decreased creatinine clearance [61,62]. Because metformin-induced lactic acidosis is associated with impaired renal function, those taking metformin should abstain for 48 hours after radiologic studies using intravenous contrast [62].

In overdose, high serum lactates are reported and severe acidemia is possible [58,60,63–71]. Treatment is largely supportive because no antidotal therapy is available. Although not routinely used, it is possible to enhance the elimination of metformin by extracorporeal techniques. The clearance of metformin using traditional hemodialysis has been reported to be 68 to 150 mL/min [72]. Hemodialysis was used in several case reports, with mixed results [66,68,69,71]. Metformin is cleared by both traditional dialysis [72,73] and by continuous renal replacement therapy using continuous veno-venous hemodialysis (CVVHD) in which the clearance was reported at 50 mL/h [74]. CVVHD may provide an alternative to traditional dialysis in the hemodynamically unstable patient. CVVHD alone [67,73] and in combination with traditional dialysis [75,76] has been used in case reports with mixed outcomes. Although enhancing the elimination of metformin, these options have the added benefit of correcting the metabolic derangements typical of the severely poisoned patient. It should also be noted that most poisoned patients have favorable clinical outcomes when managed with purely supportive efforts [13,47,58]. As with all therapeutic decisions, the risks and benefits of invasive treatment modalities must be weighed in each individual case. In a retrospective case series, Spiller and Quadrani [58] found that patients who had severe acidosis, large anion gaps, hyperglycemia, and hemodynamic instability were more likely to have serious morbidity and mortality. These data suggest that patients who develop these findings may benefit from extracorporeal elimination techniques.

Children potentially exposed to metformin do not seem to be at high risk for adverse outcomes. In a small, retrospective case series of 55 patients ingesting between 1 and 10 mg/kg, none developed hypoglycemia and all were clinically well without adverse outcomes [59].

Glitazones

Despite being available for several years, there are limited data on the glitazones in overdose. Based on case reports and the mechanism of action of these medications, hypoglycemia seems unlikely. These medications act to increase insulin sensitivity in the peripheral tissues [3,8]. Like metformin, the feedback loops remain intact in regard to insulin secretion of the pancreas, and therefore hypoglycemia does not occur. This class has been associated with hepatitis and fulminant hepatic failure with therapeutic doses [3,8].

α-glucosidase inhibitors

Acarbose is an α-glucosidase inhibitor that prevents the breakdown of carbohydrates in the gut slowing absorption [3]. This oral agent is extensively metabolized in the gut with little absorption [3,8,47]. The clinical experience with overdose is limited, but hypoglycemia seems unlikely based on the drug's mechanism of action.

Summary

The myriad of oral agents available for the treatment of diabetes complicates the approach to assessment, treatment, and disposition of the potentially poisoned patient. After initial stabilization and assessment of blood glucose, the emergency physician must make every effort to determine what class of medication the patient may have been exposed to so that complications may be anticipated and appropriate disposition decisions made.

References

[1] William A. Watson, George C. Rodgers Jr, Jessica Youniss, et al. 2004 Annual report of the American Association of Poison Control Centers Toxic Exposure Surveillance System. Am J Emerg Med 2005;23(5):589–666.
[2] Eliasson L, Renstrom E, Ammala C, et al. PKC-dependent stimulation of exocytosis by sulfonylureas in pancreatic beta cells. Science 1996;271(5250):813–5.
[3] Carlton FB Jr. Recent advances in the pharmacologic management of diabetes mellitus. Emerg Med Clin North Am 2000;18(4):745–53.

[4] Harrigan RA, Nathan MS, Beattie P. Oral agents for the treatment of type 2 diabetes mellitus: pharmacology, toxicity, and treatment. Ann Emerg Med 2001;38(1):68–78.

[5] Palatnick W, Meatherall RC, Tenenbein M. Clinical spectrum of sulfonylurea overdose and experience with diazoxide therapy. Arch Intern Med 1991;151(9):1859–62.

[6] Ciechanowski K, Borowiak KS, Potocka BA, et al. Chlorpropamide toxicity with survival despite 27-day hypoglycemia. J Toxicol Clin Toxicol 1999;37(7):869–71.

[7] Chelliah A, Burge MR. Hypoglycaemia in elderly patients with diabetes mellitus: causes and strategies for prevention. Drugs Aging 2004;21(8):511–30.

[8] Spiller HA, Sawyer TS. Toxicology of oral antidiabetic medications. Am J Health Syst Pharm 2006;63(10):929–38.

[9] Osterhoudt KC. This treat is not so sweet: exploratory sulfonylurea ingestion by a toddler. Pediatr Case Rev 2003;3(4):215–7.

[10] Seltzer HS. Drug-induced hypoglycemia. A review of 1418 cases. Endocrinol Metab Clin North Am 1989;18(1):163–83.

[11] Spiller HA, Villalobos D, Krenzelok EP, et al. Prospective multicenter study of sulfonylurea ingestion in children. J Pediatr 1997;131(1 Pt 1):141–6.

[12] Quadrani DA, Spiller HA, Widder P. Five year retrospective evaluation of sulfonylurea ingestion in children. J Toxicol Clin Toxicol 1996;34(3):267–70.

[13] Szlatenyi CS, Capes KF, Wang RY. Delayed hypoglycemia in a child after ingestion of a single glipizide tablet. Ann Emerg Med 1998;31(6):773–6.

[14] Borowski H, Caraccio T, Mofenson H. Sulfonylurea ingestion in children: is an 8-hour observation period sufficient? J Pediatr 1998;133(4):584–5.

[15] Waickus CM, de Bustros A, Shakil A. Recognizing factitious hypoglycemia in the family practice setting. J Am Board Fam Pract 1999;12(2):133–6.

[16] Shumak SL, Corenblum B, Steiner G. Recurrent hypoglycemia secondary to drug-dispensing error. Arch Intern Med 1991;151(9):1877–8.

[17] Sledge ED, Broadstone VL. Hypoglycemia due to a pharmacy dispensing error. South Med J 1993;86(11):1272–3.

[18] Goudie AM, Kaye JM. Contaminated medication precipitating hypoglycaemia. Med J Aust 2001;175(5):256–7.

[19] Ben-Chetrit E, Melmed RN. Recurrent hypoglycaemia in multiple myeloma: a case of Munchausen syndrome by proxy in an elderly patient. J Intern Med 1998;244(2):175–8.

[20] Fernando R. Homicidal poisoning with glibenclamide. Med Sci Law 1999;39(4):354–8.

[21] Owen L, Ellis M, Shield J. Deliberate sulphonylurea poisoning mimicking hyperinsulinaemia of infancy. Arch Dis Child 2000;82(5):392–3.

[22] Trenque T, Hoizey G, Lamiable D. Serious hypoglycemia: Munchausen's syndrome? Diabetes Care 2001;24(4):792–3.

[23] Hoizey G, Lamiable D, Trenque T, et al. Identification and quantification of 8 sulfonylureas with clinical toxicology interest by liquid chromatography-ion-trap tandem mass spectrometry and library searching. Clin Chem 2005;51(9):1666–72.

[24] Earle KE, Rushakoff RJ, Goldfine ID. Inadvertent sulfonylurea overdosage and hypoglycemia in an elderly woman: failure of serum hypoglycemia screening. Diabetes Technol Ther 2003;5(3):449–51.

[25] Klonoff DC. A flaw in the use of sulfonylurea screening to diagnose sulfonylurea overdosages. Diabetes Technol Ther 2003;5(3):453–4.

[26] Hirshberg B, Skarulis MC, Pucino F, et al. Repaglinide-induced factitious hypoglycemia. J Clin Endocrinol Metab 2001;86(2):475–7.

[27] Nakayama S, Hirose T, Watada H, et al. Hypoglycemia following a nateglinide overdose in a suicide attempt. Diabetes Care 2005;28(1):227–8.

[28] Nagai T, Imamura M, Iizuka K, et al. Hypoglycemia due to nateglinide administration in diabetic patient with chronic renal failure. Diabetes Res Clin Pract 2003;59(3):191–4.

[29] Fonseca VA, Kelley DE, Cefalu W, et al. Hypoglycemic potential of nateglinide versus glyburide in patients with type 2 diabetes mellitus. Metabolism 2004;53(10):1331–5.

[30] Kannisto H, Neuvonen PJ. Adsorption of sulfonylureas onto activated charcoal in vitro. J Pharm Sci 1984;73(2):253–6.

[31] Kivisto KT, Neuvonen PJ. The effect of cholestyramine and activated charcoal on glipizide absorption. Br J Clin Pharmacol 1990;30(5):733–6.

[32] Ludwig SM, McKenzie J, Faiman C. Chlorpropamide overdose in renal failure: management with charcoal hemoperfusion. Am J Kidney Dis 1987;10(6):457–60.

[33] Service FJ. Hypoglycemic disorders. N Engl J Med 1995;332(17):1144–52.

[34] Shorr RI, Ray WA, Daugherty JR, et al. Incidence and risk factors for serious hypoglycemia in older persons using insulin or sulfonylureas. Arch Intern Med 1997;157(15):1681–6.

[35] Barennes H, Valea I, Nagot N, et al. Sublingual sugar administration as an alternative to intravenous dextrose administration to correct hypoglycemia among children in the tropics. Pediatrics 2005;116(5):e648–53.

[36] Muhlhauser I, Toth G, Sawicki PT, et al. Severe hypoglycemia in type I diabetic patients with impaired kidney function. Diabetes Care 1991;14(4):344–6.

[37] Katz MD, Erstad BL. Octreotide, a new somatostatin analogue. Clin Pharm 1989;8(4): 255–73.

[38] Boyle PJ, Justice K, Krentz AJ, et al. Octreotide reverses hyperinsulinemia and prevents hypoglycemia induced by sulfonylurea overdoses. J Clin Endocrinol Metab 1993;76(3):752–6.

[39] Crawford BA, Perera C. Octreotide treatment for sulfonylurea-induced hypoglycaemia. Med J Aust 2004;180(10):540–1 [author reply 541].

[40] McLaughlin SA, Crandall CS, McKinney PE. Octreotide: an antidote for sulfonylurea-induced hypoglycemia. Ann Emerg Med 2000;36(2):133–8.

[41] Schier JG, Hirsch ON, Chu J. Octreotide as antidote for sulfonylurea-induced hypoglycemia. Ann Emerg Med 2001;37(4):417–8.

[42] Carr R, Zed PJ. Octreotide for sulfonylurea-induced hypoglycemia following overdose. The Annals of Pharmacotherapy 2002;36(11):1727–32.

[43] Green RS, Palatnick W. Effectiveness of octreotide in a case of refractory sulfonylurea-induced hypoglycemia. J Emerg Med 2003;25(3):283–7.

[44] Tenenbein M. Recent advancements in pediatric toxicology. Pediatr Clin North Am 1999; 46(6):1179–88, vii.

[45] Krentz AJ, Boyle PJ, Macdonald LM, et al. Octreotide: a long-acting inhibitor of endogenous hormone secretion for human metabolic investigations. Metabolism 1994; 43(1):24–31.

[46] Ries NL, Dart RC. New developments in antidotes. Med Clin North Am 2005;89(6): 1379–97.

[47] Spiller HA. Management of antidiabetic medications in overdose. Drug Saf 1998;19(5): 411–24.

[48] Fasano CJ, O'Malley GF. A prospective trial of octreotide vs. placebo in sulfonylurea-associated hypoglycemia. Acad Emerg Med 2006;13:180.

[49] Lheureux PE, Zahir S, Penaloza A, et al. Bench-to-bedside review: antidotal treatment of sulfonylurea-induced hypoglycaemia with octreotide. Crit Care 2005;9(6):543–9.

[50] Carstens S, Sprehn M. Prehospital treatment of severe hypoglycaemia: a comparison of intramuscular glucagon and intravenous glucose. Prehospital Disaster Med 1998;13(2–4): 44–50.

[51] Howell MA, Guly HR. A comparison of glucagon and glucose in prehospital hypoglycaemia. J Accid Emerg Med 1997;14(1):30–2.

[52] Vukmir RB, Paris PM, Yealy DM. Glucagon: prehospital therapy for hypoglycemia. Ann Emerg Med 1991;20(4):375–9.

[53] Rosenfalck AM, Bendtson I, Jorgensen S, et al. Nasal glucagon in the treatment of hypoglycaemia in type 1 (insulin-dependent) diabetic patients. Diabetes Res Clin Pract 1992; 17(1):43–50.

[54] Slama G, Alamowitch C, Desplanque N, et al. A new non-invasive method for treating insulin-reaction: intranasal lyophylized glucagon. Diabetologia 1990;33(11):671–4.

[55] Stenninger E, Aman J. Intranasal glucagon treatment relieves hypoglycaemia in children with type 1 (insulin-dependent) diabetes mellitus. Diabetologia 1993;36(10):931–5.

[56] Stumvoll M, Nurjhan N, Perriello G, et al. Metabolic effects of metformin in non-insulin-dependent diabetes mellitus. N Engl J Med 1995;333(9):550–4.

[57] Bailey CJ, Turner RC. Metformin. N Engl J Med 1996;334(9):574–9.

[58] Spiller HA, Quadrani DA. Toxic effects from metformin exposure. Ann Pharmacother 2004; 38(5):776–80.

[59] Spiller HA, Weber JA, Winter ML, et al. Multicenter case series of pediatric metformin ingestion. Ann Pharmacother 2000;34(12):1385–8.

[60] von Mach MA, Sauer O, Sacha Weilemann L. Experiences of a poison center with metformin-associated lactic acidosis. Exp Clin Endocrinol Diabetes 2004;112(4):187–90.

[61] Chan NN, Brain HP, Feher MD. Metformin-associated lactic acidosis: a rare or very rare clinical entity? Diabet Med 1999;16(4):273–81.

[62] Thomsen HS. How to avoid CIN: guidelines from the European Society of Urogenital Radiology. Nephrol Dial Transplant 2005;20(suppl 1):i18–22.

[63] Brady WJ, Carter CT. Metformin overdose. Am J Emerg Med 1997;15(1):107–8.

[64] Chang CT, Chen YC, Fang JT, et al. High anion gap metabolic acidosis in suicide: don't forget metformin intoxication–two patients' experiences. Ren Fail 2002;24(5):671–5.

[65] Gjedde S, Christiansen A, Pedersen SB, et al. Survival following a metformin overdose of 63 g: a case report. Pharmacol Toxicol 2003;93(2):98–9.

[66] Guo PY, Storsley LJ, Finkle SN. Severe lactic acidosis treated with prolonged hemodialysis: recovery after massive overdoses of metformin. Semin Dial 2006;19(1):80–3.

[67] Harvey B, Hickman C, Hinson G, et al. Severe lactic acidosis complicating metformin overdose successfully treated with high-volume venovenous hemofiltration and aggressive alkalinization. Pediatr Crit Care Med 2005;6(5):598–601.

[68] Heaney D, Majid A, Junor B. Bicarbonate haemodialysis as a treatment of metformin overdose. Nephrol Dial Transplant 1997;12(5):1046–7.

[69] Lacher M, Hermanns-Clausen M, Haeffner K, et al. Severe metformin intoxication with lactic acidosis in an adolescent. Eur J Pediatr 2005;164(6):362–5.

[70] McLelland J. Recovery from metformin overdose. Diabet Med 1985;2(5):410–1.

[71] Nisse P, Mathieu-Nolf M, Deveaux M, et al. A fatal case of metformin poisoning. J Toxicol Clin Toxicol 2003;41(7):1035–6.

[72] Lalau JD, Andrejak M, Moriniere P, et al. Hemodialysis in the treatment of lactic acidosis in diabetics treated by metformin: a study of metformin elimination. Int J Clin Pharmacol Ther Toxicol 1989;27(6):285–8.

[73] Teale KF, Devine A, Stewart H, et al. The management of metformin overdose. Anaesthesia 1998;53(7):698–701.

[74] Barrueto F, Meggs WJ, Barchman MJ. Clearance of metformin by hemofiltration in overdose. J Toxicol Clin Toxicol 2002;40(2):177–80.

[75] Barquero Romero J, Perez Miranda M. Metformin-induced cholestatic hepatitis. Gastroenterol Hepatol 2005;28(4):257–8.

[76] Panzer U, Kluge S, Kreymann G, et al. Combination of intermittent haemodialysis and high-volume continuous haemofiltration for the treatment of severe metformin-induced lactic acidosis. Nephrol Dial Transplant 2004;19(8):2157–8.

ELSEVIER
SAUNDERS

EMERGENCY
MEDICINE
CLINICS OF
NORTH AMERICA

Emerg Med Clin N Am 25 (2007) 357–373

Food Poisoning

David T. Lawrence, DO[a],
Stephen G. Dobmeier, BSN[b],
Laura K. Bechtel, PhD[b,c],
Christopher P. Holstege, MD[b,c],*

[a]Blue Ridge Poison Center, Division of Medical Toxicology, Department of Emergency
Medicine, University of Virginia, P.O. Box 800744, 1222 Jefferson Park Avenue,
4th Floor, Charlottesville, VA 22908-0774, USA
[b]Blue Ridge Poison Center, University of Virginia Health System, P.O. Box 800744,
Charlottesville, VA 22908-0774, USA
[c]Division of Medical Toxicology, Department of Emergency Medicine,
University of Virginia, P.O. Box 800744, 1222 Jefferson Park Avenue,
4th Floor, Charlottesville, VA 22908-0774, USA

Food poisoning is encountered through the world. Many of the toxins responsible for specific food poisoning syndromes are no longer limited to isolated geographic locations. With increased travel and the ease of transporting food products, it is likely that a patient may present to any emergency department with the clinical effects of food poisoning. Recognizing specific food poisoning syndromes allows emergency health care providers not only to initiate appropriate treatment rapidly but also to notify health departments early and thereby prevent further poisoning cases. This article reviews several potential food-borne poisons and describes each agent's mechanism of toxicity, expected clinical presentation, and currently accepted treatment.

Ciguatera

Background

Ciguatera poisoning is the most commonly reported marine food poisoning [1]. Ciguatoxin (CTX) is produced by the marine dinoflagellate

* Corresponding author. Division of Medical Toxicology, Department of Emergency
Medicine, University of Virginia, P.O. Box 800744, 1222 Jefferson Park Avenue, 4th Floor,
Charlottesville, VA 22908-0774.
 E-mail address: ch2xf@virginia.edu (C.P. Holstege).

Gambierdiscus toxicus. Dinoflagellates grow on algae and dead coral and are consumed by herbivorous fish [2]. The toxin is concentrated up the food chain as larger predatory fish consume multiple prey fish containing CTX. Large predatory reef fish are commonly implicated in ciguatera food poisoning and include grouper, snapper, barracuda, and sea bass [3]. CTX is generally not harmful to these fish [4], so caught toxic fish appear normal. CTX itself is colorless, odorless, and tasteless, and is not inactivated by cooking or freezing [5].

There are two types of CTX, Pacific and Caribbean [6]. They have similar actions. Contaminated fish from Pacific waters are reported to cause more neurologic symptoms, whereas Caribbean fish cause more prominent gastrointestinal symptoms [7]. Both toxins are potent heat-stable, nonprotein, lipophilic sodium channel activators [5]. CTX binds to voltage-sensitive sodium channels causing prolonged opening of these channels and an influx of sodium [8,9]. This influx causes depolarization of excitable membranes. Axonal swelling may occur [10,11]. This effect is seen in all excitable tissues (ie, neurons, skeletal muscle, and cardiac tissue) [12], but is most pronounced in sensory neurons [13,14].

Clinical presentation

There are four categories of symptoms caused by ciguatera poisoning: gastrointestinal, neuropathic, cardiovascular, and diffuse pain syndrome [15]. Victims of CTX poisoning usually have symptoms from more than one category, with neuropathic symptoms being present most commonly.

Symptoms typically appear within 4 to 6 hours following ingestion of contaminated fish [10]. This time of onset can vary considerably, however, with symptom onset ranging from several minutes to 24 hours depending on the amount ingested [10]. Symptoms typically last 2 to 5 days, with most victims fully recovered within 2 weeks. Patients may develop chronic symptoms, however, and experience paresthesias, sensory disturbances, joint and muscle aches, and fatigue lasting months [4,10]. There are rare reports of fatalities attributable to ciguatera poisoning [7].

Gastrointestinal complaints usually manifest first, and may include nausea, vomiting, and diarrhea. Neurologic symptoms follow [16]. Perioral and limb paresthesias and dysesthesias are common. Pruritus, diaphoresis, myalgias, arthralgias, muscle cramps, and weakness have all been reported [10].

There are several peculiar symptoms associated with ciguatera poisoning. Patients sometimes complain of the sensation that their teeth are falling out. Also, there is a phenomenon known as temperature reversal, wherein cold items feel hot [15]. Cold objects are described to cause a painful tingling, a burning discomfort, or an electric shock sensation [4,10]. In some cases cardiovascular symptoms have been reported, including symptomatic bradycardia [17–19], that have been hypothesized to be attributable to the effects of CTX on the muscarinic autonomic nervous system [20].

Diagnosis

Ciguatera toxicity is a clinical diagnosis. It should be suspected in patients who have symptoms consistent with ciguatera poisoning and a history of eating fish associated with CTX. There are methods for testing for CTX in fish. These tests can be valuable for confirming the diagnosis. Testing is limited by the need to have a sample of the ingested fish. Also, individuals can be affected differently by a similar amount of CTX [21,22]. There is no rapidly available test for CTX in clinical practice.

Management

The mainstay of treatment of ciguatera poisoning is supportive care and symptomatic therapy [23,24]. Patients often present dehydrated and may have electrolyte abnormalities secondary to vomiting and diarrhea [12,25]. Symptomatic bradycardia should be treated with atropine [15,18,24,26,27]. Pruritus can be treated with antihistamines [24,28].

Some authors recommend the use of activated charcoal. Given the typical delay in presentation and the frequency of vomiting, however, this is unlikely to be of benefit [10] and is not recommended.

Mannitol has been considered the treatment of choice for relieving neurologic symptoms. This practice has been supported by many reports of successful use in the past [12,16,29,30] and its mechanism is supported by several experimental papers [11,31]. It is believed that the beneficial effects are at least partially attributable to reduction of axonal edema through the osmotic effect of mannitol [11]. A recent study shows that its protective action also seems to involve an inhibition of the toxins associated with the sodium channels [31]. A study on rat nerves failed to show any improvement in conduction velocity with mannitol, however [32]. The only randomized controlled trial comparing mannitol to placebo failed to show benefit [15]. Until further data are available, given the number of reports of successful use of mannitol, it is reasonable to attempt a trial of therapy. Mannitol infusion is not without some risk, however. Mannitol is an osmotic diuretic and can worsen hypovolemia and electrolyte abnormalities caused by vomiting and diarrhea. It is important to ensure that the patient is not volume depleted before initiating therapy [10,33]. Mannitol infusions are also associated with site pain and a risk for thrombophlebitis [16]. Mannitol is most effective when administered within 48 hours. There are rare reports of improvement with delayed administration of mannitol weeks after exposure, however [16,34]. The recommended dose is 1 g/kg of 20% mannitol over 30 minutes [7,12,16]. If this is not effective or if there is recurrence of symptoms, a repeat dose may be given [7,16]. For persistent painful neuropathy, there are case reports of amitriptyline [35,36] and gabapentin being used successfully [37].

Patients who developed clinical effects from CTX should avoid alcohol and nut ingestion for at least 3 to 6 months following ciguatera exposure because these have been reported to exacerbate symptoms in recovering patients [7,10,24]. Also, patients who have had significant ciguatera poisoning should avoid fish known to harbor CTX because more significant toxicity may occur, even years later, on re-exposure. Patients should be advised that CTX can be transmitted through semen [16] and breast milk [38] and care should be taken to avoid secondarily exposing others.

Scombroid

Background

Scombroid poisoning occurs after ingestion of fish that has accumulated scombrotoxin secondary to spoilage. The fish associated with this toxicity are dark fleshed, containing large amounts of the amino acid histidine. Scombroid food poisoning develops when an individual ingests improperly refrigerated fish in which bacteria have converted histidine into histamine and histaminelike substances [39,40]. Pure histamine itself is not toxic when taken orally [41]. Therefore, scombroid is not solely caused by excess histamine ingestion [42]. There are other factors involved in toxicity, including substances that facilitate histamine absorption [42–44] and urocanic acid that acts as a mast cell degranulator adding to the histamine-related symptoms [45]. Fish commonly implicated include those in the Scombridae and Scomberesocidae families, such as tuna, mackerel, and bonito [46]. Nonscombroid fish, such as mahi-mahi, bluefish [41,47], anchovies, sardines [46], swordfish [48], and escolar [49], have also caused this syndrome.

Clinical presentation

Patients who ingest scombroid present with signs and symptoms of a histamine reaction: flushing, erythematous or urticarial rash, headache, dizziness, crampy abdominal pain, nausea, vomiting, diarrhea, shortness of breath, and wheezing [39,50,51]. In severe cases it can lead to hypotension and even hemodynamic collapse [46,52,53]. The ingested causative fish usually does not smell or taste spoiled, but the victims often report an unusual peppery or metallic taste [48,49]. Symptoms begin within an hour and usually last less than 12 hours.

Scombroid poisoning may be worse in patients taking isoniazid. Isoniazid acts as a histaminase inhibitor. Patients taking isoniazid may have more severe or prolonged reaction to scombroid poisoning [54–56].

Diagnosis

The diagnosis is accomplished by observing the clinical syndrome of scombroid toxicity with a history of eating causative fish. Although the treatment of scombroid is similar to that of an acute type I allergic reaction, it is important to not label these as allergic reactions. These patients do not have seafood allergies [50,57] and should not be told to avoid seafood.

Evidence suggests that victims of scombroid poisoning have elevated plasma and urinary histamine levels [58,59]. This finding may aid in confirming cases but is not useful in guiding emergency clinical decisions. The fish may also be tested to aid in confirming the diagnosis, but this can be misleading because histamine levels can vary greatly even within the same cut of fish [57].

Management

The cornerstone of treatment is with antihistamines [60,61]. Intravenous H1 and H2 blockers (ie, diphenhydramine and cimetidine, respectively) should be administered [40,62,63]. Bronchodilators (ie, albuterol) can be helpful if the patient experiences bronchospasm. Severe cases, with hypotension and respiratory distress, require aggressive treatment with intravenous fluids, airway control, and possibly epinephrine [51,61]. Scombroid poisoning is a self-limited illness; symptoms typically resolve within 12 hours [39].

Tetrodotoxin

Background

Tetrodotoxin (TTX) is found in the order Tetraodontidae, which includes the toad fish, blow fish, balloon fish, porcupine fish, and puffer fish [64]. These fish contain various amounts of TTX, with the highest concentrations found within the liver, ovaries, intestines, and skin [65]. TTX has also been found in other animals, including certain mollusks, the horseshoe crab, the Californian newt, and the blue-ringed octopus [66].

TTX poisoning has been encountered throughout history. One of the earliest recorded depictions of poisoning attributable to TTX was by Captain James Cook on September 7, 1774 [67].

> Without the least suspicion of its being of a poisonous quality we had ordered it for supper...only the Liver and Roe was dressed of which the two Mr. Fosters and myself did but taste. About 3 or 4 o'clock in the morning we were seized with an extraordinary weakness in all our limbs attended with a numbness or sensation like to that caused by exposing ones hands or feet to a fire after having been pinched by a frost, I almost lost the sense of feeling nor could I distinguish between light and heavy bodies, a quart pot full of water and a feather was the same in my hand.

TTX can be found in a number of foods [68,69]. It is best described following ingestion of fugu. Fugu is considered a delicacy in some parts of the world, especially Japan. Despite legislation addressing fugu preparation and marketing that has lead to a decrease in the number of deaths from fugu, tetrodotoxin poisoning continues to be encountered owing to sale by unlicensed cooks and unskilled preparation of puffer fish [1,69,70].

TTX was first isolated in 1909 by a Japanese scientist, Dr. Yoshizumi Tahara. TTX is heat stable and is not damaged by freezing. TTX is a specific high-affinity blocking ligand of voltage-dependent Na^+ channels [71]. TTX binds competitively to a site on the external surface of the channel, named toxin site 1. Binding of TTX inhibits sodium flux through these ion channels rendering excitable tissues, such as nerves and muscle, nonfunctional.

Clinical presentation

The severity and speed of clinical effects vary depending on the amount ingested [1]. A grading system has been described based on presenting signs and symptoms (Box 1) [65]. Paresthesias are common and typically the first symptom to be reported, usually beginning within an hour after ingestion [64,65]. Paresthesias initially affect the tongue, lips, and mouth, and progress to involving the extremities [72]. Gastrointestinal symptoms may be seen and include nausea and vomiting, and less often diarrhea. Muscle weakness, headache, ataxia, dizziness, urinary retention, floating sensations, and feelings of doom may occur [69]. An ascending flaccid paralysis can develop. Other reported effects include diaphoresis, pleuritic chest pain, fixed dilated pupils, dysphagia, aphonia, seizures, bradycardia, hypotension, and heart blocks [69]. Death can occur within hours secondary to respiratory muscle paralysis or dysrhythmias. Clinical effects in the mildest of cases resolve within hours, whereas the more severe cases may not resolve for days.

Diagnosis

The diagnosis is accomplished by observing the clinical syndrome of TTX toxicity with a history of eating causative fish. Confirmation of TTX poisoning in human urine or blood samples can be performed. Confirmation is performed using high-performance liquid chromatography with tandem mass spectrometry detection methods. TTX is rapidly metabolized and

---

Box 1. Clinical grading system for tetrodotoxin poisoning

Grade 1. Perioral numbness and paresthesias, with or without gastrointestinal symptoms

Grade 2. Numbness of tongue, face, and other areas (distal); early motor paralysis and incoordination; slurred speech; normal reflexes

Grade 3. Generalized flaccid paralysis; respiratory failure; aphonia; fixed dilated pupils; patient still conscious

Grade 4. Severe respiratory failure with hypoxia; hypotension; bradycardia; cardiac arrhythmias; unconsciousness may occur

---

Data from Isbister GK, Son J, Wang F, et al. Puffer fish poisoning: a potentially life-threatening condition. Med J Aust 2002;177(11–12):650–3.

primarily excreted through the urine. Urine analysis is therefore the preferred method.

Management

Treatment is supportive; there is no specific antitoxin. Symptomatic patients who have grade 2 or greater clinical effects should be admitted to the hospital for observation until peak effects have passed. Those who have respiratory failure should be intubated and placed on mechanical ventilation. Vasopressor support may be necessary for hypotension refractory to intravenous fluids [69]. Atropine has been used for symptomatic bradycardia. One report documented dramatic improvement following dialysis in a uremic patient. It was hypothesized that TTX is dialyzable because it has a low molecular weight, is water soluble, and is not significantly protein bound [73].

Botulism

Background

Botulism is a progressive paralytic illness caused by botulinum toxin [74]. Botulinum toxin is an extremely potent neurotoxin considered to be the most potent biologic poison [75]. It is produced by the bacteria *Clostridium botulinum*. There are seven distinct subtypes of clostridial neurotoxins (A, B, C1, D, E, F, and G), of which only A, B, E, and rarely F cause illness in humans [76].

There are several syndromes caused by botulinum toxin: food-borne botulism, infant botulism, wound botulism, and adult intestinal botulism. Food-borne botulism is caused by ingestion of preformed botulinum toxin. In improperly preserved foods botulinum spores can germinate and proliferate and elaborate their toxin; this process is favored by an anaerobic, low-sodium, and nonacidic medium [77]. The toxin is inactivated by heating at 85°C for 5 minutes.

Infant botulism is the most common form of botulism encountered. It occurs when botulism spores are ingested and germinate in the gastrointestinal tract. The bacteria then produces toxin that is absorbed into the body [78]. Although classically associated with ingestion of honey, infant botulism is usually contracted by ingesting dust containing *C botulinum* spores [79]. The soil in southeastern Pennsylvania, Utah, and California has the greatest chance of containing these spores and most cases are from these states [80]. Infant botulism can present subtly. Constipation is often the initial symptom [81] and may precede neurologic symptoms by days. Symptoms can progress to poor feeding, weak cry, ptosis, weakness, and respiratory insufficiency [78,79]. Infants can also get botulism from the ingestion of preformed toxin [82] and subsequent signs and symptoms can rapidly progress, confusing the diagnosis.

Wound botulism occurs when *C botulinum* spores contaminate wounds. They can germinate and produce toxin that is systemically absorbed

[83,84]. This syndrome is treated the same as food-borne botulism. Administration of antibiotics and drainage or debridement of infected tissue must also be performed [84,85].

Adult intestinal botulism is similar to infant botulism. It occurs in adults who have altered intestinal flora because of antibiotic use, abdominal surgery, achlorhydria, or inflammatory bowel disease [76,86,87].

After botulinum toxin is systemically absorbed it attacks cholinergic presynaptic nerve endings. The toxin cannot cross the blood–brain barrier and therefore only affects the peripheral nervous system [88]. The toxin is taken up into the nerve by endocytosis and prevents the fusion of the synaptic vesicle with the nerve terminus. Ultimately, the nerve cannot release acetylcholine and neurotransmission is interrupted [88,89].

Clinical presentation

With food-borne botulism, the onset of symptoms is variable and delayed. Because of the delay it can be challenging to identify the source. Symptoms may appear as early as 2 hours postingestion, with most patients developing symptoms within 36 hours [89]. Signs and symptoms may not be noticed for up to 8 days, however [90]. It is thus prudent to carefully observe any asymptomatic individuals who have eaten food that has caused symptoms in others. If there is any sign of toxicity, treatment should be started immediately [76].

The presenting symptoms follow a stereotypical pattern of descending weakness [89]. This pattern begins with cranial nerve dysfunction manifested as dysphagia, diplopia, and dysarthria. On examination, ptosis, gaze paralysis, and facial palsy are most often noted [90]. It progresses as a descending motor paralysis affecting the upper limbs, then the lower limbs. In severe cases the intercostals and diaphragm are affected, possibly necessitating mechanical ventilation [88]. Dry mouth is a common initial complaint [90]. This symptom is caused by inhibition of muscarinic cholinergic function, which can also cause dilated pupils and constipation [88]. Food-borne botulism also may have gastrointestinal symptoms, including nausea, vomiting, constipation, and less commonly diarrhea [86,87,89]. These symptoms may precede neurologic symptoms.

Botulism does not affect the central nervous system. Mentation therefore is normal [90]. Peripheral sensory involvement is also lacking [89]. These findings are helpful in distinguishing botulism from other neurologic conditions. Patients tend to be afebrile [90].

The paralysis caused by botulinum toxin persists until the cleaved proteins are regenerated. If a patient's condition progresses to the point of requiring mechanical ventilation, the patient may become ventilator-dependent for several months [90]. For this reason it is important to recognize botulism and initiate treatment with antitoxin as early as possible. Antitoxin treatment does not reverse any paralysis that has already occurred but arrests the progression, thus limiting disability and possibly preventing the need for intubation [88].

A classic pentad for diagnosing botulism consists of nausea and vomiting, dysphagia, diplopia, dry mouth, and dilated and fixed pupils [91]. In a study of 705 patients who had botulism, 68% of patients had at least three symptoms on admission, whereas only 2% had all five symptoms [92]. Patients often do not present with all classic clinical effects.

Diagnosis

The diagnosis of botulism toxicity must be initially made by the clinician using history-taking skills and physical examination skills. The local public health department should be called immediately with any suspected cases. Public health officials can then help orchestrate definitive testing and appropriate treatments. Given the delay in symptom onset, it may be difficult to identify the causative agent.

Management

The first step is supportive care, with attention to airway protection and ventilatory support. The definitive treatment of botulism is the administration of botulinum antitoxin [76]. The standard antitoxin is a horse-derived serum with antibodies against subtypes A, B, and E. The antitoxin works by binding to and neutralizing any botulinum toxin that is free in the serum. It is important to initiate antitoxin therapy as soon as possible because the toxin must be neutralized before it is able to bind irreversibly to nerve terminus. This therapy is empiric, based on clinical suspicion, because no confirmatory tests are readily available [88,90].

Botulinum antitoxin administration should be considered in any patient who has a clinical presentation suspicious for botulism, especially when a group of two or more present with suggestive symptoms. Suspicious cases should be reported immediately to the local or state health department, or the Centers for Disease Control and Prevention should be contacted directly to arrange antitoxin delivery [88]. The antitoxin is a horse serum–derived product resulting in a significant chance of an allergic reaction. Historically, the incidence of allergic reactions has been reported to be 9%. It is important to be well prepared in advance to treat any anaphylactic reaction. Skin testing is recommended before administering the antitoxin. Further delaying treatment to perform the skin test may not be feasible in some cases, however. Depending on the clinical scenario, the benefit of treating the illness as rapidly as possible may outweigh the risk for taking the additional time to skin test. Additionally, the rate of adverse reactions has declined to about 1% since the recommended dose was reduced to one vial [88] and skin testing may not predict an adverse reaction. In one study more than half the patients who had an acute reaction had a negative skin test [93].

Other antidotes

The equine-derived antitoxin is not recommended to treat infant botulism, in part because of the high rate of adverse reactions and fear of sensitizing infants against horses and horse-derived products [94]. Recently, a human-derived immune globulin (BabyBIG) has been introduced and should be used to treat infant botulism. It is effective for types A and B [95]. In addition to infants, BabyBIG can be considered for those who have had a serious reaction to the trivalent antibody and were not able to receive the full treatment or in those who have known severe allergy to equine-derived products. Currently this antidote is only available from the California State Health Department (510-540-2646) [88].

The US Army possesses an antitoxin against all seven (A–G) serotypes. It is an equine-derived immunoglobulin that has been cleaved by pepsin discarding the Fc (immunogenic portion) and leaving the F(ab′)2 fragments specific for botulinum toxin [88]. This therapy has a lower chance of adverse allergic reaction but a skin test is still advised before administering this product.

Monosodium glutamate

Monosodium glutamate (MSG) is added to many foods as a flavor enhancer [96]. MSG is described to cause a complex grouping of clinical effects appearing 15 to 20 minutes after ingestion. These effects consist of a sensation of burning or warmth, pressure or tightness, and numbness or tingling confined to the face, neck, and upper chest and arms. It disappears within 2 hours of exposure [97]. MSG has also been implicated in causing asthma exacerbations and migraine headaches [97,98].

MSG is the sodium salt of glutamate and is rapidly broken down to free glutamate in the gastrointestinal tract. Glutamate is a nonessential amino acid. It is used as a fuel—as much as 95% of ingested glutamate is used as energy by the intestinal mucosa [99]—and is a substrate for glutathione synthesis [98,99]. Glutamate also serves the major excitatory neurotransmitter in the brain [100] and has effects on pulmonary [101] and vascular tissue [102]. Exogenous glutamate does not cross an intact blood–brain barrier. The effects of ingested glutamate therefore do not include central nervous system effects [99,103].

Despite case reports of MSG sensitivity, numerous double-blind studies have failed to find a link between MSG consumption and symptoms [104–106]. Studies that have shown a link between MSG consumption and symptoms have given subjects pure MSG on an empty stomach, a different scenario than what is actually encountered [107]. When MSG is consumed with carbohydrates and protein, it fails absorb quickly enough to cause an increase in serum glutamate [107]. At this point it is difficult to definitively attribute the various symptoms attributed to MSG to consumption of foods containing MSG.

Studies have also been unable to firmly establish a relationship between MSG and asthma [98,99,108]. MSG is reported to be a migraine trigger [98]. It is proposed that cerebral vasospasm is the cause [102], although there are no clinical data supporting this hypothesis [98].

Because there is currently disagreement in the literature regarding the association of MSG and adverse clinical effects, it is advisable for those who experience symptoms to avoid MSG.

Oxalate

Ingestion of plants high in oxalic acid can cause several adverse reactions. There are two distinct types of oxalate salts, insoluble and soluble [109]. Insoluble oxalate salts are found in several ornamental plants, including the genera *Philodendron* and *Dieffenbachia* [110]. These are not considered edible plants. There are reports of these being mistakenly ingested with adverse outcome. Soluble oxalate salts are found in several edible plants, including spinach, rhubarb, swiss chard, and beet greens [109,111].

Insoluble salts are not systemically absorbed. Rather, calcium oxalate crystals, called raphides, present in these plants penetrate the mucosa causing localized irritation, swelling, and possibly extreme pain [112]. Most reactions are self-limited [113]. There are reports of serious adverse outcomes, however, including airway obstruction [114]. There is also a report of esophagitis leading to an aortoesophageal fistula [115]. A fatality caused by *Dieffenbachia* ingestion, attributable to asphyxiation from edema of the glottis, was reported in a canine [116]. Treatment is primarily supportive. Standard treatments used in managing allergic reactions are typically ineffective [114]. Topical application of eugenol can reduce edema associated with insoluble oxalate exposure [117].

Soluble oxalate salts are readily absorbed through the gastrointestinal system. Oxalic acid combines with the body's calcium to form calcium oxalate salts. This phenomenon can result in hypocalcemia [109,111,118], which may lead to tetany, arrhythmias, coma, and death. These calcium oxalate crystals can deposit in multiple tissues, particularly the kidneys, digestive tract, and brain [109]. Nephropathy and renal failure are commonly seen with significant oxalate poisoning [109,118,119]. This observation is attributable in part to deposition of calcium oxalate crystals. Two patients suffered renal failure after drinking star fruit juice [119], with the connection to oxalate content in the star fruit juice confirmed in a rat model [120]. High dietary oxalate consumption has also been associated with kidney stone formation. Patients suffering from kidney stones should be advised to restrict consumption of these foods [121]. Oxalate crystal deposition in the brain can lead to cerebral edema, encephalitis, and focal necrosis [109,122]. This development can be especially dangerous in patients who have renal failure. There are multiple reports of star fruit ingestions causing seizures and other signs of neurotoxicity in patients who have renal failure

[123–125]. Treatment is primarily supportive. Symptomatic hypocalcemia must be treated with intravenous calcium [109]. Adequate hydration must be assured to allow adequate urine output.

Grayanotoxin

There are numerous reports of outbreaks of people suffering toxicity following ingestion of honey contaminated by grayanotoxin [126,127]. This toxicity is a result of honey produced by bees using pollen primarily from grayanotoxin-containing rhododendron species [128].

Most reports of grayanotoxin-contaminated honey originate from Turkey, because of the large number of Rhododendrons in that country [126,127]. Rhododendrons are found in many regions, however, including parts of North America, Europe, Japan, Nepal, and Brazil [127]. Reports have also been published of the development of symptoms after ingesting honey imported from endemic areas [128]. Emergency personnel from different regions may encounter patients with this toxic syndrome.

Grayanotoxins bind to sodium channels when they are in their open state. This binding modifies the channels and they are unable to be inactivated [129,130]. Patients who have grayanotoxin toxicity can present with dizziness, weakness, excessive sweating, vomiting, paresthesias, blurred vision, hypotension, syncope, and convulsions [126–128,131–133]. Cardiotoxic effects may develop, including sinus bradycardia, nodal rhythms, and complete atrioventricular block with hypotension [126–128,131]. Other conduction abnormalities, such as a transient Wolff-Parkinson-White pattern, have been observed [132]. Patients usually experience symptoms within 1 to 2 hours, with a range of 30 minutes to 3 hours for symptom onset [128]. Treatment is primarily supportive. Hypotension and bradycardia reportedly respond to intravenous fluids and atropine [128,131].

Summary

The food toxins reviewed in this article have the potential to cause significant illness and even death. Prompt recognition and treatment can be helpful in minimizing clinical effects. With increased travel and the ease of transporting foods, victims of these poisonings could present to any emergency department.

References

[1] Isbister GK, Kiernan MC. Neurotoxic marine poisoning. Lancet Neurol 2005;4(4):219–28.
[2] Gillespie NC, Lewis RJ, Pearn JH, et al. Ciguatera in Australia. Occurrence, clinical features, pathophysiology and management. Med J Aust 1986;145(11–12):584–90.
[3] Hokama Y, Yoshikawa-Ebesu J. Ciguatera fish poisoning: a foodborne disease. J Toxicol Toxin Rev 2001;20(2):85–139.

[4] Butera R, Prockop LD, Buonocore M, et al. Mild ciguatera poisoning: Case reports with neurophysiological evaluations. Muscle Nerve 2000;23(10):1598–603.

[5] Pearn J. Neurology of ciguatera. J Neurol Neurosurg Psychiatr 2001;70(1):4–8.

[6] Lehane L, Lewis RJ. Ciguatera: recent advances but the risk remains. Int J Food Microbiol 2000;61(2–3):91–125.

[7] Lewis RJ. Ciguatera: Australian perspectives on a global problem. Toxicon 2006;48(7): 799–809.

[8] Bidard JN, Vijverberg HPM, Frelin C, et al. Ciguatoxin is a novel of type of Na channel toxin. J Biol Chem 1984;259(13):8353–7.

[9] Dechraoui M-Y, Naar J, Pauillac S, et al. Ciguatoxins and brevetoxins, neurotoxic polyether compounds active on sodium channels. Toxicon 1999;37(1):125–43.

[10] Palafox N, Buenconsejo-Lum L. Ciguatera fish poisoning: review of clinical manifestations. J Toxicol Toxin Rev 2001;20(2):141–60.

[11] Mattei C, Molgo J, Marquais M, et al. Hyperosmolar mannitol reverses the increased membrane excitability and the nodal swelling caused by Caribbean ciguatoxin-1 in single frog myelinated axons. Brain Res 1999;847(1):50–8.

[12] Pearn JH, Lewis RJ, Ruff T, et al. Ciguatera and mannitol: experience with a new treatment regimen [see comment]. Med J Aust 1989;151(2):77–80.

[13] Cameron J, Flowers AE, Capra MF. Effects of ciguatoxin on nerve excitability in rats (Part I). J Neurol Sci 1991;101(1):87–92.

[14] Cameron J, Flowers AE, Capra MF. Electrophysiological studies on ciguatera poisoning in man (Part II). J Neurol Sci 1991;101(1):93–7.

[15] Schnorf H, Taurarii M, Cundy T. Ciguatera fish poisoning: a double-blind randomized trial of mannitol therapy. Neurology 2002;58(6):873–80.

[16] Ting JY, Brown AF. Ciguatera poisoning: a global issue with common management problems. Eur J Emerg Med 2001;8(4):295–300.

[17] Hung Y-M, Hung S-Y, Chou K-J, et al. Persistent bradycardia caused by ciguatoxin poisoning after barracuda fish eggs ingestion in southern Taiwan. Am J Trop Med Hyg 2005;73(6):1026–7.

[18] Chan TYK, Wang AYM. Life-threatening bradycardia and hypotension in a patient with ciguatera fish poisoning. Trans R Soc Trop Med Hyg 1993;87(1):71.

[19] Bagnis R, Kuberski T, Laugier S. Clinical observations on 3,009 cases of ciguatera (fish poisoning) in the South Pacific. Am J Trop Med Hyg 1979;28(6):1067–73.

[20] Sauviat M-P, Marquais M, Vernoux J-P. Muscarinic effects of the Caribbean ciguatoxin C-CTX-1 on frog atrial heart muscle. Toxicon 2002;40(8):1155–63.

[21] Glaziou P, Legrand A-M. The epidemiology of ciguatera fish poisoning. Toxicon 1994; 32(8):863–73.

[22] Centers for Disease Control and Prevention. Ciguatera fish poisoning—Texas, 1998, and South Carolina, 2004. MMWR Morb & Mortal Wkly Rep 2006;55(34):935–7.

[23] Bourdy G, Cabalion P, Amade P, et al. Traditional remedies used in the Western Pacific for the treatment of ciguatera poisoning. J Ethnopharmacol 1992;36(2):163–74.

[24] de Haro L, Pommier P, Valli M. Emergence of imported ciguatera in Europe: report of 18 cases at the Poison Control Centre of Marseille. J Toxicol Clin Toxicol 2003;41(7): 927–30.

[25] Lehane L. Ciguatera update. Med J Aust 2000;172(4):176–9.

[26] Barton ED, Tanner P, Turchen SG, et al. Ciguatera fish poisoning. A southern California epidemic. West J Med 1995;163(1):31–5.

[27] Geller RJ, Benowitz NL. Orthostatic hypotension in ciguatera fish poisoning. Arch Intern Med 1992;152(10):2131–3.

[28] Goodman A, Williams TN, Maitland K. Ciguatera poisoning in Vanuatu. Am J Trop Med Hyg 2003;68(2):263–6.

[29] Palafox NA, Jain LG, Pinano AZ, et al. Successful treatment of ciguatera fish poisoning with intravenous mannitol. JAMA 1988;259(18):2740–2.

[30] Williamson J. Ciguatera and mannitol: a successful treatment [comment]. Med J Aust 1990; 153(5):306–7.

[31] Birinyi-Strachan LC, Davies MJ, Lewis RJ, et al. Neuroprotectant effects of iso-osmolar d-mannitol to prevent Pacific ciguatoxin-1 induced alterations in neuronal excitability: a comparison with other osmotic agents and free radical scavengers. Neuropharmacology 2005;49(5):669–86.

[32] Purcell CE, Capra MF, Cameron J. Action of mannitol in ciguatoxin-intoxicated rats. Toxicon 1999;37(1):67–76.

[33] Beadle A. Ciguatera fish poisoning. Mil Med 1997;162(5):319–22.

[34] Eastaugh J. Delayed use of intravenous mannitol in Ciguatera (fish poisoning). Ann Emerg Med 1996;28(1):105–6.

[35] Davis RT, Villar LA. Symptomatic improvement with amitriptyline in ciguatera fish poisoning. N Engl J Med 1986;315(1):65.

[36] Bowman PB. Amitriptyline and ciguatera. Med J Aust 1984;140(13):802.

[37] Perez CM, Vasquez PA, Perret CF. Treatment of Ciguatera poisoning with Gabapentin. N Engl J Med 2001;344(9):692–3.

[38] Blythe DG, de Sylva DP. Mother's milk turns toxic following fish feast [see comment]. JAMA 1990;264(16):2074.

[39] Kerr GW, Parke TR. Scombroid poisoning—a pseudoallergic syndrome. Journal of the Royal Society of Medicine 1998;91(2):83–4.

[40] McInerney J, Sahgal P, Vogel M, et al. Scombroid poisoning. Ann Emerg Med 1996;28(2): 235–8.

[41] Etkind P, Wilson ME, Gallagher K, et al. Bluefish-associated scombroid poisoning. An example of the expanding spectrum of food poisoning from seafood. JAMA 1987;258(23): 3409–10.

[42] Lange WR. Scombroid poisoning. Am Fam Physician 1988;37(4):163–8.

[43] Foo LY. Scombroid poisoning—recapitulation on the role of histamine. N Z Med J 1977; 85(588):425–7.

[44] Bjeldanes LF, Schutz DE, Morris MM. On the aetiology of scombroid poisoning: cadaverine potentiation of histamine toxicity in the guinea-pig. Food Cosmet Toxicol 1978; 16(2):157–9.

[45] Lehane L, Olley J. Histamine fish poisoning revisited. Int J Food Microbiol 2000;58(1–2): 1–37.

[46] Borade PS, Ballary CC, Lee DKC. A fishy cause of sudden near fatal hypotension. Resuscitation 2007;72(1):158–60.

[47] Pugno PA, Kaufman D, Feder HM Jr. Bluefish: a newly discovered cause of scombroid poisoning. J Fam Pract 1983;17(6):1071–2.

[48] Russell FE, Maretic Z. Scombroid poisoning: mini-review with case histories. Toxicon 1986;24(10):967–73.

[49] Feldman KA, Werner SB, Cronan S, et al. A large outbreak of scombroid fish poisoning associated with eating escolar fish (*Lepidocybium flavobrunneum*). Epidemiol Infect 2005; 133(1):29–33.

[50] Attaran RR, Probst F. Histamine fish poisoning: a common but frequently misdiagnosed condition. Emerg Med J 2002;19(5):474–5.

[51] Sanchez-Guerrero IM, Vidal JB, Escudero AI. Scombroid fish poisoning: a potentially life-threatening allergic-like reaction. J Allergy Clin Immunol 1997;100(3):433–4.

[52] Grinda J-M, Bellenfant F, Brivet FG, et al. Biventricular assist device for scombroid poisoning with refractory myocardial dysfunction: a bridge to recovery. Crit Care Med 2004;32(9):1957–9.

[53] Iannuzzi M, D'ignazio N, Bressy L, et al. Severe scombroid fish poisoning syndrome requiring aggressive fluid resuscitation in the emergency department. Minerva Aneestesiol 2006;72:1–3.

[54] Uragoda CG, Kottegoda SR. Adverse reactions to isoniazid on ingestion of fish with a high histamine content. Tubercle 1977;58(2):83–9.

[55] Uragoda CG, Lodha SC. Histamine intoxication in a tuberculous patient after ingestion of cheese. Tubercle 1979;60(1):59–61.

[56] Morinaga S, Kawasaki A, Hirata H, et al. Histamine poisoning after ingestion of spoiled raw tuna in a patient taking isoniazid. Intern Med 1997;36(3):198–200.

[57] Lerke PA, Werner SB, Taylor SL, et al. Scombroid poisoning. Report of an outbreak. West J Med 1978;129(5):381–6.

[58] Bedry R, Gabinski C, Paty M-C. Diagnosis of scombroid poisoning by measurement of plasma histamine. N Engl J Med 2000;342(7):520–1.

[59] Morrow JD, Margolies GR, Rowland J, et al. Evidence that histamine is the causative toxin of scombroid-fish poisoning. N Engl J Med 1991;324(11):716–20.

[60] Kim R. Flushing syndrome due to mahimahi (scombroid fish) poisoning. Arch Dermatol 1979;115(8):963–5.

[61] Smart DR. Scombroid poisoning. A report of seven cases involving the Western Australian salmon, *Arripis truttaceus*. Med J Aust 1992;157(11–12):748–51.

[62] Eckstein M, Serna M, DelaCruz P, et al. Out-of-hospital and emergency department management of epidemic scombroid poisoning. Acad Emerg Med 1999;6(9):916–20.

[63] Blakesley ML. Scombroid poisoning: prompt resolution of symptoms with cimetidine. Ann Emerg Med 1983;12(2):104–6.

[64] Ahasan HA, Mamun AA, Karim SR, et al. Paralytic complications of puffer fish (tetrodotoxin) poisoning. Singapore Med J 2004;45(2):73–4.

[65] Isbister GK, Son J, Wang F, et al. Puffer fish poisoning: a potentially life-threatening condition. Med J Aust 2002;177(11–12):650–3.

[66] Yin HL, Lin HS, Huang CC, et al. Tetrodotoxication with nassauris glans: a possibility of tetrodotoxin spreading in marine products near Pratas Island. Am J Trop Med Hyg 2005;73(5):985–90.

[67] Doherty MJ. Captain Cook on poison fish. Neurology 2005;65(11):1788–91.

[68] Sierra-Beltran AP, Cruz A, Nunez E, et al. An overview of the marine food poisoning in Mexico. Toxicon 1998;36(11):1493–502.

[69] How CK, Chern CH, Huang YC, et al. Tetrodotoxin poisoning. Am J Emerg Med 2003;21(1):51–4.

[70] Tetrodotoxin poisoning associated with eating puffer fish transported from Japan–California, 1996. MMWR Morb Mortal Wkly Rep 1996;45(19):389–91.

[71] Waxman SG, Cummins TR, Dib-Hajj S, et al. Sodium channels, excitability of primary sensory neurons, and the molecular basis of pain. Muscle Nerve 1999;22(9):1177–87.

[72] Kanchanapongkul J. Puffer fish poisoning: clinical features and management experience in 25 cases. J Med Assoc Thai 2001;84(3):385–9.

[73] Lan MY, Lai SL, Chen SS, et al. Tetrodotoxin intoxication in a uraemic patient. J Neurol Neurosurg Psychiatr 1999;67(1):127–8.

[74] Sobel J, Tucker N, Sulka A, et al. Foodborne botulism in the United States, 1990–2000. Emerg Infect Dis 2004;10(9):1606–11.

[75] Ravichandran E, Gong Y, Saleem FHA, et al. An initial assessment of the systemic pharmacokinetics of botulinum toxin. J Pharmacol Exp Ther 2006;318(3):1343–51.

[76] Sobel J. Botulism. Clin Infect Dis 2005;41(8):1167–73.

[77] Villar RG, Elliott SP, Davenport KM. Botulism: the many faces of botulinum toxin and its potential for bioterrorism. Infect Dis Clin N Am 2006;20(2):313–27.

[78] Fox CK, Keet CA, Strober JB. Recent advances in infant botulism. Pediatr Neurol 2005;32(3):149–54.

[79] Thompson JA, Filloux FM, Van Orman CB, et al. Infant botulism in the age of botulism immune globulin. Neurology 2005;64(12):2029–32.

[80] Scarfone RJ, Puchalski AL. Why so sleepy? Pediatr Ann 2001;30(10):614–8.

[81] Maria GT, Michael PG. Association between honey consumption and infant botulism. Pharmacotherapy 2002;22(11):1479–83.

[82] Armada M, Love S, Barrett E, et al. Foodborne botulism in a six-month-old infant caused by home-canned baby food. Ann Emerg Med 2003;42(2):226–9.

[83] Passaro DJ, Werner SB, McGee J, et al. Wound botulism associated with black tar heroin among injecting drug users. JAMA 1998;279(11):859–63.

[84] Brett MM, Hallas G, Mpamugo O. Wound botulism in the UK and Ireland. J Med Microbiol 2004;53(6):555–61.

[85] Werner SB, Passaro D, McGee J, et al. Wound botulism in California, 1951–1998: recent epidemic in heroin injectors. Clin Infect Dis 2000;31(4):1018–24.

[86] Lindstrom M, Korkeala H. Laboratory diagnostics of botulism. Clin Microbiol Rev 2006; 19(2):298–314.

[87] Robinson RF, Nahata MC. Management of botulism. Ann Pharmacother 2003;37(1):127–31.

[88] Horowitz BZ. Botulinum toxin. Crit Care Clin 2005;21(4):825–39.

[89] Cherington M. Botulism: update and review. Semin Neurol 2004;24(2):155–63.

[90] Arnon SS, Schechter R, Inglesby TV, et al. Botulinum toxin as a biological weapon: medical and public health management. JAMA 2001;285(8):1059–70.

[91] Wainwright RB, Heyward WL, Middaugh JP, et al. Food-borne botulism in Alaska, 1947-1985: epidemiology and clinical findings. J Infect Dis 1988;157(6):1158–62.

[92] Varma JK, Katsitadze G, Moiscrafishvili M, et al. Signs and symptoms predictive of death in patients with foodborne botulism–Republic of Georgia, 1980-2002 [see comment]. Clin Infect Dis 2004;39(3):357–62.

[93] Black RE, Gunn RA. Hypersensitivity reactions associated with botulinal antitoxin. Am J Med 1980;69(4):567–70.

[94] Ketcham EM, Gomez HF. Infant botulism: a diagnostic and management challenge. Air Med J 2003;22(5):6–11.

[95] Arnon SS, Schechter R, Maslanka SE, et al. Human botulism immune globulin for the treatment of infant botulism. N Engl J Med 2006;354(5):462–71.

[96] Scinska-Bienkowska A, Wrobel E, Turzynska D, et al. Glutamate concentration in whole saliva and taste responses to monosodium glutamate in humans. Nutr Neurosci 2006; 9(1–2):25–31.

[97] Kenney RA. The Chinese restaurant syndrome: an anecdote revisited. Food Chem Toxicol 1986;24(4):351–4.

[98] Freeman M. Reconsidering the effects of monosodium glutamate: a literature review. J Am Acad Nurse Pract 2006;18(10):482–6.

[99] Beyreuther K, Biesalski HK, Fernstrom JD, et al. Consensus meeting: monosodium glutamate—an update. Eur J Clin Nutr 2007;61(3):304–13.

[100] Bellisle F. Glutamate and the UMAMI taste: sensory, metabolic, nutritional and behavioural considerations. A review of the literature published in the last 10 years. Neurosci Biobehav Rev 1999;23(3):423–38.

[101] Woessner KM, Simon RA, Stevenson DD. Monosodium glutamate sensitivity in asthma. J Allergy Clin Immunol 1999;104(2):305–10.

[102] Merritt JE, Williams PB. Vasospasm contributes to monosodium glutamate-induced headache. Headache 1990;30(9):575–80.

[103] Tarasoff L. Another case of glutamania? Food Chem Toxicol 1995;33(1):72–8.

[104] Geha RS, Beiser A, Ren C, et al. Review of alleged reaction to monosodium glutamate and outcome of a multicenter double-blind placebo-controlled study. J Nutr 2000;130(4S Suppl):1058S–62S.

[105] Tarasoff L, Kelly MF. Monosodium: a double-blind study and review. Food Chem Toxicol 1993;31(12):1019–35.

[106] Rosenblum I, Bradley JD, Coulston F. Single and double blind studies with oral monosodium glutamate in man. Toxicol Appl Pharmacol 1971;18(2):367–73.

[107] Yang WH, Drouin MA, Herbert M, et al. The monosodium glutamate symptom complex: assessment in a double-blind, placebo-controlled, randomized study. J Allergy Clin Immunol 1997;99(6 Part 1):757–62.

[108] Stevenson DD. Monosodium glutamate and asthma. J Nutr 2000;130(4S Suppl): 1067S–73S.

[109] Sanz P, Reig R. Clinical and pathological findings in fatal plant oxalosis. A review. Am J Forensic Med Pathol 1992;13(4):342–5.

[110] Watson J, Jones R, Siston A, et al. Outbreak of food-borne illness associated with plant material containing raphides. Clin Toxicol 2005;43(1):17–21.

[111] James LF. Oxalate toxicosis. Clin Toxicol 1972;5(2):231–43.

[112] Gardner DG. Injury to the oral mucous membranes caused by the common houseplant, dieffenbachia: a review. Oral Surg Oral Med Oral Pathol 1994;78(5):631–3.

[113] Pedaci L, Krenzelok EP, Jacobsen TD, et al. Dieffenbachia species exposures: an evidence-based assessment of symptom presentation. Vet Hum Toxicol 1999;41(5):335–8.

[114] Cumpston KL, Vogel SN, Leikin JB, et al. Acute airway compromise after brief exposure to a Dieffenbachia plant. J Emerg Med 2003;25(4):391–7.

[115] Snajdauf J, Mixa V, Rygl M, et al. Aortoesophageal fistula—an unusual complication of esophagitis caused by Dieffenbachia ingestion. J Pediatr Surg 2005;40(6):e29–31.

[116] Loretti AP, da Silva Ilha MR, Ribeiro RES. Accidental fatal poisoning of a dog by *Dieffenbachia picta* (dumb cane). Vet Hum Toxicol 2003;45(5):233–9.

[117] Dip EC, Pereira NA, Fernandes PD. Ability of eugenol to reduce tongue edema induced by *Dieffenbachia picta* Schott in mice. Toxicon 2004;43(6):729–35.

[118] Farre M, Xirgu J, Salgado A, et al. Fatal oxalic acid poisoning from sorrel soup [see comment]. Lancet 1989;2(8678–79):1524.

[119] Chen CL, Fang HC, Chou KJ, et al. Acute oxalate nephropathy after ingestion of star fruit. Am J Kidney Dis 2001;37(2):418–22.

[120] Fang HC, Chen CL, Wang JS, et al. Acute oxalate nephropathy induced by star fruit in rats. Am J Kidney Dis 2001;38(4):876–80.

[121] Lewandowski S, Rodgers AL. Idiopathic calcium oxalate urolithiasis: risk factors and conservative treatment. Clin Chim Acta 2004;345(1–2):17–34.

[122] Heye N, Zimmer C, Terstegge K, et al. Oxalate-induced encephalitis after infusions of sugar surrogates. Intensive Care Med 1991;17(7):432–4.

[123] Tsai M-H, Chang W-N, Lui C-C, et al. Status epilepticus induced by star fruit intoxication in patients with chronic renal disease. Seizure 2005;14(7):521–5.

[124] Tse KC, Yip PS, Lam MF, et al. Star fruit intoxication in uraemic patients: case series and review of the literature. Intern Med J 2003;33(7):314–6.

[125] Yu-Chin Lily W, Ber-Ming L, Robert BS, et al. Management of star fruit—induced neurotoxicity and seizures in a patient with chronic renal failure. Pharmacotherapy 2006;26(1): 143–6.

[126] Gunduz A, Turedi S, Uzun H, et al. Mad honey poisoning. Am J Emerg Med 2006;24(5): 595–8.

[127] Onat FY, Yegen BC, Lawrence R, et al. Mad honey poisoning in man and rat. Rev Environ Health 1991;9(1):3–9.

[128] Yilmaz O, Eser M, Sahiner A, et al. Hypotension, bradycardia and syncope caused by honey poisoning. Resuscitation 2006;68(3):405–8.

[129] Maejima H, Kinoshita E, Seyama I, et al. Distinct sites regulating grayanotoxin binding and unbinding to D4S6 of Nav1.4 sodium channel as revealed by improved estimation of toxin sensitivity. J Biol Chem 2003;278(11):9464–71.

[130] Yuki T, Yamaoka K, Yakehiro M, et al. State-dependent action of grayanotoxin I on Na+ channels in frog ventricular myocytes. J Physiol 2001;534(3):777–90.

[131] Ozhan H, Akdemir R, Yazici M, et al. Cardiac emergencies caused by honey ingestion: a single centre experience. Emerg Med J 2004;21(6):742–4.

[132] Biberoglu K, Biberoglu S, Komsuoglu B. Transient Wolff-Parkinson-White syndrome during honey intoxication. Isr J Med Sci 1988;24(4–5):253–4.

[133] Ergun K, Tufekcioglu O, Aras D, et al. A rare cause of atrioventricular block: mad honey intoxication. Int J Cardiol 2005;99(2):347–8.

ELSEVIER
SAUNDERS

EMERGENCY
MEDICINE
CLINICS OF
NORTH AMERICA

Emerg Med Clin N Am 25 (2007) 375–433

Plant Poisoning

Blake Froberg, MD, Danyal Ibrahim, MD, R. Brent Furbee, MD, FACMT*

*Indiana Poison Center, Methodist Hospital, Clarian Health Partners,
I-65 at 21st Street, Indiana University School of Medicine,
Indianapolis, IN 46206-1367, USA*

Each year over 100,000 exposures to toxic plants are reported to poison centers around the country [1]. Most of these exposures are of minimal toxicity largely because of the fact that they involve pediatric ingestions, which are of low quantity. The more serious poisonings usually involve adults who have mistaken a plant as edible or have deliberately ingested the raw plant or tea made from the plant to derive perceived medicinal or toxic properties. Plants have been used since the times of antiquity for various reasons, such as hallucinogens, abortifacients, and antiarthritics. The plants within this manuscript have been chosen because they have been documented to cause fatalities or account for emergency medicine visits.

There is a poor correlation between taxonomy and toxicity. Members of the same family may have different toxic effects or sometimes, no toxicity at all. Not infrequently, a single plant may contain several different toxins. In this discussion, plants are grouped by their toxins rather than on the basis of their taxonomy.

Plant identification is often a daunting task. If a specimen is available, local nurseries may be of help in identification. Poison centers are usually a good starting point in the identification of plants and management of their ingestion. Most centers have botanical consultants and other resources that are of assistance in the event of plant exposures. As discussed in this article, there are few antidotes for plant exposures. With the exception of the plants containing the cardiac glycosides and those that have cholinergic and anticholinergic presentations, treatment is usually supportive.

* Corresponding author.
E-mail address: bfurbee@clarian.org (R.B. Furbee).

0733-8627/07/$ - see front matter © 2007 Elsevier Inc. All rights reserved.
doi:10.1016/j.emc.2007.02.013

Toxalbumins (ricin, abrin)

Ricinus communis (castor bean) has had commercial importance as the source of castor oil, which has been used as a laxative and machine lubricant. Castor beans are generally the size of a peanut, mottled gray to brown in color. They, like the seeds of *Abrus precatorium*, are often used to make necklaces and bracelets. In several countries, castor beans are used medicinally as cathartics, emetics, and for the treatment of leprosy and syphilis. Although the castor bean was known to be poisonous for centuries, its major toxic component, ricin, was not isolated until 1905 [2]. *Ricinus*, *Abrus*, and *Jatropha* spp differ somewhat in appearance and taxonomy but contain toxins that are structurally and functionally similar. Ricin and abrin are generally considered to be the most potent (by weight) of plant toxins, though the plants containing them no longer account for major morbidity or mortality [3]. This is probably because most exposures are oral and, therefore, of much lower toxicity than the exceedingly rare parenteral exposure. Ricin has recently been on the news because of its association with terrorist activity, including in London (2001), South Carolina (2003), and Washington (2004).

Plants

Plants that contain toxalbumins are: *R communis* (castor bean, castor oil plant, palma cristi) (Fig. 1), *Abrus precatorius* (jequirty, roseary pea, prayer bean, crab's eye, mieniemienie, indian bead, Seminole bead, weather plant) (Fig. 2), and *Jatropha curcas* (coral plants, physic nuts, barbados nuts).

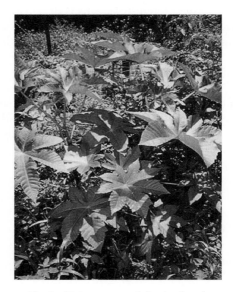

Fig. 1. *Ricinus communis* (castor bean).

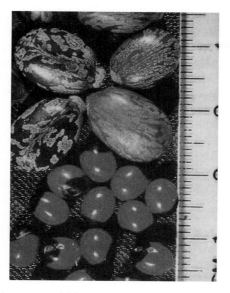

Fig. 2. *Ricinus communis/abrus precartonius* (castor bean/jequirty pea).

Also, suspected plants are: *Hura crepitans, Robinia pseudoacacia, Momordica charantia*, and some species of *Sophora* [4].

Location

R communis is found throughout the southern United States but may be grown as an ornamental in the northern states. *Jatropha* and *Abrus* species have a more limited tropical range. Both may be found in Florida.

Toxic parts

All parts of the plant are toxic, especially the seeds. There is general agreement that if these seeds are left with the husk intact (unchewed), toxicity will not occur as they pass through the gastrointestinal tract.

Description

R communis (see Fig. 1) grows to 5 to 15 feet at maturity and has a palmate leaf. Seeds grow in clusters near the top of the plant and are covered with a spiney husk (see Fig. 2). *Jatropha* spp has a similar appearance. *Abrus precatorius* grows as a vine with compound leaves and tendrils. The seeds measure 0.3 cm by 0.8 cm and are scarlet with a black "eye" (see Fig. 2).

Mechanism of toxicity

Toxalbumins are proteins that bind to carbohydrates. Olsnes and colleagues [5] identified the molecular structure of both ricin and abrin in

1974. Both compounds consist of two peptide chains that are cross-linked by two disulfide bonds. The B chain, or "haptomer," binds to galactose containing receptors on the cell surface. The A chain, or "effectomer," then penetrates the cell and is transported into the cytoplasm to the ribosomes where it interrupts protein synthesis (Fig. 3). Wheat germ and barley have a similar "ribosome-inactivating protein," but due to their lack of a cell-penetrating B chain, they are not cytotoxic [6]. The cytotoxic properties of these compounds are being explored as a means of suppressing tumor cell growth [7] and in research to determine binding sites within nuclei [6]. Ricin, when parenterally administered to animals, has been shown to increase cardiac output, cause hemorrhage and necrosis of the heart, induce vasospasm of coronary arteries [8], and depress systolic and diastolic cardiac function [9]. Because these effects were demonstrated with purified toxin, other constituents of the seeds may contribute to the clinical picture. *R communis* seeds also contain a hemaglutinin, which does not appear to cause hemolysis when administered by the oral route [5].

Clinical presentation (oral)

The toxicity of castor bean is largely dependent upon the route of administration. By far the most common exposure is by way of the oral route. The most consistent presentation is that of gastrointestinal upset. In a review of 103 case reports from 1900 to 1985, Challoner and McCarron [10] found the signs and symptoms listed in Table 1.

Clinical presentation (parenteral)

Ricin, when administered by the parenteral route, is considerably more toxic as exemplified in animal studies. A case report by Knight [11] in 1979

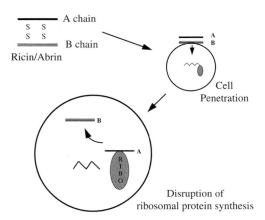

Fig. 3. The B chain of ricin attaches to the cell wall. Once inside, the A chain attaches to the ribosome and disrupts protein synthesis.

Table 1
Relative frequency of the signs and symptoms associated with castor bean poisoning

Symptoms/signs	Patients reporting (%)
Vomiting	84%
Diarrhea	83%
Dehydration	35%
Shock	27%
Abdominal pain	13%
Abnormal kidney function tests	9%
Leg cramps	6%
Abnormal liver function tests	5%
Acrocyanosis	5%
Hematuria	5%
Miosis	3%
Gastrointestinal bleeding	3%
Hemolysis	3%

seemed to confirm the parenteral toxicity of this compound. The case report is based upon a coroner's inquest, and premortem details are incomplete. A 49-year-old Bulgarian broadcaster was brought to a London hospital after being jabbed in the posterior thigh with an umbrella while standing on a street corner. His initial complaint was fever and malaise. A circular area of inflammation with a central punctate lesion of 2 mm diameter was noted on his posterior thigh. The following day, his white blood cell count was 33,000 per cm^3, and a tentative diagnosis of sepsis was made. He died on the third day. Postmortem examination revealed a platinum-iridium sphere beneath the puncture wound. It had been cross-drilled allowing for a volume of 0.28 cm^3. Based upon that information and the clinical course of an experimental animal injected with ricin, the diagnosis of ricin poisoning was made by a Government Chemical Defense official at Porter Down. No confirmation of the toxin could be made. In later years, however, circumstantial evidence seemed to support the claim. A more recent case of parenteral poisoning was reported by Fine and colleagues [12], which bears resemblance to the case reported by Knight. A 36-year-old chemist injected approximately 2 mg/kg ricin intramuscularly. The patient initially suffered from headache and rigors. His heart rate was 120, and blood pressure was 140/80 on admission. Two 3-cm erythematous patches marked the injection sites. His white blood cell count, amylase, aspartate aminotransferase, and alanine aminotransferase were mildly elevated. He remained intermittently febrile for 8 days and was released in good health after 10 days. Thus, parenteral injection of ricin in humans is not well documented, although its toxicity is thought to be severe. The clinical presentation of an oral exposure should not be confused with that of the potentially fatal parenteral exposure.

A precatorius (jequirty pea) seems to cause gastrointestinal irritation. The mechanism of action of abrin is similar to that of ricin. Clinical reports indicate that, like castor bean, gastrointestinal irritation is the most frequent presentation associated with ingestion [13]. Reports of fatalities are from literature dating from the 1950s or earlier.

Jatropa seed has been reported to cause vomiting (64%), abdominal pain (52%), muscle twitching, nausea, salivation, and sweating. In the Phillipines, where *Jatropa* spp exposures are common, 98% of patients in one study were discharged in 24 to 48 hours with only supportive care [14]. *Jatropha* spp are grown as ornamental plants in the southern United States.

Allergic reactions

Several anaphylactic reactions to castor bean have been reported [15,16] in castor oil workers and in nonindustrial settings. Because several of these cases were reported in the distant past, they may serve to confuse the true clinical picture of castor bean ingestion.

Laboratory studies

There are currently no clinically useful determinations for ricin or abrin. Electrolyte status, complete blood cell count, liver function [17], and creatine phosphokinase should be monitored.

Management of oral exposures

Since the early 1900s, warnings have persisted about the potential lethality of castor beans [18]. Medical literature has perpetuated the idea that, if chewed, a single bean may kill a child, and perhaps as few as 8 beans could prove fatal to an adult. Rauber and Heard [19,20] reviewed medical literature from circa 1900 to 1984. Of 751 exposures to castor bean, there were 14 deaths for an overall mortality rate of 1.8%. Challoner and McCarron [10] reviewed a portion of those data and some more recent cases and established an overall mortality of 3.4% with only 1 death occurring since 1950. A review of the reported deaths indicates that the treatment, which in the early 1900s included oubain, cocaine, camphor, 20% fructose, digitalis, and strychnine, might have contributed to the mortality. Other fatalities seem to have been due to inadequate or no rehydration [16,20]. Based upon available information, the management of asymptomatic nonsuicidal patients who have consumed only a few seeds (*R communis, A precatorius, Jatropha* spp) should consist of oral administration of activated charcoal and close home monitoring. Hospital admission is indicated for patients who have developed symptoms or for asymptomatic patients who cannot be closely watched at home. Symptomatic patients should be given activated charcoal. The dose of activated charcoal is 50 to 100 g in 8 ounces of tap water for adults and 1 gm/kg or 25 to 50 g in 4 ounces of water for children. Aggressive fluid resuscitation and other supportive care is the mainstay of management of the more serious exposures. Cathartics are not indicated, and extracorporeal elimination is of no benefit.

Management of parenteral exposures

At present, there are insufficient data to make specific recommendations beyond supportive care. No antidote exists for oral or parenteral exposures. A vaccine to ricin has recently been developed and is currently undergoing clinical studies because of the concern regarding use by terrorists.

Cicutoxin

The first reports of toxic effects from *Cicuta* spp occurred in 1697. Stockbridge [21] reported the first case of poisoning in the United States in 1814. In a review of deaths reported to poison centers between 1986 and 1996, Krenzelok and colleagues [3] found reports of 19 deaths. Of these, *Cicuta* spp accounted for more than any other plant. Exposure to *Cicuta* and *Oenanthe* spp may be accidental as in most pediatric cases, but more commonly, the fatal cases involve misidentification of the plant as a foodstuff or as a hallucinogen.

Plants

Plants containing cicutoxin are: *Cicuta maculata* (water hemlock), *Cicuta douglasii* (western water hemlock), and *Oenanthe crocata* (hemlock water dropwort) (Figs. 4–6).

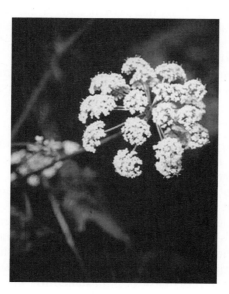

Fig. 4. *Circuta* spp flower (water hemlock).

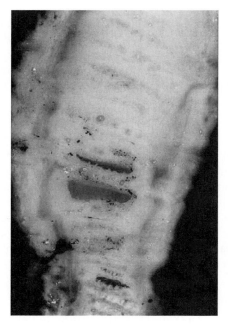

Fig. 5. *Cicuta* spp root (water hemlock).

Location

Water hemlock grows in the eastern half of the United States and Canada. *C douglasii* (western water hemlock) grows in the western United States. *O crocata* is considered to be a European plant, but is reported to have been transplanted into the Washington, DC area [22]. These plants are found in or immediately adjacent to water. They are most frequently encountered in lakes or streams, but may be found in marshy areas.

Description (Cicuta *spp)*

These plants are generally found growing out of the water or close enough for their roots to make contact with the water. Both varieties form a low-growing bush that may be 3 to 4 feet tall. Stems are hollow and have a carrot-like odor. Flowers, which occur during the summer months, are small and white in flat-topped clusters or "umbels." Leaves of the eastern variety are sharply toothed like the western water hemlock, but *C maculata* has a longer, thinner leaf. *C douglasii* produces a more ovate leaf. Both plants have thick whitish roots which, when sliced sagitally, possess transverse stripes. The stripes may form small chambers late in the growing season. The roots have been mistaken for wild carrots. They are 5 to 6 in long, white, and, when cut, have a strong carrot-like odor.

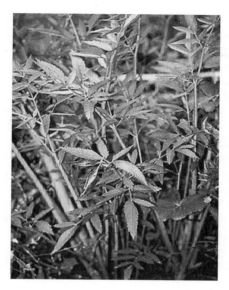

Fig. 6. *Cicuta* spp (water hemlock).

Although the roots are characterized as having transverse chambers, they are frequently solid. Roots of *Oenanthe* spp are also said to secrete a yellowish sap when cross-sectioned [23]. Water hemlock bears a striking resemblance to other "umbellifores," which are nontoxic. *Heracleum lanatum* (cow parsnip) and *Daucus carota* (Queen Anne's lace) may be distinguished by their location and physical differences in the stem. Mistaking a toxic member of the Apiaceae family for a nontoxic one has been a fatal error for several foragers over the years [24–27]. Almost yearly, one to two deaths are reported to poison centers in the United States due to the ingestion of these plants.

Toxic parts

All parts of the plants are toxic, especially the roots.

Mechanism of toxicity

Though nausea and vomiting are considered to be the most consistent findings, seizure activity followed by cardiac arrest is the common sequence in fatal exposures [28]. An exact mechanism for the proconvulsant activity of cicutoxin has not been determined. Starreveld and Hope [29] suggested that seizure activity might be due to cholinergic overstimulation of the reticular formation or basal ganglia. Nelson and colleagues [30] performed a series of experiments in mice to explore the efficacy of anticholinergic agents in the prevention of cicutoxin-induced seizures. They found that anticholinergic agents failed to protect the animals, whereas pretreatment with cholinergic agents did not appear to lower seizure threshold.

By 1979, a more appealing theory for cicutoxin's proconvulsant activity had arisen. Carlton and colleagues [31] suggested that cicutoxin (Fig. 7) is structurally similar to picrotoxin, an indirect antagonist at GABA$_A$ receptors. GABA receptors serve as ion channels to allow the passage of chloride ions into the neuron (Fig. 8). This hyperpolarizes the neuron moving it away from its threshold for firing. Many anticonvulsants, such as the benzodiazepines and barbiturates, act as indirect agonists at the GABA receptor. By preventing the action of GABA, picrotoxin hyperpolarizes the neuron, moving it closer to its threshold for firing. If cicutoxin acts on the GABA receptor at the picrotoxin site, seizure activity would be expected as it is with picrotoxin. This would also be consistent with Nelson's findings that seizures were better controlled in animals treated with diazepam or barbiturates than with other agents [30,32].

Clinical presentation

Case reports of *Cicuta* spp [24,28,29,33–35] and *Oenanthe* spp [23,36–39] ingestions are similar in presentation. Ingestion is followed by nausea, vomiting, and diaphoresis. Although these signs and symptoms have led some authors to speculate about increased cholinergic activity as the mechanism for seizure activity [29], the frequent reports of mydriasis [33–35] detract from this theory. The initial convulsion often occurs within the first hour. Repeated convulsions with intermittent lethargy ensue for the next several hours. Fatalities usually occur within 10 hours and are almost invariably associated with repeated seizure activity. *O crocata* poisoning has been estimated to be 70% fatal in one small series [38].

Rhabdomyolysis and renal failure have been reported [31]. Although some toxins may cause rhabdomyolysis directly, the presence of prolonged seizure activity that was reported in this patient may be the etiology.

Laboratory studies

Although clinically useful means of determining cicutoxin or oenanthotoxin are not available, methods of identification are described by King and colleagues [37] for the latter. These methods included ultraviolet absorption; thin-layer chromatography; high-pressure liquid chromatography; and mass spectrometry, which may be useful for later confirmation of exposure.

$$HOCH_2(CH_2)_2\text{-}(C \equiv C)_2\text{-}(CH = CH)_3\text{-}\overset{\displaystyle \overset{OH}{|}}{C}HCH_2CH_2CH_3$$

Cicutoxin

Fig. 7. Structure of cicutoxin.

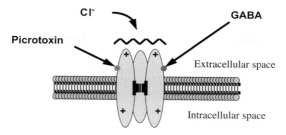

Fig. 8. When picrotoxin attaches to the GABA receptor, the chloride ionophore closes preventing hyperpolarization of the interior of the neuron.

Management

Asymptomatic patients should be given activated charcoal and observed for 4 hours postingestion. If no symptoms occur, they may be released. The dose of activated charcoal is 50 to 100 g in 8 ounces of tap water for adults and 1 gm/kg or 25 to 50 g in 4 ounces of water for children. Activated charcoal should not be given to a comatose patient until the patient's airway is protected.

Symptomatic patients frequently arrive after seizures have occurred. The patient's airway should be secured first. Diazepam or phenobarbital are most appropriate for seizure control and should be used aggressively. Phenytoin has no clear role in management of cicutoxin-induced seizures. Because of vomiting, and occasionally diarrhea, fluid replacement is often required. Creatine phosphokinase should be monitored because of the possibility of rhabdomyolysis. In addition to maintaining urine output, urine alkalinization may be of benefit in patients who have rhabdomyolysis [40]. Hemodialysis plus charcoal hemoperfusion has been performed in one case [41]; however clearance of cicutoxin was not measured, and the favorable outcome is consistent with many of the cases managed without extracoporeal elimination [34]. At this time, hemodialysis/hemoperfusion have not been shown to be beneficial. Seizure control and supportive care are the mainstay of therapy.

Cardiac glycosides

The medicinal properties of the cardiac glycosides were known to the ancient Egyptians as well as the Romans who used it as an emetic, heart tonic, and diuretic [42]. In 1785, William Withering published *An Account of the Foxglove and Some of Its Medical Uses: With Practical Remarks on Dropsy and Other Diseases* thus popularizing its use. In 1890, Sir Thomas Fraser introduced *Strophanthus* and its digitalis-like effects. Worldwide, these plants have been used as abortifacients, and in the treatment of leprosy, venereal disease, malaria, and as a suicide agent [43]. More than 200 naturally occurring cardiac glycosides have been identified to date. *Digitalis* spp ingestion is seldom reported. *Convallaria majalis* (lily of the valley) exposures are associated with minimal morbidity and, in a recent review of 10 years of data from regional poison centers, have had no associated mortality [41]. Of the many plants containing cardiac glycosides, *Nerium oleander* is responsible for the greatest number of toxic exposures each year [44]. For that reason, this discussion is focused on that plant.

Plants

Plants containing cardiac glycosides are: *Digitalis purpurea*, *D lanata* (foxglove) (Fig. 9); *N oleander* (oleander) (Fig. 10); *Strophanthus gratus* (oubain); *Thevetia peruviana* spp (yellow oleander) (Fig. 11); *Convallaria majalis* (lily of the valley) (Fig. 12); and *Urginea maritima*, *U. indica* (squill). Other plants thought to contain cardiac glycosides: *Asclepias* (milkweed); *Calotropis* (crown flower) [45]; *Euonymus europaeus* (spindle tree); *Cheiranthus*, *Erysimum* (wall flower); and *Hellaborus niger* (henbane).

Location

Oleander is native to the Mediterranean and Asia, but thrives in both tropical and subtropical areas around the world. In the United States, where it is planted as an ornamental, it can be found from the Southeast to the Southwest. It may be grown in northern states, but does not survive freezing

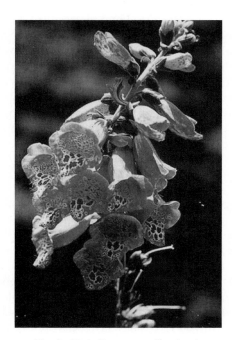

Fig. 9. *Digitalis purpurea* (foxglove).

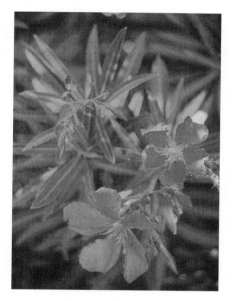

Fig. 10. *Nerium oleander* (oleander).

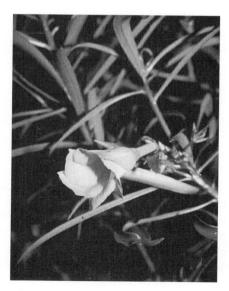

Fig. 11. *Thevia peruviana* (yellow oleander).

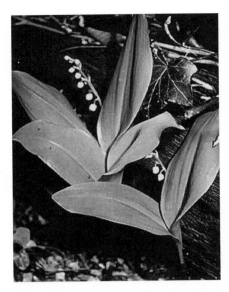

Fig. 12. *Convalleria majalis* (lily of the valley).

conditions. *Digitalis* spp and *Convallaria majalis* may be found throughout North America.

Description

N *oleander* is a shrub that may grow to 30 feet in some locations. The leaves are usually 6 in long and 1 in wide. The leaves are leathery with a smooth margin and overall lanceolate shape. Flowers of *N oleander* are red, white, or pink. Leaves of *Thevetia peruviana* are smaller but similar in shape, and they are yellow/orange.

Toxic parts

All parts of the plant are toxic. Seeds are said to contain more glycoside than other parts of the plant.

Mechanism of toxicity

Oleandrin (*N. oleander*) and thevetin (*T peruviana*) are structurally similar to digitoxin (Fig. 13). Because of this and the similarity of clinical presentation, the three are considered to act in similar fashion. The toxin attaches to the α subunit of the Na^+/K^+-ATPase pump to inhibit its action. Because this pump exchanges intracellular sodium ions for extracellular potassium ions, inhibition leads to an overall increase in intracellular sodium ions. Rises in intracellular sodium concentration result in secondary rises in intracellular calcium levels, explaining the positive inotropic effect of

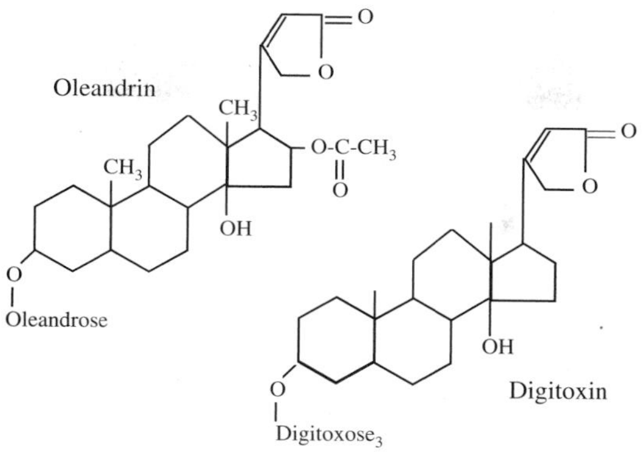

Fig. 13. Structures of oleandrin and digitoxin.

cardiac glycosides. In toxic amounts, the rises in intracellular sodium and calcium depolarize the cell after repolarization to cause late afterdepolarizations and increased automaticity typical of cardiac glycoside poisoning. Depolarization of baroreceptors innervated by the ninth cranial nerve triggers afferent reflexes, which increase vagal tone and produce bradycardia and heart blocks [46]. Severe poisoning results in hyperkalemia as the ability to pump potassium into the muscle is curtailed.

Clinical presentation

Gastrointestinal irritation is common with ingestion of *N. oleander or T peruviana*. The latter was studied as a potential antiarrhythmic agent in the 1930s, but was not marketed because it caused more gastrointestinal irritation than digitalis [47]. Saravanapavananthan and colleagues [48] reviewed 170 cases of *T peruviana* ingestion and found that vomiting was the most common presenting complaint (68.2%). Other symptoms are shown in Table 2.

Electrocardiographic effects have occurred in up to 61.8% of patients in one study (Table 3) [48].

PR prolongation, QT shortening, P- or T-wave flattening may occur [49]. Hyperkalemia occurs in more serious poisonings [49–51]. Central nervous system (CNS) depression may occur as a direct effect of the toxin [51],

Table 2
Relative frequency of signs and symptoms associated with oleander poisoning

Symptom	%
Dizziness	35.9
Diarrhea	38.0
Abdominal pain	5.9
Pain/numbness in tongue, throat, lips	4.1
No symptoms	12.9

Table 3
Relative frequency of dysrhythmias associated with oleander poisoning

Electrocardiographic change	%
AV block	52.4
Bradycardia	49.5
T-wave changes	35.2
ST depression	23.8
Ventricular ectopy	6.6
Atrial ectopy	2.8

but is frequently associated with bradycardia and hypotension. Death has been reported [48,49].

Laboratory studies

Osterloh and colleagues [50] described cross-reactivity of oleander glycosides on radioimmunoassay for digoxin. The test may serve as confirmation of the presence of cardiac glycosides; however, clinical symptoms are more indicative of toxicity. Postmortem serum concentrations are known to increase and do not predict the premortem levels [49].

Management

In general, management of cardiac glycoside toxicity from plants is the same as for digitalis toxicity. Airway control and other basic life support measures are the first concern. Gastric decontamination with activated charcoal should follow those measures. The dose of activated charcoal is 50 to 100 g in 8 ounces of tap water for adults and 1 gm/kg or 25 to 50 g in 4 ounces of water for children. Hyperkalemia may be treated with such agents as insulin and dextrose infusions, nebulized albuterol, and/or sodium bicarbonate infusion. Ventricular tachyarrhythmias may be managed with lidocaine, and bradyrythmias may respond to atropine or ventricular pacing.

Large doses of Fab-antidigoxin antibodies correct both rhythm and hyperkalemia in dogs poisoned by oleander [52]. Shumaik and colleagues [53] reported the use of digoxin-specific Fab fragments in the treatment of a 37-year-old man who had ingested *N oleander* leaves. Other reports of their use have supported those findings [51,54]. Indications for Fab fragments are shown in Box 1.

Grayanotoxins

Rhododendrons and azaleas were introduced into Europe from Asia in the mid-1700's to early 1800's. Both are parts of the 500 to 1000 natural species with numerous hybrids. Exact species identification can be difficult. The toxic components of this genus vary, and their presence in a given plant is difficult to predict. Although ingestion of leaves, flowers, nectar, or the use

---

Box 1. Indications for Fab fragments

1. Hyperkalemia (K+>5.5 mEq/L)
2. Refractory ventricular dysrhythmias
3. Hemodynamically significant bradydysrhythmia unresponsive to atropine
4. Severely symptomatic elderly patients should be treated aggressively with Fab fragments

---

of the leaves in the production of tea will produce toxicity, most poisonings result from consuming honey made from nectar of these plants. Honey poisonings are less common today, because honey from several different sources is combined before marketing. The earliest description of poisoning by these plants appears in the Anabasis, a description of the unsuccessful military expedition of Cyrus the Younger to overthrow Artaxerxes II (401–400 BC). The following is an account of the incident that took place in what is now northeastern Turkey on the coast of the Black Sea:

> The number of bee hives was extraordinary, and all of the soldiers that ate of the honey combs lost their senses, vomited, and were affected with purging, and none of them was able to stand upright; such as had eaten only a little were like men greatly intoxicated, and such as had eaten much were like mad men and some like persons at the point of death. They lay upon the ground, in consequence, in great numbers, as if there had been a defeat; and there was general dejection. The next day, no one of them was found dead; and they recovered their senses about the same hour they had lost them on the preceding day.

Several other recent accounts of the toxicity of "mad honey" are available [55].

Plants

Plants containing grayanotoxins are: *Rhododendron* spp (rhododendrons, azaleas), *Kalmia angustifolia (sheep laurel)*, *Kalmia latifolia* (mountain laurel), and *Pieris* spp (Andromeda). Grayanotoxin I may also be found in honey made from the nectar of these plants (Fig. 14).

Location

Native to the temperate parts of the world, they are grown widely as ornamentals. *R occidentale*, *R macrophyllum*, and *R albiflorum* are of special interest on the West coast in the production of honey. Reports of contaminated honey have also occurred in the East where rhododendrons as well as *Kalmia latifolia* (mountain laurel) and *K angustifolia* (sheep laurel) may serve as a source of grayanotoxin.

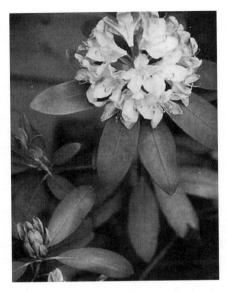

Fig. 14. *Rhododendron* spp (rhododendron).

Description

Leaves are evergreen, oblong, leathery, and have a smooth margin. They appear in whorls about the branch. Because of the many species, the leaf size is variable but generally ranges from 1 to 5 in. The flowers are white to pink (rhododendrons), and white, pink, magenta, crimson, or orange (azaleas).

Toxic parts

The entire plant is toxic.

Mechanism of toxicity

In 1955, it was discovered that the members of the Ericaceae family contained structurally similar compounds that were responsible for their toxicity. These compounds, which were formerly known as andromedotoxin, acetylandromedol, and rhodotoxin, are now termed *Grayanotoxin I* (Fig. 15) [56]. Grayanotoxin II and III are toxic derivatives of Grayanotoxin I. Animal studies initially indicated that these toxins were capable of producing respiratory depression, bradycardia, hypotension, and seizure activity [57]. Subsequent studies in squid axons have shown that Grayanotoxin I acts by attaching to the sodium channels of cell membranes and changing both open and closed channels to a modified open state. This increases sodium conductance dramatically and leads to cellular depolarization [58,59]. It seems that a single molecule of grayanotoxin is sufficient to activate a sodium channel [60]. This effect is thought to explain, in part, the CNS and cardiac

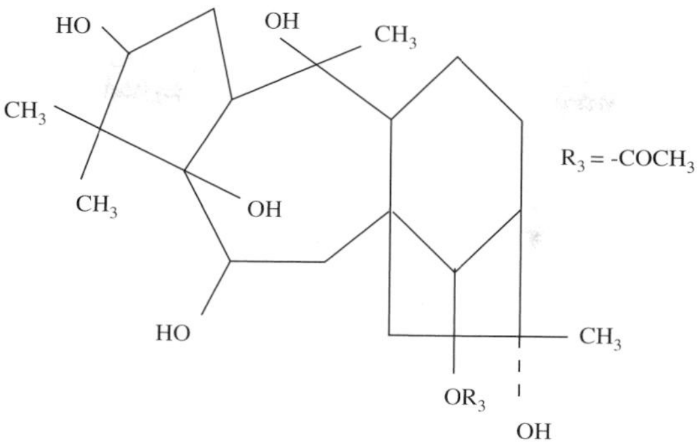

Grayanotoxin I

Fig. 15. Structure of grayanotoxin I.

manifestations of grayanotoxin poisoning. Masutani and colleagues [61] noted in their study of grayanotoxin effects on frog skeletal muscle, that grayanotoxin seems to contain four hydroxyl groups essential for its biologic activity. These are also present in veratridine (false and white hellebore), batrachotoxin (poison dart frog), and aconitine (monkshood).

The rises in intracellular sodium concentrations in the heart, baroreceptor cells, and brain cells mimic the effects of cardiac glycosides to produce increased automaticity, enhanced vagal tone (heart blocks, bradyrhythmias, and so forth), and CNS changes. Because $Na+/K+$-ATPase is not inhibited, hyperkalemia is notably absent.

Clinical presentation

Although most exposures are of little consequence [62], serious cardiotoxicity has been reported. Vomiting, loss of consciousness, and seizure were observed in a 27-year-old female who had ingested 75 mL of honey she had purchased in Turkey. She was hypotensive and bradycardic. Her only laboratory abnormality was a mild leukocytosis. Dysrhythmias included sinus node arrest, AV-escape beats, second-degree AV block, and intraventricular conduction block. The patient recovered after insertion of a cardiac pacemaker [63].

Laboratory studies

Thin-layer chromatography has been used to identify these compounds [64].

Management

Initial management should include the administration of activated charcoal if the ingestion has occurred within the last 2 hours. The dose of activated charcoal is 50 to 100 g in 8 ounces of tap water for adults and 1 gm/kg or 25 to 50 g in 4 ounces of water for children. Supportive care is usually sufficient for management; however, bradycardia may be treated with atropine or cardiac pacemaker. Although experimental agents, such as tetrodotoxin [65], have been used to reverse the effects of Grayanotoxin I, no clinically available antidote exists. Lidocaine or other sodium channel–blocking antiarrhythmics (group I) would seem appropriate for ventricular arrhythmias.

Veratrum alkaloids

Veratrum alkaloids are found in the various species of *Veratrum* and *Zigadenus* found throughout the United States and in parts of Canada. Historically these plants have been used as sources of medicines and insecticide. Their toxicity was noted in sneezing powders, made from pulverized roots of these plants. Inhalation or ingestion has resulted in several signs and symptoms including hypotension or bradydysrhythmia. Teratogenicity in farm animals, particularly sheep, has been widely reported.

Plants

Plants containing veratrum alkaloids are: *Veratrum album* (white hellebore) (Fig. 16), *V californicum* (corn lily, skunk cabbage), *V viride* (false hellebore), and *Zigadenus* spp (death camus) (Fig. 17) [66,67].

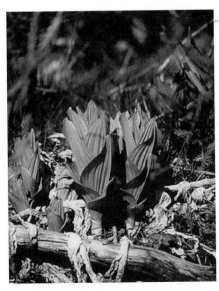

Fig. 16. *Veratrum* spp (false hellabore).

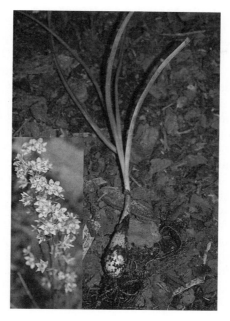

Fig. 17. *Zigadenus* spp (death camus).

Location

V viride is found in Canada and the eastern United States from New England to Georgia. Related species are found in western United States (*V californicum*), Alaska and Europe (*V album*), and Asia (*V japonicum*) [68]. False hellebore tends to grow in low-lying, swampy areas, whereas white hellebore is found in alpine meadows [56].

Description

Veratrum plants are tall (2–7 feet) perennial herbs. Broad, longitudinally plicated leaves are spirally arranged on a stout stem. White to yellowish green pedicellate flowers line the terminal 30 to 60 cm of the stem. These plants also contain a highly seeded fruit [56].

Zigadenus spp is a genus of the lily family. It is found throughout the United States and Canada. Flowers are pale yellow, pink, or white. The leaves are long, thin, and grass-like. The root is a bulb that is similar in appearance to and often mistaken for wild onion. *Zigadenus*, however, lacks an onion-like odor [66,69].

Toxic parts

The entire plant contains toxic veratrum alkaloids; however, the bulb and flowers most commonly cause poisoning. Fruit seeds and leaves rarely cause human toxicity.

Mechanism of toxicity

The veratrum alkaloids, which are chemically similar to steroids, include protoveratrines (Fig. 18), veratridine, and jervine [68]. These agents were introduced in the 1950s as antihypertensive agents; however, they were found to have a narrow therapeutic index and their use was discontinued [68,70]. Of these steroidal alkaloids, veratridine is the most potent [60]. The primary activity of these compounds is to attach to voltage-sensitive sodium channels in conductive cells and increase sodium permeability raising intracellular sodium concentration–like grayantoxins. Veratrine affects only a limited number of the sodium channels, but those affected reactivate 1000 times more slowly than the unaffected channels (ie, slow recovery). These alkaloids also appear to block inactivation of sodium channels and change the activation threshold of the sodium channels so that some remain open even at their resting potential [60]. Again, the rise in intracellular sodium concentrations leads to increased automaticity, enhanced vagal tone without hyperkalemia, and occasional neurotoxicity. High doses given to animals result in cardiac arrest [71].

Clinical presentation

Poisoning with veratrum alkaloids most typically occurs after accidental ingestion of the plant secondary to confusion with an edible species [68]. Toxicity also results from inhalation of sneezing powders prepared from pulverized white hellebore root [72]. Nausea and vomiting are most commonly seen after ingestion of the veratrum alkaloids. Clinically significant bradycardia and hypotension are also generally seen. Other reported toxic effects have included abdominal pain and distention, salivation, respiratory depression, yellow or green scotomata, paresthesias, increased muscle tone,

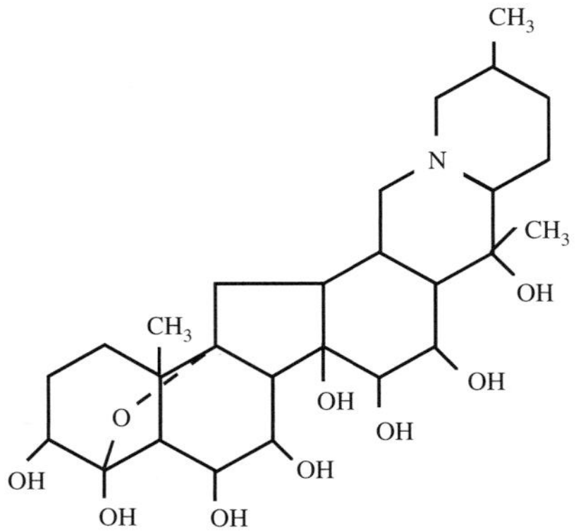

Protoverine

Fig. 18. Structure of protoverine.

rigors, and rarely, seizures [68,70,72–74]. Various electrocardiographic changes have also been reported with veratrum poisoning. Marinov and colleagues [75] reported a characteristic electrocardiographic pattern in 10 of 12 patients poisoned with *V album* that included PR and QT interval shortening, ST segment depression, T-wave morphology changes, and bundle branch block. Quatrehomme and colleagues [76] noted nausea and vomiting followed by hypotension. In contrast to Marinov's observations, Quatrehomme and colleagues reported QT prolongation.

Characteristic facial deformities (cyclopia, cleft lip and palate, microphthalmia) and limb defects (bowed fibulae, shortened tibia, excessive flexure of the knees) occur in offspring of pregnant sheep who ingest plants containing veratrum alkaloids. Jervine and other steroidal alkaloids found in the *Veratrum* spp are responsible for these birth defects [77].

Laboratory studies

There is no clinically useful laboratory study to confirm veratrum alkaloid exposure.

Management

Initial management should include the administration of activated charcoal if the ingestion has occurred within the last 2 hours. The dose of activated charcoal is 50 to 100 g in 8 ounces of tap water for adults and 1 gm/kg or 25 to 50 g in 4 ounces of water for children. Bradycardia usually responds to atropine administration. Hypotension may or may not respond to the atropine. Crystalloid fluids or vasopressors, such as dopamine, have been used to support blood pressure. Symptoms generally resolve in 24 to 48 hours or less, and deaths are rare [68].

Aconitine

Members of this genus grow throughout the world. Exposures are commonly associated with the overzealous consumption of herbal preparations containing aconitine. Though several fatal poisonings have been reported, aconitine is still readily available at many nutrition or herbal medicine stores.

Plants

Plants containing aconitine are: *Aconitum napellus* (monkshood) (Fig. 19), *A vulparia* (Wolfsbane). Several species are also used in herbal preparations including *A carmichaeli* ("chuanwu") and *A kusnezoffii* ("caowu") [78]. The latter two appear to account for more fatalities than ingestion of monk's hood. *Delphinium* spp (Larkspur) have similar toxicity [79].

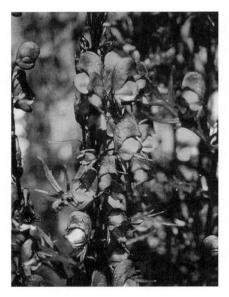

Fig. 19. *Aconitum napellus* (monkshood).

Location

A napellus and *A vulparia* grow in meadow areas of the mountainous areas from Arizona into Canada. *Aconitum* spp are cultivated as perennial ornamentals. *Delphinium* spp are found throughout the United States and Canada where they are also grown as ornamentals.

Description

Plants grow to 3 to 4 feet. The leaves are palmately divided into five lobes, which are divided into narrow segments. Flowers, which are dark blue to purple or purple and white, are composed of five petal-like sepals, one of which covers the top of the flower. The latter forms a hood-like structure over the flower, hence the name. These plants, though perennial, dry up and appear dead soon after the onset of summer heat.

Toxic parts

All parts are toxic (roots, flowers, leaves, stems) [80].

Mechanism of toxicity

Like grayanotoxins and veratrum alkaloids, aconitine affects its toxicity through action on sodium channels. Aconitine (Fig. 20) seems to increase sodium entry into muscle, nerve, baroreceptors, and Purkinje fibers to produce a positive inotropic effect, enhanced vagal tone, neurotoxicity, and increased

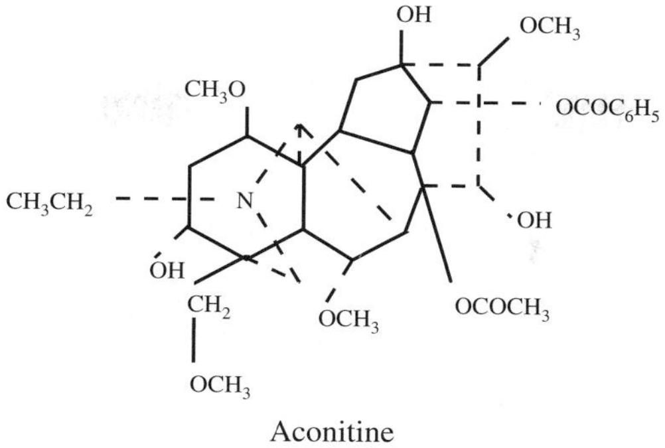

OH
OCH3
CH3O
OCOC6H5
CH3CH2
N
OH
OH
CH2
OCH3
OCOCH3
OCH3
Aconitine

Fig. 20. Structure of aconitine.

automaticity and torsade de pointes [81]. During late repolarization of the Purkinje fiber (late phase 4), aconitine attaches to a limited number of the sodium channels and increases Na^+ influx [71,82,83] causing *late* (or delayed) afterdepolarizations (Fig. 21) and increased automaticity (eg, premature ventricular beats). However, aconitine-induced sodium accumulation may also lead to *early* afterdepolarization during late phase 2 or early phase 3 of the action potential (Fig. 22). These early afterdepolarizations produce lengthening of the QT interval and are thought to explain reports of torsade de pointes in patients poisoned with aconite [82–85]. Bifascicular ventricular tachycardia, a dysrhythmia most frequently associated with digitalis toxicity, has also be reported in patients poisoned with aconite [86].

Clinical presentation

Most case reports of aconitine poisoning have come from ingestion of herbs containing aconitine [78,87]. Following exposure, onset of symptoms

1
"Triggered Activity"
0
2
3
Na+
4
PVC

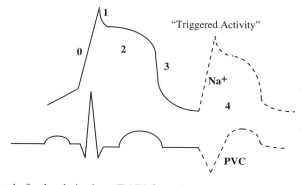

Fig. 21. Delayed afterdepolarizations (DAD) formation. Increasing sodium concentration in phase 4 leads to refiring of the Purkinje cell and DADs. These are manifest as premature ventricular contractions.

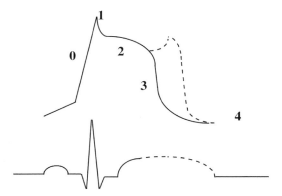

Fig. 22. Early afterdepolarization (EAD) formation frequently occurs when positive ions such as K + are held within the cell. The cell re-fires in late phase 2 or early phase three. When this occurs, an EAD is produced and results in QT prolongation, and sometimes, torsade de pointes.

has been reported in one series of cases to occur between 3 minutes to 2 hours, with a median of 30 minutes [85]. Symptoms may persist for 30 hours [88]. Neurologic complaints include initial visual impairment, dizziness, limb paresthesias, weakness [89], and ataxia [80]. Coma may follow. Chest discomfort, dyspnea, tachycardia, and diaphoresis may also occur [89]. Hyperglycemia, hypokalemia, bradycardia (with hypotension), atrial and nodal ectopic beats, supraventricular tachycardia, bundle branch block, intermittent bigeminy, ventricular tachycardia, ventricular fibrillation, and asystole have been reported [80,82,89,90]. Death is usually due to ventricular arrhythmia [89,91]. Ingestion of delphinium root has also resulted in ventricular dysrhythmias and cardiac arrest [79,89,91].

Laboratory studies

The presence of aconitine has been demonstrated by high-performance liquid chromatography at autopsy [91].

Management

Neurologic complaints require supportive care. The paramount concern is management of lethal arrhythmias. Ventricular tachycardia has failed to respond to several antiarrhythmic agents, including lidocaine, disopyramide, bretylium, amiodarone, potassium, and phenytoin. Tai and colleagues [86] reported successful use of flecainide following lidocaine failure in a single case. Yeih and colleagues [92] reported successful use of amiodarone following lidocaine failure in a case report. No antiarrhythmic agents have demonstrated clear superiority. In animal studies, Adaniya and colleagues [82] demonstrated the ability of magnesium to suppress early afterdepolarizations and polymorphic ventricular tachycardia. Although some authors [93] differentiate between polymorphic ventricular tachycardia and torsade de pointes, Adaniya and colleagues [82] seem to use the two terms interchangeably.

Nicotine and related compounds

Pyridine/piperidine alkaloids including nicotine, coniine, anabasine, cystisine, arecoline, lobeline, and many others have a similar mechanism of action. Plants containing these alkaloids are widely distributed today, but are thought to have originated in South America. *Nicotiana rustica*, which contains up to 18% nicotine, is thought to have been the first tobacco export from the New World. Much more potent than *N tabacum* (0.5%–9% nicotine), it is still smoked in Turkey and serves as a source for commercial nicotine production [94]. *N tabacum* is planted throughout the Southeast as the source of cigar and cigarette tobacco. Because the toxicity of smoked tobacco has been widely discussed elsewhere, only dermal and gastrointestinal absorption are addressed in this article. Small quantities of nicotine are also found in plants from the family Solanaceae such as tomatoes, potatoes, and eggplant. This is of little consequence in terms of poisoning [95,96]. Several of the *Nicotiana* and *Lobelia* species are cultivated as flowering plants. Of the uncultivated plants in this group, *N glauca* (tree tobacco) and *Conium maculatum* (poison hemlock) are the most common sources of poisoning.

Plants

Nicotine

Plants containing nicotine are: *N tabacum* (tobacco), *N glauca* (tree tobacco) (Fig. 23), *N trigonophylla* (desert tobacco), and *N attenuata* (coyote tobacco).

Conine

Conium maculatum (poison hemlock) contains conine (Figs. 24 and 25).

Lobeline, lobelamine

Plants containing lobeline/iobelamine are: *Lobelia inflata* (indian tobacco), *L cardinalis*, and other species.

Other plants with nicotine or related compounds: *Aethusa cynaprium* (fool's parsley) contains coniine. *Laburnum anagyroides* (golden chain tree), *Sophora secundiflora* (mescal bush bean), *S tomentosa* (necklace pod *Sophora*), *and Gymnocladus dioicus* (Kentucky coffee bean) all contain cystisine. *Areca catechu* (betel palm/betel nut) contains arecoline [94].

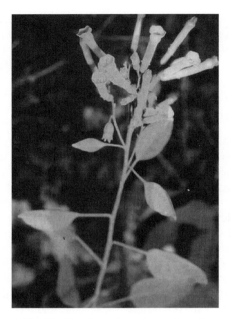

Fig. 23. *Nicotiana glauca* (tree tobacco).

Location

Conium maculatum

Poison hemlock grows throughout the United States and southern Canada except in desert regions. It is frequently found along roadways or railroads.

Nicotiana glauca

Tree tobacco is common from the Southeast to the Southwest, where it may grow to 10 feet or higher. It will grow in the desert but is commonly found along ditches in those areas. Where water is more plentiful, it has a wider range.

Description

Conium maculatum

This biennial may reach 10 feet in height. The leaves are pinately divided three to four times and have a fern-like appearance similar to parsley, for which it is sometimes mistaken. The flower is umbrella-shaped and strikingly similar to that of *Daucus carota* (Queen Anne's lace) or *Cicuta* spp (water hemlock). The stem is hollow and has red to purple speckles along

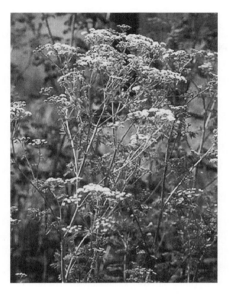

Fig. 24. *Conium maculatum* flowers (poison hemlock).

its length. The crushed stems are said to smell like mouse urine; however, that observation is extremely subjective and should not be used to identify the plant. Its taproot is occasionally mistaken for parsnip. This plant is reputed to be the source of poison used in the execution of Socrates [32].

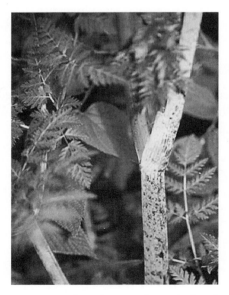

Fig. 25. *Conium maculatum* leaves and stem (poison hemlock).

Nicotiana glauca

Early growth has a shrub-like appearance and may be mistaken for collard greens due to the grayish cast of the green leaves. The leaves are oval with a smooth margin with a rubbery texture and grow up to 6 in in length. The flowers are approximately 2 in long by 1/2 in wide, bright yellow, with a tubular shape.

Toxic parts

All parts of both plants are poisonous. The seeds and roots of *C maculatum* are especially toxic.

Mechanism of toxicity

Nicotine, coniine (Fig. 26), anabasine, lobeline, and related pyridine/piperidine alkaloids cause similar toxicity. Their primary action is activation and then blockade of nicotinic acetylcholine receptors. Activation of nicotinic receptors in the cortex, thalamus, interpeduncular nucleus, and other locations in the central nervous system account for coma and seizures. Nicotine has been shown to enhance fast excitatory neural transmission in the CNS by triggering presynaptic cholinergic receptors, which increase presynaptic calcium and stimulate both cholinergic and glutaminergic transmission [97]. Nicotinic receptor activation facilitates the release of many neurotransmitters, including acetylcholine, norepinephrine, dopamine, serotonin, beta-endorphins, and others.

Activation of nicotinic receptors at autonomic ganglia produce varied effects in the sympathetic and parasympathetic nervous system. These most commonly include nausea, vomiting, diarrhea, bradycardia, tachycardia, and miosis [98]. Nicotine alkaloids act as depolarizing neuromuscular blocking agents and produce fasciculations and paralysis.

Clinical presentation

Ingestion or dermal exposure to nicotine and related compounds can result in any or all of the signs and symptoms listed in Box 2.

Nicotine

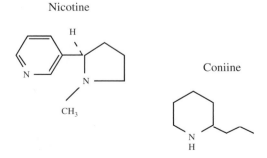

Coniine

Fig. 26. Structure of nicotine and coniine.

Box 2. Muscarinic and nicotinic effects of nicotine and related compounds

Muscarinic
Salivation
Lacrimation
Urination
Gastrointestinal cramping
Emesis
Miosis
Bronchospasm
Bradycardia

Nicotinic
Weakness
Fasciculations
Paralysis
Tachycardia
Coma
Seizures

Though rare, severe poisonings do occur [99], one of the more commonly reported poisonings results from the ingestion of cigarettes. The ingestion of a single cigarette (up to 2.0 mg nicotine absorbed) is enough to cause symptoms in a small child. Smolinske and colleagues [100] reported three severely poisoned children who had ingested a minimum of 1.4 mg/kg. Twenty-five asymptomatic children ingested less than 1 mg/kg. Curry and colleagues [101] reported nine cases of ingestion of *N glauca*, which had been mistaken for collard and turnip greens. Three fatalities occurred. Symptoms included leg cramps, paresthesias, dizziness, and headache. Onset was within 1 hour, and resolution in the surviving patients ranged from 3 hours to several hours. Mellick and colleagues [102] reported two cases of *N glauca* ingestion resulting in neuromuscular blockade and eventual complete recovery. Frank and colleagues [103] reported a *C maculatum* ingestion in a 4-year-old, which resulted in miosis, vomiting, and coma. The onset of symptoms was 30 minutes after ingestion with resolution in approximately 9 hours. Drummer and colleagues [96] reported three fatalities from *C maculatum*. Foster and colleagues [104] reported the accidental ingestion of *C maculatum* by a 14-year-old child that resulted in respiratory failure, asphyxia, and eventual death. Another child who ingested a smaller amount of the same *C maculatum* plant had symptoms of nausea, malaise, and tingling of the extremities and survived. The 2002 American Association of Poison Control Center Annual Report describes a 13-year-old child that

developed ascending paralysis, had a seizure, and then died after ingestion of
C maculatum that was mistaken for parsley [105].

Green tobacco sickness commonly occurs in the tobacco-growing states.
Workers handling leaves can absorb nicotine through the skin. It occurs
almost exclusively in workers who are cropping leaves from the plant [98].
Symptoms comprise nausea, vomiting, diarrhea, diaphoresis, and weakness,
which usually resolve with symptomatic treatment.

The use of betel quid, which is popular in India, Southeast Asia, and the
East Indies [94], has been reported in people who have immigrated to the
United States from those countries. The quid is a betel nut wrapped in a betel
vine leaf and smeared with a paste of burnt lime [106]. It contains arecoline
and several other cholinergic pyridine alkaloids.

Rhabdomyolysis has been reported from the ingestion of *C maculatum*,
although the reports are somewhat confusing in that "hemlock poisoning"
is attributed to exposure to both *Cicuta* and *Conium* species [107,108].

Laboratory studies

Nicotine and conine and other alkaloids may be measured in urine by
various methods, including gas chromatography [109], mass spectrometry
[96], and thin-layer chromatography [110].

Management

Activated charcoal should be administered for ingestions that have
occurred in the previous 2 hours. The dose of activated charcoal is 50 to
100 g in 8 ounces of tap water for adults and 1 gm/kg or 25 to 50 g in 4 ounces of water for children. In patients who have dermal exposure, as in the
case of green tobacco sickness, the skin should be thoroughly washed
with soap and water. Atropine may be used to block muscarinic symptoms,
such as bronchospasm, vomiting, diarrhea, or bradycardia. There is no standard dose in this situation, and the amount given should be titrated to reverse muscarinic symptoms without inducing anticholinergic toxicity.
Convulsions are best treated with benzodiazepines or barbiturates. Nicotinic
symptoms such as weakness, fasciculations, or paralysis cannot be reversed,
but supportive care is generally sufficient to manage the patient, with some
patients requiring ventilatory support. There are no clinically useful antidotes for the nicotinic effects. Patients should be monitored for rhabdomyolysis and its subsequent renal impairment. Due to the usual rapid
onset of symptoms, patients who present and remain asymptomatic and
who are not suicidal may be released after 4 hours of observation.

Anticholinergics

Several plants and mushrooms exhibit anticholinergic properties. The
best known of these are the members of the Solanaceae family. Of the

anticholinergic plants, the genera *Atropa*, *Datura*, and *Hyoscyamus* produce hyoscyamine (atropine). Other members of this group produce scopolamine. The members of both groups are listed, but for the sake of this discussion, *Datura* spp is the primary focus, because they account for more hospitalizations than the other plants.

The first recorded *Datura* poisoning occurred in 1676 during the Bacon Rebellion when soldiers under Captain John Smith made a salad of *Datura stramonium* leaves and began to hallucinate. The name "Jamestown weed" was given to this plant, and its name has been corrupted over the years to "Jimson weed."

Plants

Plants that have anticholinergic properties are: *Atropa bella-donna* (deadly nightshade), *Datura metaloides* (sacred datura) (Figs. 27 and 28), *D stramonium* (Jimson weed) (Fig. 29), *D arborea* (trumpet lily), *D candida*, *D suaveolens* (angel trumpet), other *Datura* spp, *Hyoscyamus niger* (henbane), *Lycium barbarum* (matrimony vine) and *Mandragora officinarum* (mandrake) (Figs. 27–29).

Location

Datura metaloides is a perennial southwestern plant that grows well in desert areas. *D stramonium* grows as an annual on recently disturbed

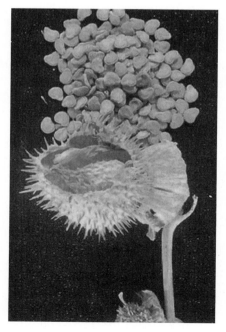

Fig. 27. *Datura metaloides* (sacred datura seeds).

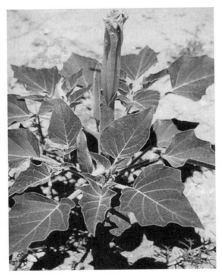

Fig. 28. *Datura metaloides* (sacred datura).

ground throughout the United States. It is frequently found in soybean fields.

Description

D meteloides

D meteloides is a stout bushy plant with thick stems. The large leaves are oval with wavy edges. The foliage has a pungent odor. Seeds are found in

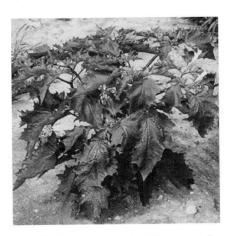

Fig. 29. *Datuna stramonium* (jimson weed).

spiney pods approximately 1.5 in long. The flowers are 6 to 8 in long and white with purple edges.

D stramonium

Similar to *D metaloides*, Jimson weed has a dark purple stem and is a taller plant.

Toxic parts

The entire plant is toxic. The flowers, fruits, and seeds are especially toxic.

Mechanism of toxicity

The members of the genus *Datura* contain varying amounts of hyoscyamine (atropine) and scopalamine (Fig. 30). Young plants tend to contain mostly scopalamine, but as they mature, hyoscyamine predominates. The toxicity of these compounds results from competitive blockade of acetylcholine at peripheral and central muscarinic receptors.

Clinical presentation

Onset of symptoms is usually within 30 to 60 minutes of ingestion and may last for 24 to 48 hours. Both central and peripheral syndromes may be seen. Levy [111] described 27 cases in which every patient had altered mental status and mydriasis.

Central anticholinergic syndrome

Central nervous system excitation often manifests as agitation and hallucinations. CNS depression and coma may follow. Hallucinations are generally visual but may be auditory. Speech has a characteristic mumbling quality and is often incomprehensible. Patients frequently answer questions with appropriate one-word answers, but if prompted (and able) to speak in

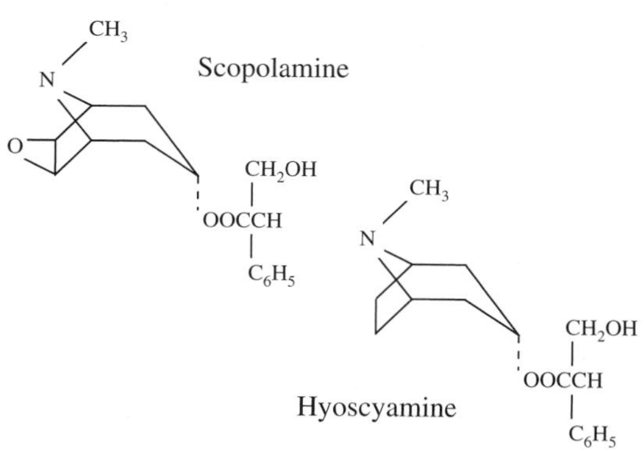

Fig. 30. Structures of scopolomine and hyoscyamine.

sentences, the fragmented speech pattern becomes obvious. Undressing behavior is not uncommon.

Peripheral anticholinergic syndrome

Tachycardia and mydriasis are common findings. Flushed skin may be more difficult to detect. Fever is occasionally noted. Bowel sounds may be depressed or absent, but usually persist. Bladder motility may be decreased as well. Although dry mucous membranes may be associated with hyperventilation, dry axillae in association with the other signs indicates anticholinergic poisoning and helps distinguish it from increased adrenergic activity.

Datura accounts for many admissions to critical care units each year. Although children are occasionally poisoned, the most frequent exposure occurs in patients who have ingested seeds or a tea brewed from the seeds in an attempt to induce hallucinations. Death is rare and may result more as the result of impaired judgment than direct toxicity. A few death reports do seem to indicate potentially fatal toxicity in high-dose exposures [112,113]. Petechial hemorrhages of the endocardium and hyperemia and edema of the lungs were reported in both cases.

Laboratory studies

Atropine may be detected by radioimmunoassay, gas chromatography/ mass spectrometry, thin-layer chromatography [114], and liquid chromatography. Scopolamine has been analyzed in plasma and urine by radioreceptor assay and gas chromatography/mass spectrometry [109].

Management

Decontamination is best accomplished with the administration activated charcoal if the ingestion has occurred within the previous 2 hours. The dose of activated charcoal is 50 to 100 g in 8 ounces of tap water for adults and 1 gm/kg or 25 to 50 g in 4 ounces of water for children. Tachycardia rarely requires treatment. Patients should be monitored for urine output and bladder distention. A nasogastric tube should be inserted in patients who have decreased gut motility. Hypotension should be treated with intravenous isotonic fluids. Dopamine may be used if hypotension persists after the patient's intravascular volume has been restored, but this is unusual. The combination of impaired diaphoresis with agitation may lead to severe hyperthermia, which must be aggressively treated with sedation/paralysis and active cooling. Rhabdomyolysis is common and explains renal failure and other complications seen in severe *Datura* toxicity. Because of their anticholinergic activity, phenothiazines and diphenhydramine should be avoided. Haloperidol does not seem to be effective for resolution of central anticholinergic effects [115]. Benzodiazepines are, on the other hand, effective in the treatment of agitation.

Several authors have advocated the use of intravenous physostigmine for patients who have central anticholinergic effects [111,115,116]. Physostigmine inhibits acetylcholinesterase, thus increasing the amount of acetylcholine available to the muscarinic receptors. While benzodiazepines may be used to sedate agitated patients, physostigmine may restore the patient's level of consciousness to its baseline. It is particularly helpful in differentiating anti-cholinergic poisoning from other causes of altered mental status. It should not be used unless peripheral anticholinergic signs accompany a clinical picture of central anticholinergic poisoning. Seizure activity, bradycardia, heart blocks, and asystole have followed use of physostigmine [117,118]. Because of the potential for greater risks than benefits, consultation with a poison center or medical toxicologist regarding administration of physo-stigmine for anticholinergic plant ingestion is recommended before use.

Saponin glycosides

Phytolacca americana (pokeweed) contains several potentially toxic compounds. Saponin glycosides, which play a defensive role for these plants, account for gastrointestinal injury and are found in other species that are listed below. In addition to these glycosides, *P americana* also con-tains proteins that have mitogenic, hemaglutinin [119], and antiviral [120] properties.

Plants

Plants containing saponin glycosides are: *P americana* and synonym, *Phytolacca decandra* (pokeweed, poke, pigeonberry, inkberry, pocan, garget redwood, cancer-root, jalap, scoke, American nightshade) (Fig. 31).

Other plants containing saponin glycosides are: *Glycyrrhiza glabra* (Licorice), *Panax ginseng* (Ginseng), *Hedera helix* (English ivy), and *Aleur-ites* spp (Tung tree).

Location

It is found throughout the eastern half of the United States from the southern states into Canada. It has been introduced into some parts of the Southwest [69].

Description

Phytolacca americana grows up to 9 feet tall by late summer. It tends to grow in areas of partial sunlight where the ground is untended. The leaves are eliptic-lanceolate and 6 to 12 in in length with alternating attachment. The stems and stalks are red. The white flowers are 1/4 in in clusters. The berries grow to 1/4 in diameter by fall when they are deep purple. They

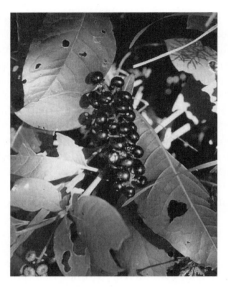

Fig. 31. *Phytolacca americana* (pokeberry).

are found in clusters of 20 to 30 berries. The root is large, tan with a rough surface, and has multiple branches.

Toxic parts

All parts of the plant, especially the roots, are toxic.

Mechanism of toxicity

The toxic components of pokeweed are triterpene saponins, which include phytolaccatoxin, phytolaccagenin (Fig. 32), and a proteinaceous mitogen

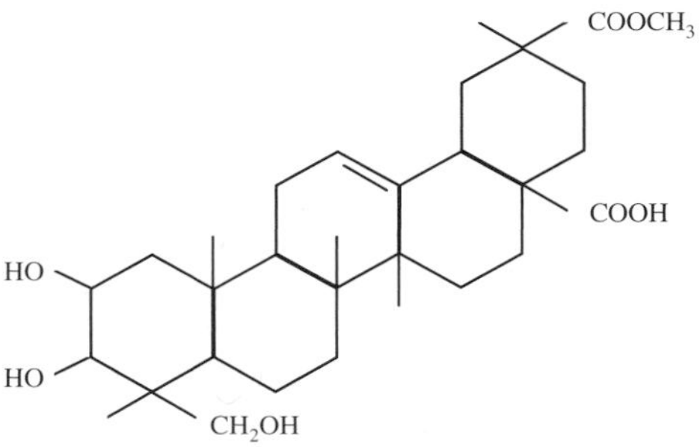

Phytolaccagenin

Fig. 32. Structure of phytolaccagenin.

[121]. Phytolaccatoxin, phytolaccagenin, and saponin glycosides produce gastrointestinal irritation, which causes vomiting and diarrhea with a foaming or "soapy" consistency. In 1964, Farnes and colleagues [122] reported the mitogenic properties of pokeweed. In 1966, Barker and colleagues [123] reported several children who had varying exposure to *P americana*. Those who had ingested pokeberries or who had abrasions or scratches on their hands when they handled the berries developed increased numbers of circulating plasmablasts and proplasmacytes as well as mature plasma cells for up to 2 weeks following the exposure. They subsequently reported eosinophilia, thrombocytopenia, and abnormal platelet morphology in similarly exposed children [124]. Waxdal [119] isolated five separate proteins designated Pa-1 through Pa-5, which had varying amounts of mitogenic activity. Pa-1 was the most mitogenic and was also the most potent hemaglutinin. These proteins are thought to account for the mitogenic properties of pokeweed on both thymus-dependent (T) cells and thymus independent (B) lymphocytes. A pokeweed antiviral protein has also been reported. This protein seems to remove an adenine residue from RNA of eukaryotic ribosomes interfering with protein synthesis. It has been found to inhibit herpes simplex infection of certain cell lines and repress human immunodeficiency virus 1 replication in T cells at concentrations that do not inhibit cellular protein synthesis [120]. The utility of these findings remains under study.

Clinical presentation

Exposure to pokeweed is frequently reported [26,117,125]. The leaves are prepared as a salad; berries are used for teas [121], and roots have been mistaken for horseradish [126], parsnips, or other vegetables. Various parts of the plant are used as herbal medications for rheumatism, antihelmenths, emetics, laxatives, and for the treatment of a host of other maladies. The most frequent route of exposure is oral, but plasmacytosis has been noted after berries have come into contact with broken skin [123,124,127].

Ingestion of pokeleaves as a salad has been a common source of gastroenteritis. The traditional preparation is of poke salad involves "parboiling" the immature leaves. Parboiling is a process of boiling the leaves in water, discarding the water, reboiling the leaves, and rinsing them after the second boiling. This however is sometimes insufficient to remove the toxins [128].

Nausea, vomiting, and stomach cramps were reported in over 80% of patients in one report [128]. Lower-dose exposure to berries may only result in mild diarrhea and may be delayed up to 12 hours after exposure [129]. Loss of consciousness has been reported after ingestion of pokeberry tea. This was accompanied by salivation, vomiting, urinary incontinence, and hypotension, suggesting it may have been due to a vasovagal event [130]. Heme positive stools have also been observed [126,131]. Cardiac effects have included hypotension, bradycardia, tachycardia, and Mobitz type I heart block [132], which was felt by the authors to represent a vagal effect. The dysrhythmia occurred during an episode of extreme nausea and resolved when the patient was treated with promethazine. Roberge and colleagues [133] also reported ventricular fibrillation in a single patient who had heart disease. The authors felt that the ischemic changes on her electrocardiogram (precordial ST–T-wave depression, Q waves in leads II and III) were most likely related to her accelerated heart rate and dysrhythmia because saponin glycosides are not thought to be directly cardiotoxic. Other signs of poisoning include an initial burning in the mouth and throat, diaphoresis, and generalized weakness. Visual disturbances and coma have also been reported, although these may be related to hypotension [130]. Although most reports of death are from the distant past, there has been one recent report in the American Association of Poison Control Centers Annual Report data. In the 2000 American Association of Poison Control Centers Annual Report, there is a case of an 18-year-old that accidentally ingested a *P americana* root. The individual had emesis 90 minutes after the ingestion and ventricular fibrillation leading to death approximately 2 hours after the exposure [134]. Hematopoetic effects resolve in a matter of weeks [123,124].

Laboratory studies

Specific tests for *Phytolacca* derived toxins are not clinically useful. Diagnosis is based on history and, when possible, plant identification. Electrocardiographic findings are nonspecific. Complete blood cell count may occasionally show atypical lymphocytes, plasma cells, thrombocytopenia, or eosinophilia a few days after exposure [123,124].

Management

Supportive care is the mainstay of therapy. Gastric decontamination may be accomplished with the administration of activated charcoal if ingestion has been within 2 hours of presentation. The dose of activated charcoal is 50 to 100 g in 8 ounces of tap water for adults and 1 gm/kg or 25 to 50 g in 4 ounces of water for children. Nausea and vomiting may be treated antiemetics. Hypotension, which may result from gastrointestinal losses or vagal stimulation, should be treated initially with fluids. Dysrhythmias should be treated in the usual fashion, although resolution of hypovolemia and vagal stimulation are presumably sufficient to treat abnormal cardiac rhythms [132,133].

Catechol phenols (urushiol) and noncatechol phenols (resorcinol)

Urushiol and noncatechol phenols like resorcinol are oleoresins found in plants of the family Anacardiaceae (72 genera of flowering plants bearing fruits that are drupes) [135,136]. The oleoresins elicit an allergic skin reaction on contact in higher primates including human [137–140]. Historically, urushiol-based lacquers, which were used to produce traditional lacquer-wares in Japan approximately 7000 BC, were made from the sap of the lacquer tree (*Rhus verniciflua*). The name urushiol is derived from the Japanese word *urushi*, denoting the sap (kiurushi) of the lacquer tree [141]. Plants of the family Anacardiaceae cause more allergic contact dermatitis than all other plant families combined [139,140]. Toxicodendron, a genus of this family, comprises the most allergic members in North America including poison ivy, poison oak, and poison sumac [138,142–148]. The main allergens in toxicodendrons are catechols-like urushiol (1,2–dihydroxybenzene) (Fig. 33) [149–151]. Urushiol oleoresin is a slightly yellow liquid that avidly binds to skin. On exposure to oxygen, it turns dark brown within 10 minutes and black by 24 hours [152]. The cashew nut tree (*anacardium occidentale*), mango (*mangifera indica*), and the Brazilian pepper tree (*schinus terebinthifolius*), common throughout the tropics, are also implicated, albeit less frequently, in allergic contact dermatitis in the United States [132,148,153]. The main allergens in those trees are noncatechol phenols like resorcinols (1,3–dihydroxybenzene) (Fig. 34). Urushiol, a catechol, possesses greater allergenicity than noncatechol phenols [154]. Urushiol-induced contact dermatitis affects approximately 10 to 50 million Americans per year. Outdoor activities and occupations (agriculture, forestry, and firefighting) expose individuals to a significant risk of contracting Toxicodendron dermatitis with consequent lost-time injuries and treatment cost [155,156].

Plants

There are two species of poison ivy (*Toxicodendron radicans and Toxicodendron rydbergii*) and poison oak (*Toxicodendron diversilobum and Toxicodendron toxicarium*) and one species of poison sumac (*Toxicodendron vernix*) that are common to North America (Figs. 35 and 36) [139,157].

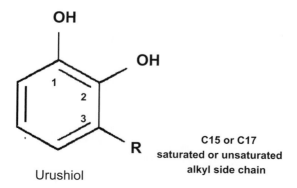

Fig. 33. Structure of urushiol.

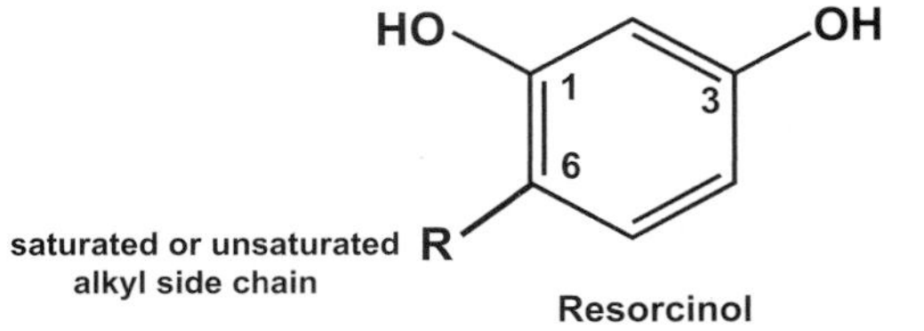

HO⟍ ⟍OH

saturated or unsaturated **R**
alkyl side chain

Resorcinol

Fig. 34. Structure of resorcinol.

Location

Toxicodendron radicans (common or Eastern poison ivy) is found in the Eastern half of the United States and southern Canada. It grows as weeds (along roads, trails and streams) or shrub-like. It also climbs as a woody vine. *Toxicodendron rydbergii* (Northern or Western poison ivy) is found in the Western half of the United States (except California) and in northern border states. It grows as nonclimbing shrubs. *Toxicodendron diversilobum* (Western poison oak) is found in the Pacific coast of the United States. It grows as a shrub and climbing woody vine. *Toxicodendron toxicarium* (Eastern poison oak) is found in the southeastern United States. It grows in sandy soils as a shrub but can also climb. Toxicodendron vernix (poison sumac) is found in the eastern third of the United States. It grows as a bush in damp and swampy areas [139,148,157].

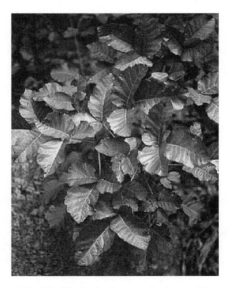

Fig. 35. *Toxicodendron* spp (poison oak).

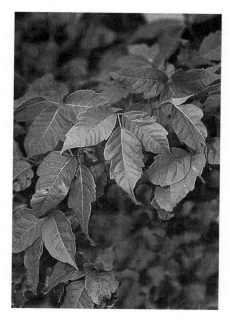

Fig. 36. *Toxicodendron* spp (poison ivy).

Toxic parts

The urushiol oil in all Toxicodendron species is found in the stems, roots, leaves, and skin of its fruits. Usually a break in the plant skin is required for plants to release the urushiol. Urushiol is nonvolatile and dries up quickly retaining its antigenic potential. When the oil is transferred to the human skin, as little as 2 mg is sufficient to cause dermatitis in the sensitized individual. Toxicodendrons undergo seasonal variations. In the fall, the leaves turn red and accumulate higher concentration of urushiol. In the winter and fall, as the leaves dry up, the nonleaf remaining parts of the plant retain its urushiol content and thus remain a significant potential contact hazard [139,148,157].

Description

Toxicodendron plants are ubiquitous throughout North America. They are rarely found above 5000 feet elevation. They have pinnately or alternate compound leaves, possessing three or more leaflets. The plants show a wide spectrum of variation in appearance. They grow as woody creeping or climbing vines, shrubs, or trees. A single plant can have leaves with smooth, toothed, or lobed edges. Flowers and fruit arise uniquely in an axillary position in the angle between the leaf and twig. The leaf stalk leaves a characteristic "V"-shaped scar after it falls off. The green fruits turn off-white as they ripen. Poison ivy and poison oak grow along roads, trails, or streams. They possess three (sometimes five) leaflets per leaf giving rise to the adage, "leaves of three, let them be." Poison ivy leaves are 3 to 12 cm long and classically have pointed tips and are ovate (widest point below the center). It can grow as a shrub up to 4 feet, as a creeping vine (4–10 in high) or climbing vine. It reproduces by creeping rootstocks or by seeds. Virginia creeper (*Parthenocissus quinquefolia*) belongs to the grape family and is nontoxic. It has a similar appearance and growth habitat and often grows together with poison ivy. Poison oak leaves are 3 to 15 cm long and usually have round ends. Western poison oak grows as a dense shrub in open sunlight or as a climbing vine in shaded areas. Eastern poison oak grows as an erect shrub up to 3 feet tall. Poison oak reproduces by creeping rootstocks or by seeds. Poison sumac contains leaves that are pinnate, are 25 to 50 cm long, and have 7 to 13 leaflets. It grows as a woody bush up to 3 m tall. Poison sumac grows exclusively in wet and flooded soils [139,147,148,157–160].

Mechanism of toxicity

Urushiol molecules consist of catechols (1,2–dihyroxybenzene) substituted at position 3 with an alkyl side chain that has 15 or 17 carbon atoms (see Fig. 33). The alkyl group may be saturated or unsaturated. The urushiol oleoresin is a variable mixture of the saturated and unsaturated urushiol molecules depending on the toxicodendrons species. Poison ivy and poison sumac contain mostly C15 alkyl side chains (pentadecylcatechols), but poison oak contains mostly catechols with C17 side chains (heptadecylcatechols). Catechols and their alkyl side chains are immunologically inert on their own. However, combining them to produce urushiol converts them into potent immune sensitizers. The allergenicity of the particular urushiol resin is dependent on the degree of unsaturation of the alkyl chain at position 3 of the catechol. Placement at position 6 induces tolerance [136,137,161–166]. Urushiol-induced allergic contact dermatitis is mediated by a T-lymphocyte–mediated delayed type IV hypersensitivity reaction [136,167–174]. On initial skin contact, urushiol catechols bind and penetrate the skin. They are converted to quinine intermediates (hapten) that bind to host proteins on Langerhans cells (antigen-presenting cells) in the epidermis and become antigens. As a result, cytokines are released by keratinocytes, Langerhans cells, and macrophages in the skin. The cytokines in turn activate Langerhans cells to take-up and process the antigens and emigrate to regional lymph nodes. The Langerhans cells mature into dendritic cells that process and re-express the antigens on their surface for presentation to naïve T cells in the regional lymph node. Upon antigen presentation, T cells with receptors specific to the antigen get activated and clonally expanded to produce urushiol-specific effector and memory T lymphocytes. Urushiol-specific T lymphocytes recirculate in the periphery where it may contact the antigen again. This is the induction phase of allergic contact hypersensitivity pathogenesis, which confers the naïve host "sensitization" to urushiol [174]. After subsequent contact with urushiol, antigen-specific memory and effector (clonal) T cells are activated in the skin with the induction of their inflammatory cytokines. This elicits a cell-mediated cytotoxic immune response that ultimately produces the clinical manifestation of contact dermatitis: erythema, edema, vesicles, pain, and pruritis. This elicitation phase of allergic contact hypersensitivity pathogenesis not only is urushiol-specific, but also dose-dependent (ie, the severity of the inflammatory response is proportional to the amount and duration of exposure) [175–177].

Clinical presentation

Over 70% of the United States population reacts to poison ivy allergens after patch testing. But, only 50% reacts to plants in their habitat. In areas where toxicodendron plants are less common, the prevalence is approximately 20%. Tolerance is conferred in approximately 10% to 15%. Peak frequency for sensitization occurs between 8 and 14 years of age. Genetic susceptibility has been demonstrated. Break in the plant skin is required to release urushiol. Therefore, lightly brushing against uninjured leaves is benign. Urushiol may be spread by contaminated clothing, pets, sawdust, lacquered furniture, or smoke aerosols. Urushiol-containing smoke aerosols can cause severe dermatitis and respiratory tract inflammation, especially in forest firefighters [178]. After contact with urushiol, a sensitized individual typically develops an erythematous pruritic eruption within 2 days (4–96 hours) of the exposure. However, dermatitis may occur up to 3 weeks after primary contact or within hours of secondary contact. Streaks of erythema and edematous papules typically precede vesicles and bullae. If the urushiol load is lower, only erythematous edematous reaction may be seen. However, significant exposure will produce bullae, edema, and severe pain. Vesicle and bulla fluid contain no urushiol as demonstrated by patch testing, and thus it does not propagate the rash. Variation in skin thickness (especially stratum corneum) and urushiol load at various body parts likely cause variable time appearance of clinical manifestations. In addition, contact with dormant urushiol on fingernails, pets, and inanimate objects may cause symptoms to appear within few weeks after the initial exposure. Without treatment, the dermatitis lasts approximately 3 weeks. More severe reactions especially in susceptible individuals take longer to resolve and can last up to 6 weeks [138–140,142–148,179–181]. In "black-spot poison ivy dermatitis," an uncommon manifestation of toxicodendron exposure, urushiol acts as both an irritant and allergen [182,183]. Oxidized resin can be found on the skin, resulting in a black discoloration. This results in an acute irritant contact dermatitis that is superimposed on an acute allergic contact dermatitis [184]. This form of dermatitis is uncommon because most people wash off the resin as soon as it is noted. Uncommon complications of toxicodendron exposure include erythema multiforme [185–187] and nephritis [188], thought to be immune complex–mediated. Hyperpigmentation following urushiol-induced dermatitis occurs more commonly in dark skin. Secondary polymicrobial bacterial infections have been reported in urushiol-induced dermatitis [189,190]. Though less commonly reported than skin and inhalation exposures, ingestions of toxicodendron plants do occur. A syndrome of systemic contact dermatitis with skin manifestations of inflammation has been described following both intentional and unintentional toxicodendron ingestions [191,192].

Laboratory studies

The black spot test maybe used in the field to identify urushiol-containing plants [152]. Urushiol turns dark brown within 10 minutes of exposure to oxygen and black by 24 hours. Patch testing is used to diagnose delayed allergic reactions such as contact dermatitis. An allergen, in this case urushiol oleoresin, is applied to a patch, which is then placed on the skin. Patch testing for toxicodendron allergy has limited clinical utility. Only 50% of individuals who have positive skin patch test actually react to poison ivy in the field. Furthermore, patch testing with urushiol oleoresin carries a 10% to 20% risk of sensitizing an individual to the oleoresin. Therefore, patch testing is not recommended for diagnostic purposes [193–195].

Management

Urushiol oil is degraded in water. The oleoresin can be removed in a significant amount only if it is washed off as soon as the exposure to the toxicodendron is recognized. After 10 minutes, only 50% can be removed; after 15 minutes, only 25%; after 30 minutes, only 10%; and after 60 minutes, none of the urushiol can be removed [195]. Postexposure decontamination products have shown some effectiveness in reducing the dermatitis if applied to the skin within 2 hours of exposure. Vesicles, bullae, and weepy lesions are best treated with lukewarm baths, wet-to-dry soaks, or mild shake lotions (calamine). An astringent such as Burow's solution (aluminum subacetate) works well to cool and dry the weeping lesions. Topical antihistamines, anesthetics, and antibiotics should be avoided to prevent sensitization. Topical steroids are more effective if applied in the early stages of the erythema and pruritis before the appearance of vesicles. Steroid topicals with moderate potency are recommended. Abrupt discontinuation can cause a rebound inflammation. Immunosuppressive topical treatment with tacrolimus (inhibits T-cell activation in skin) has been shown to be a safer and effective alternative to topical corticosteroids in atopic dermatitis [195a]. However, its effectiveness in urushiol-induced dermatitis has not been studied. Systemic corticosteroids are effective when indicated. It is recommended in moderate to severe urushiol-induced dermatitis. Doses are usually 1 to 2 mg/kg per day, slowly tapered over 2 to 3 weeks. If the corticosteroid course is short, then rebound dermatitis is likely to follow [145,146,148,160,180,195].

Prevention

Urushiol penetrates latex but not vinyl gloves. Hyposensitiztion strategies for Anacardiaceae sensitized individuals have not been effective [148,161, 195–198]. Barrier creams like ivy-block (an organoclay compound, 5% quaternium-18 bentonite lotion) have been tested and shown to be effective [199,200]. This product has been approved by the US Food and Drug Administration for prevention of Toxicodendron dermatitis.

Oxalates

There are many plants that contain oxalates. The oxalates contained in plants are found in two different forms insoluble oxalates, usually calcium oxalate, or soluble oxalates or oxalic acid. One family of oxalate-containing plants is the Aracea family, which comprises over 109 genera [201]. *Dieffenbachia* is one genus within the Aracea family that is of particular historical significance. *Diffenbachia* species have been used for their toxic effects for hundreds of years. They have acquired the common name of "dumb cane" and "mother-in-law's tongue" secondary to their local irritative effect when chewed [202]. In the Caribbean, *Diffenbachia* spp were used to punish slaves by rubbing the plant stalks on their tongues, resulting in mucosal swelling, pain, and the inability to talk [202]. They were used in a similar manner on the same islands to sabotage crime witnesses, rendering them unable to testify in court [202]. Several plants, including spinach and rhubarb, that contain soluble oxalates are common to the human diet and are not well known for toxic effects.

Plants

A list of more common oxalate-containing plants includes: *Dieffenbachia* spp (dumb cane, mother-in-law's tongue) (Fig. 37), *Philodendron* spp, *Caladium* spp, *Colocasia* spp (elephant's ear, taro), *Arisaema* spp (jack-in-the-pulpit), *Rheum rhabarbarum* (rhubarb), and *Spinacea oleracea* (spinach).

Locations

Dieffenbachia spp, *Philodendron* spp, *Colocasia* spp, and *Caladium* spp can all be found in the tropical regions of the Americas. They are all now common ornamental houseplants in the United States. Both the *Rheum* and *Spinacea* spp originated in Asia but now are cultivated in commercial and residential gardens in the United States.

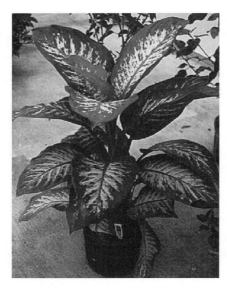

Fig. 37. *Dieffenbachia* spp (dumbcane).

Toxic parts

Dieffenbachia spp, *Philodendron* spp, *Colocasia* spp, *Caladium* spp, and *Arisaema* spp: all parts are toxic except the tubers of *Colocasia esculenta*. Rhubarb's leaf blades are toxic. Spinach has leaves that contain soluble calcium oxalates.

Description

Dieffenbachia spp are shrubby plants with large oval-shaped leaves. Leaves may be completely green or green with ivory mottling. *Philodendron* spp have climbing vines with triangular or heart-shaped leaves, which are green, red, or white in color. *Caladium* spp are stemless with multicolored (green, red, and white) heart-shaped leaves. *Colocasia* have large heart-shaped leaves that may grow up to 65 cm in size. Rhubarb has a thick reddish leaf stalk and large fan-shaped leaves. Spinach has oval-shaped leaves that grow in a rosette formation.

Mechanism of toxicity

The plants that contain insoluble oxalates have a different form of toxicity than the plants that contain soluble oxalates. Insoluble oxalate is in the form of calcium oxalate that forms needle-shaped crystals or raphides. In certain plants, such as the *Dieffenbachia* spp, these raphides are contained in oval-shaped cells called idioblasts. The idioblast cells have an opening on both ends of the cell. When mechanical force is applied to the idioblasts, the rahpides fire out of the cell and are propelled a distance of 2 to 3 cell lengths. The mechanical force of these calcium oxalate crystals causes local cell damage [202–204]. There is also evidence that there may be some other toxic component within the idioblasts. Research has failed to identify the exact nature of this other toxic substance; however theories include a proteinaceous substance, a substance with a proteolytic property, or a substance that affects bradykinin activity [203,204].

Soluble oxalates, or oxalic acids, produce its toxicity in a different manner. Oxalic acid can bind with ionized calcium leading to systemic hypocalcemia. Hypocalcemia has been documented by this method in livestock, but has not been well documented in humans. Oxalic acid can also bind with calcium in the urine, leading to nephrolithiasis. Nephrolithiasis by this mechanism is thought to be more common in people who have a diet high in oxalic acid–containing foods and whose gastrointestinal tract absorbs more oxalic acid [205–207].

Clinical presentation

Most exposures to calcium oxalate–containing plants result in no effects. The Pittsburgh Poison Center did a retrospective review of *Dieffenbachia* and *Philodendron* exposures called to their center over a 2-year period. There were a total of 188 exposures with 4 resulting in local oral symptoms that were either self-limited or resolved with minimal treatment [208]. The clinical effects of calcium oxalate–containing plants are the results of local irritation. Swelling, pain, and oral ulcers can occur as a consequence of chewing or eating these plants [209,210]. An irritant contact dermatitis can occur after handling plants with calcium containing raphides [201,211]. *Philodendron* spp can cause an allergic contact dermatitis in susceptible individuals. Chemosis, tearing, and pain has been reported after ocular exposure to the juice of *Dieffenbachia* spp [212].

Ingestion of plants containing soluble oxalates can theoretically lead to hypocalcemia leading to tremor, tetany, and seizures. This clinical scenario has not been well documented in humans, and an older case reports that attributes death to this plant overlooks confounding factors that may have caused or contributed to the death [213]. An older publication warns about the dangers of rhubarb toxicity, but fails to cite references [214]. Chronic ingestion of soluble oxalates can lead to an increase in nephrolithiasis and associated symptoms [205–207].

There are three case reports in the literature that attribute severe toxicity and/or death to *Dieffenbachia* or *Philodendron* species. The following two cases involve patients who have significant periods of time outside of the hospital between the exposure and serious outcome. These nonobserved time periods allow for possible confounding variables and thus difficulty in concluding the relationship between the plant and the outcome. The only reported death was from an 11-month-old boy who died from cardiac arrest 17 days after he was found chewing on a *Philodendron* plant. The child had original symptoms consistent with local oral mucosa irritation and was admitted to the hospital. His condition improved after 5 days and he was discharged from the medical facility. Fifteen days after the ingestion, he was readmitted to the hospital, and an endoscopy on day 16 showed esophageal erosions and an esophageal stricture. The child died of cardiac arrest in the hospital on day 17. The reporting physicians concluded that his cardiac arrest was caused by vagotonia related to his esophageal injury [215]. There is a report of a 12-year-old child that had an aortoesophageal fistula as a complication of esophagitis caused by the intentional ingestion of a *Dieffenbachia* leaf. The child had an initial endoscopy that showed grade 2 esophagitis of the entire esophagus. After a 2-week hospitalization, the child was discharged home on nasogastric tube feeds. Five weeks after the ingestion, the child had an endoscopy that showed improvement of the esophagitis. Two days after the endoscopy, the patient had an acute gastrointestinal bleed. The child required emergent surgery and was found to have an aortoesophageal fistula [216].

A 69-year-old man suffered from airway edema and glossitis requiring emergency tracheostomy approximately 1 hour after oral exposure to a *Dieffenbachia* plant. The man had mistaken the plant for sugar cane. The patient was treated with methylprednisolone, albuterol, and diphenhydramine, and his condition resolved after 3 days [204].

Laboratory studies and imaging

There are no readily available tests to confirm oxalate–containing plant exposure. Electrolyte status and calcium levels may be useful in a patient who is symptomatic and has ingested a large amount of soluble oxalates. A patient who has obvious oral burns and symptoms of dysphagia should undergo endoscopy. A patient who has ocular symptoms should undergo slit-lamp examination.

Management

Treatment for calcium oxalate–containing plants consists of symptomatic care. For oral exposure with local pain, systemic pain medications or viscous lidocaine may be beneficial. Local oral edema may respond to an H2-antagonist such as diphenhydramine. Oral edema along with airway compromise should be treated aggressively with systemic steroids, an H2-antagonist, and consideration of endotracheal intubation or tracheostomy if necessary. In the one reported case in the literature with severe airway compromise, the patient was also treated with nebulized albuterol and racemic epinephrine, both with unclear results [204]. Patients who have significant oral symptoms, oral lesions, and/or dysphagia should be considered for endoscopy.

Contact dermatitis from raphide-containing plants may respond to topical or systemic steroids. Symptomatic care with an H2-antagonist may also be beneficial. Corneal irritation from raphide-containing plants may be treated with a cycloplegic or steroidal eye drop [212].

Summary

Patients who have exposures to potentially toxic plants frequent emergency departments. It is important for health care providers to realize that most of these exposures are of minimal toxicity. The more serious poisonings usually involve adults who have either mistaken the plant as edible or have deliberately ingested the plant to derive perceived medicinal or toxic properties. There are multiple potential mechanisms of toxicity following plant exposure. Health care providers should be aware of the plants endogenous to their region.

References

[1] Watson WA, Litovitz TL, Rodgers GC Jr, et al. 2004 Annual report of the American Association of Poison Control Centers Toxic Exposure Surveillance System. Am J Emerg Med 2005;23(5):589–666.

[2] Balint GA. Ricin: the toxic protein of castor oil seeds. Toxicology 1974;2:77–102.

[3] Krenzelok EP, Jacobsen TD, Aronis JM. Hemlock ingestions: the most deadly plant exposures [abstract]. J Toxicol Clin Toxicol 1996;34(5):601–2.

[4] Lampe KF. Changes in therapy in *Abrus* and *Ricinus* poisoning suggested by recent studies in their mechanism of toxicity. Clin Toxicol 1976;9:21.

[5] Olsnes S, Refsnes K, Pihl A. Mechanism of action of the toxic lectins abrin and ricin. Nature 1974;249:627–31.

[6] Lord JM, Roberts LM, Robertus JD. Ricin: structure, mode of action, and some current applications. FASEB J 1994;8:201–8.

[7] Fitzgerald D, Pastan I. Targeted toxin therapy for the treatment of cancer. J Natl Cancer Inst 1989;81:1455–63.

[8] Zhang L, Hsu CH, Robinson CP. Effects of ricin administration to rabbits on the ability of their coronary arteries to contract and relax *in vitro*. Toxicol Appl Pharmacol 1994;129: 16–22.

[9] Ma L, Hsu CH, Patterson E, et al. Ricin depresses cardiac function in the rabbit heart. Toxicol App Pharm 1996;138:72–6.

[10] Challoner KR, McCarron MM. Castor bean intoxication. Ann Emerg Med 1990;19(10): 1177–83.

[11] Knight B. Ricin–a potent homicidal poison. Br Med J 1979;350–1.

[12] Fine DR, Shepheard HA, Griffiths GD, et al. Sub-lethal poisoning by self-injection with ricin. Med Sci Law 1992;32(1):70–2.

[13] Hart M. Hazards to health: jequirty-bean poisoning. N Engl J Med 1963;268(16):885–6.

[14] Makalinao IR. A descriptive study on the clinical profile of Jatropa seed poisoning. Vet Hum Toxicol 1993;35(4):330.

[15] Lockey SD. Anaphylaxis from an Indian necklace. JAMA 1968;206(13):2900–1.
[16] Ratner B, Gruehl HL. Respiratory anaphylaxis (asthma) and ricin poisoning induced with castor bean dust. Am J Hygeine 1929;10:236–44.
[17] Garnier R, Hoffelt J, Carlier P, et al. Acute veratrine intoxication with home-made gentian wine–clinical and anaytical findings. Vet Hum Toxicol 1982;24(4):294.
[18] Meldrum WP. Poisoning by castor oil seeds. BMJ 1900;1:317.
[19] Rauber A, Heard J. Castor bean toxicity re-examined: a new perspective. Vet Hum Toxicol 1985;27(6):498–502.
[20] Rauber AP, Heard JH. The great castor bean panic. Vet Hum Toxicol 1985;28(4):308.
[21] Stockbridge J. Account of the effect of eating, a poisonous plant called *Cicuta maculata*. Boston Medical Surgical Journal 1814;3:334–7.
[22] Lampe KF, McCann MA. The AMA handbook of poisonous and injurious plants. Chicago: Chicago Review Press; 1985.
[23] Mitchell M, Routledge PA. Poisoning by hemlock water dropwort. Lancet 1977;1:423–4.
[24] Applefeld JJ, Caplan ES. A case of water hemlock poisoning. JACEP 1979;8(10):401–3.
[25] CDC. Water hemlock poisoning–Maine, 1992. MMWR Morb Mortal Wkly Rep 1994; 43(13):229–31.
[26] Litovitz TL, Felberg L, Skoloway RA, et al. 1994 annual report of the American Association of Poison Control Centers Toxic Exposure Surveillance System. Am J Emerg Med 1995;13(5):551–97.
[27] Withers LM, Cole FR, Nelson RB. Water-hemlock poisoning [letter]. N Engl J Med 1975; 281:566–7.
[28] Landers D, Seppi K, Blauer W. Seizures and death on a white river float trip: report of water hemlock poisoning. West J Med 1985;142:637–40.
[29] Starreveld E, Hope CE. Cicutoxin poisoning (water hemlock). Neurology 1975;25(August): 730–4.
[30] Nelson RB, North DS, Kaneriya M, et al. The influence of biperiden, benztropine, physostigmine and diazepam on the convulsive effects of *Cicuta douglasii*. Proc West Pharmacol Soc 1978;21:137–9.
[31] Carlton BE, Tufts E, Girard DE. Water hemlock poisoning complicated by rhabdomyoslysis and renal failure. Clin Toxicol 1979;14(1):87–92.
[32] Nelson RB, Cole FR. The convulsive profile of *Cicuta douglasii* (water hemlock). Proc West Pharmacol Soc 1976;19:193–7.
[33] Costanza DJ, Hoversten VW. Accidental ingestion of water hemlock: report of two patients with acute and chronic effects. Calif Med 1973;119(May):78–82.
[34] Egdahl A. A case of poisoning due to eating poison-hemlock (*Cicuta maculata*). Archives of Internal Medicine 1911;7:348–56.
[35] Robson P. Water hemlock poisoning. Lancet 1965;2:1274–5.
[36] Ball MJ, Flather ML, Forfar JC. Hemlock water dropwort poisoning. Postgrad Med J 1987;63:363–5.
[37] King LA, Lewis MJ, Parry D, et al. Identification of oenanthotoxin and related compounds in hemlock water dropwort poisoning. Hum Toxicol 1985;4:355–64.
[38] Mitchell MI, Routledge PA. Hemlock water dropwort poisoning–a review. Clin Toxicol 1978;12(4):417–26.
[39] Mutter L. Poisoning by western water hemlock. Can J Public Health 1976;67:368.
[40] Curry SC, Chang D, Conner D. Drug and toxin-induced rhabdomyolysis. Ann Emerg Med 1989;18:1068–84.
[41] Knutsen OH, Paszkowski P. New aspects in the treatment of water hemlock poisoning. Clin Toxicol 1984;22(2):157–66.
[42] Gilman A, Rall T, Nies A, et al. Goodman and Gilman's the pharmacological basis of therapeutics. New York: Macmillan Publishing Company; 1990.
[43] Langford SD, Boor PJ. Oleander toxicity: an examination of human and animal toxic exposures. Toxicology 1996;109:1–13.

[44] Shaw D, Pearn J. Oleander poisoning. Med J Aust 1979;2:267–9.

[45] Radford DJ, Gillies AD, Hinds JA, et al. Naturally occurring cardiac glycosides. Med J Aust 1986;144:539–40.

[46] Ayachi S, Brown A. Hypotensive effects of cardiac glycosides in spontaneously hypertensive rats. J Pharmacol Exp Ther 1980;213:520–4.

[47] Middleton WS, Chen KK. Clinical results from oral administration of thevetin, a cardiac glycoside. Am Heart J 1936;11:75–88.

[48] Saravanapavananthan N, Ganeshamoorthy J. Yellow oleander poisoning–study of 170 cases. Forensic Sci Int 1988;36:247–50.

[49] Haynes BE, Bessen HA, Wightman WD. Oleander tea: herbal draught of death. Ann Emerg Med 1985;14(4):350–3.

[50] Osterloh J, Herold S, Pond S. Oleander interference in the digoxin radioimmunoassay in a fatal ingestion. JAMA 1982;247:1596–7.

[51] Safadi R, Levy I, Amitai Y, et al. Beneficial effect of digoxin-specific Fab antibody fragments in oleander intoxication. Arch Intern Med 1995;155:2121–5.

[52] Clark RF, Selden B, Curry SC. Digoxin-specific Fab fragments in the treatment of oleander toxicity in a canine model. Ann Emerg Med 1991;20(10):1073–7.

[53] Shumaik G, Wu AW, Ping AC. Oleander poisoning: treatment with digoxin-specific Fab antibody fragments. Ann Emerg Med 1988;17(7):732–5.

[54] Bartell S, Anchor A. Use of digoxin-specific antibody fragments in suicidal oleander toxicity [abstract]. J Toxicol Clin Toxicol 1996;34(5):600.

[55] Lampe KF. Rhododendrons, mountain laurel, and mad honey. JAMA 1988;259(13):2009.

[56] Frohne D, Pfander HJ. A colour atlas of poisonous plants: a handbook for pharmacists, doctors, toxicologists, and biologists. London: Solfe Publishing, Ltd.; 1983.

[57] Moran NC, Dresel PE, Perkins ME, et al. The pharmacological actions of andromedotoxin, an active principle from *Rhododendron maximum*. J Pharmacol Exp Ther 1954;110: 415–32.

[58] Seyama I, Narahashi T. Modulation of sodium channels of squid nerve membranes by Grayanotoxin I. J Pharmacol Exp Ther 1981;219:614–24.

[59] Yakehiro M, Yamamoto S, Baba N, et al. Structure-activity relationship for D-ring derivatives of grayanotoxin in the squid giant axon. J Pharm Exp Toxicol 1993;265(3): 1328–32.

[60] Catterall WA. Neurotoxins that act on voltage-sensitive sodium channels in excitable membranes. Annu Rev Pharmacol Toxicol 1980;20:15–43.

[61] Masutani T, Seyama I, Narahashi T, et al. Structure-activity relationship for grayanotoxin derivatives in frog skeletal muscle. J Pharmacol Exp Ther 1981;217:812–9.

[62] Klein-Schwartz W, Litovitz T. Azalea toxicity: an overrated problem? Clin Toxicol 1985; 23(2–3):91–101.

[63] Gossinger H, Hruby K, Haubenstock A. Cardiac arrhythmias in a patient with grayanotoxin-honey poisoning. Vet Hum Toxicol 1983;25(5):328–9.

[64] Puschner B, Holstege DM, Lamberski N. Grayanotoxin poisoning in three goats. J Am Vet Med Assoc 2001;218:573–5.

[65] Narahashi T, Seyama I. Mechanism of nerve membrane depolarization caused by grayanotoxin I. J Physiol 1974;242:471–87.

[66] Heilpern KL. *Zigadenus* poisoning. Ann Emerg Med 1995;25(2):259–62.

[67] Wagstaff DJ, Case AA. Human poisoning by *Zigadenus*. Clin Toxicol 1987;25(4): 361–7.

[68] Jaffe AM, Gephardt D, Courtemanche L. Poisoning due to ingestion of *Veratrum viride* (False Hellebore). J Emerg Med 1990;8:161–7.

[69] Schmutz EM, Hamilton LB. Plants that poison. 1st edition. Flagstaff (AZ): Northland Publishing; 1979.

[70] Crummet D, Bronstein D, Weaver Z. Accidental *Veratrum viride* poisoning in three "ramp" foragers. N C Med J 1985;46(9):469–71.

[71] Pennec JP, Aubin M. Effects of aconitine and veratrine on the isolated perfused heart of the common eel (*Anguilla anguilla L.*). Comp Biochem Physiol C 1984;77(2):367–9.

[72] Fogh A, Kulling P, Wickstrom E. Veratrum alkaloids in sneezing-powder a potential danger. J Toxicol Clin Toxicol 1983;20(2):175–9.

[73] Kulig K, Rumack BH. Severe veratrum alkaloid poisoning [abstract]. Vet Hum Toxicol 1982;24(4):294.

[74] Nelson DA. Accidental poisoning by *Veratrum japonicum*. JAMA 1954;156(1):33–5.

[75] Marinov A, Koev P, Mircher N. [Electrocardiographic studies in patients with acute hellebore (Veratrum album) intoxication]. Vutr Boles 1987;26:36–9 [in Bulgarian].

[76] Quatrehomme G, Bertrand F, Chauvet C, et al. Intoxication from Veratrum album. Hum Exp Toxicol 1993;12(2):111–5.

[77] Keeler RF, Binns W. Teratogenic compounds of *Veratrum californicum* (Durand). Comparison of cyclopian effects of steroidal alkaloids from the plant and structurally related compounds from other sources. Teratology 1968;1:5–10.

[78] Chan TYK, Chan JCN, Tomlinson B, et al. Chinese herbal medicines revisited: a Hong Kong perspective. Lancet 1993;342:1532–4.

[79] Tomassoni AJ, Snook CP, McConville BJ, et al. Recreational use of delphinium–an ancient poison revisited [abstract]. J Toxicol Clin Toxicol 1996;34(5):598.

[80] Fatovich DM. Aconite: a lethal Chinese herb. Ann Emerg Med 1992;21(3):309–11.

[81] Chan TYK, Tse LKK, Chan J, et al. Aconitine poisoning due to Chinese herbal medicines: a review. Vet Hum Toxicol 1994;36(5):452–5.

[82] Adaniya H, Hayami H, Hiraoka M, et al. Effects of magnesium on polymorphic ventricular tachycardias induced by aconitine. J Cardiovasc Pharmacol 1994;24:721–9.

[83] Sawanobori T, Hirano Y, Hiraoka M. Aconitine-induced delayed afterdepolarization in frog atrium and guinea pig papillary muscles in the presence of low concentrations of Ca^{++}. Jpn J Physiol 1987;37:59–79.

[84] Leichter D, Danilo P, Boyden P, et al. A canine model of torsade de pointes. Pacing & Clinical Electrophysiology 1988;11:2235–45.

[85] Tai YT, But PPH, Young K, et al. Cardiotoxicity after accidental herb-induced aconite poisoning. Lancet 1992;340:1254–6.

[86] Tai YT, Lau CP, But PP, et al. Bidirectional tachycardia induced by herbal aconite poisoning. Pacing Clin Electrophysiol 1992;15:831–9.

[87] Chan TYK. Aconitine poisoning: a global perspective. Vet Hum Toxicol 1994;36(4):326–8.

[88] Chan TYK, Critchley JAJH. The spectrum of poisonings in Hong Kong: an overview. Vet Hum Toxicol 1994;36(2):135–7.

[89] Tai YT, Lau CP, But PPH. Three fatal cases of herbal aconite poisoning. Vet Hum Toxicol 1994;36(3):212–5.

[90] Chan TYK. Aconitine poisoning following the ingestion of Chinese herbal medicines: a report of eight cases. Aust N Z J Med 1993;23:268–71.

[91] Dickens P, Tai YT, But PPH, et al. Fatal accidental aconitine poisoning following ingestion of Chinese herbal medicine: a report of two cases. Forensic Sci Int 1994;67:55–8.

[92] Yeih DF, Chiang FT, Huang SK. Successful treatment of aconitine induced life threatening ventricular tachyarrhythmia with amiodarone. Heart 2000;84(4):E8.

[93] Jackman WM, Friday KJ, Anderson JL, et al. The long QT syndrome: a critical review, new clinical observations and a unifying hypothesis. Prog Cardiovasc Dis 1988;31(2):115–72.

[94] Kunkel DB. Tobacco and friends. Emerg Med 1985;142–58.

[95] Domino E, Hornbach E, Demana T. The nicotine content of common vegetables. N Engl J Med 1993;329(6):437.

[96] Drummer OH, Roberts AN, Bedford PJ, et al. Three deaths from hemlock poisoning. Med J Aust 1995;162:592–3.

[97] McGehee DS, Heath MJS, Gelber S, et al. Nicotine enhancement of fast excitatory synaptic transmission in CNS by presynaptic receptors. Science 1995;269:1692–6.

[98] Hipke ME. Green tobacco sickness. South Med J 1993;86(9):989–92.

[99] Litovitz TL, Normann SA, Veltri JC. 1985 annual report of the American Association of Poison Control Centers National Data Collection System. Am J Emerg Med 1986;4(5): 427–58.

[100] Smolinske SC, Spoerke DG, Spiller SK, et al. Cigarette and nicotine chewing gum toxicity in children. Hum Toxicol 1988;7:27–31.

[101] Curry S, Bond R, Kunkel D. Acute nicotine poisonings after ingestions of tree tobacco. Vet Hum Toxicol 1988;30(4):369.

[102] Mellick LB, Makowski T, Mellick GA, et al. Neuromuscular blockade after ingestion of tree tobacco (Nicotiana glauca). Ann Emerg Med 1999;34(1):101–4.

[103] Frank BS, Michelson WB, Panter KE, et al. Ingestion of poison hemlock (Conium maculatum). West J Med 1995;163:573–4.

[104] Foster PF, McFadden R, Trevino R, et al. Successful transplantation of donor organs from a hemlock poisoning victim. Transplantation 2003;76(5):874–6.

[105] Watson WA, Litovitz TL, Rodgers GC Jr, et al. 2002 annual report of the American Association of Poison Control Centers Toxic Exposure Surveillance System. Am J Emerg Med 2003;21(5):353–421.

[106] Taylor RFH, Al-Jarad N, John LME, et al. Betel-nut chewing and asthma. Lancet 1992; 339:1134–6.

[107] Rizzi D, Basile C, Di Maggio A, et al. Rhabdomyolysis and acute tubular necrosis in coniine (hemlock) poisoning [letter]. Lancet 1989;2:1461–2.

[108] Scatizzi A, Di Maggio A, Rizzi D, et al. Acute renal failure due to tubular necrosis caused by waildfoul-mediated hemlock poisoning. Ren Fail 1993;15(1):93–6.

[109] Baselt RC, Cravey RH. Disposition of toxic drugs and chemicals in man. Foster City (CA): Chemical Toxicology Institued; 1995.

[110] Cromwell BT. The separation, micro-estimation and distribution of the alkaloids of hemlock (Conium maculatum L.). Biochem J 1956;64:259–66.

[111] Levy R. Jimson seed poisoning–a new hallucinogen on the horizon. JACEP 1977;6(2): 58–61.

[112] Michalodimitrakis M. Discussion of "Datura stramonium: a fatal poisoning". J Forensic Sci 1984;29:961–2.

[113] Ulrich RW, Bowerman DL, Levisky JA, et al. Datura stramonium: a fatal poisoning. J Forensic Sci 1982;27(4):948–54.

[114] Smith EA, Meloan CE, Pickell JA, et al. Scopolamine poisoning from homemade "Moon Flower" wine. J Anal Toxicol 1991;15(4):216–9.

[115] Ramakrishnan SS. Pitfalls in the treatment of Jimson weed intoxication. Am J Psychiatry 1994;151(9):1396–7.

[116] Hanna JP, Schmidley JW, Braselton WE. Datura delirium. Clin Neuropharmacol 1992; 15(2):109–13.

[117] Litovitz TL, Clark LR, Soloway RA. 1993 annual report of the American Association of Poison Control Centers Toxic Exposure Surveillance System. Am J Emerg Med 1994; 12(5):546–84.

[118] Pentel P, Peterson C. Asystole complicating physostigmine treatment of tricyclic antidepressant overdose. Ann Emerg Med 1980;9:588–90.

[119] Waxdal MJ. Isolation, characterization, and biological activities of five mitogens from pokeweed. Biochemistry 1974;13(18):3671–7.

[120] Hur Y, Hwang DJ, Zoubenko O, et al. Isolation and characterization of pokeweed antiviral protein mutations in Saccharomyces cerevisiae: identification of residues important for toxicity. Proc Natl Acad Sci U S A 1995;92:8448–52.

[121] Lewis WH, Smith PR. Poke root herbal tea poisoning. JAMA 1979;242(25):2759–60.

[122] Farnes P, Barker BE, Brownhill LE. Mitogenic activity in *Phytolacca americana* (pokeweed). Lancet 1964;2:1100.

[123] Barker BE, Farnes P, LaMarche PH. Peripheral blood plasmacytosis following systemic exposure to Phytolacca americana (Pokeweed). Pediatr 1966;38:490–3.

[124] Barker BE, Farnes P, LaMarche PH. Haematological effects of pokeweed [letter]. Lancet 1967;38:437.

[125] Litovitz TL, Felberg L, White S, et al. 1995 annual report of the American Association of Poison Control Centers Toxic Exposure Surveillance System. Am J Emerg Med 1996;14(5): 487–537.

[126] Goldfrank L, Kirstein R. The feast. Hosp Physician 1976;12(8):34–8.

[127] Kell SO, Rosenberg SA, Conlon TJ, et al. A peek at poke: mitogenicity and epidemiology. Vet HumToxicol 1982;24(4):294.

[128] CDC. Plant poisonings–New Jersey. MMWR Morb Mortal Wkly Rep 1981;30(6): 65–7.

[129] Edwards N. Pokeberry pancake breakfast-or-it's gonna be a great day. Vet Hum Toxicol 1982;(Suppl):135–8.

[130] Jaeckle KA, Freemon FR. Pokeweed poisoning. South Med J 1981;74(5):639–40.

[131] Stein ZLG. Pokeweed-induced gastroenteritis. Am J Hosp Pharm 1979;36:1303.

[132] Hamilton RJ, Shih RD, Hoffman RS. Mobitz type I heart block after pokeweed ingestion. Vet Hum Toxicol 1995;37(1):66–7.

[133] Roberge R, Brader E, Martin M, et al. The root of evil–pokeweed intoxication. Ann Emerg Med 1986;15(4):470–3.

[134] Litovitz TL, Klein-Schwartz W, White S, et al. 2000 Annual report of the American Association of Poison Control Centers Toxic Exposure Surveillance System. Am J Emerg Med 2001;19(5):337–95.

[135] Symes WF, Dawson CR. Separation and structural determination of the olefinic components of poison ivy urushiol, cardanol and cardol. Nature 1953;171(4358):841–2.

[136] Baer H. Chemistry and immunochemistry of poisonous Anacardiaceae. Clin Dermatol 1986;4(2):152–9.

[137] Baer H, Watkins RC, Kurtz AP, et al. Delayed contact sensitivity to catechols. 3. The relationship of side-chain length to sensitizing potency of catechols chemically related to the active principles of poison ivy. J Immunol 1967;99(2):370–5.

[138] Baer RL. Poison ivy dermatitis. Cutis 1986;37(6):434–6.

[139] Fisher AA. The notorious poison ivy family of Anacardiaceae plants. Cutis 1977;20(5): 570–82.

[140] Gayer KD, Burnett JW. Toxicodendron dermatitis. Cutis 1988;42(2):99–100.

[141] Munson JR. A medical history of poison ivy (Rhus toxicodendron). Trans Stud Coll Physicians Phila 1966;34(1):26–32.

[142] Sanders SH, Taub SJ. Contact dermatitis due to poison ivy, oak, and sumac. Eye Ear Nose Throat Mon 1965;44(10):99–100.

[143] Peterson WC Jr. Poison ivy (Rhus dermatitis). Minn Med 1968;51(5):671–2.

[144] Guin JD. Poison ivy (Rhus) dermatitis. J Indiana State Med Assoc 1978;71(8):774–5.

[145] Resnick SD. Poison-ivy and poison-oak dermatitis. Clin Dermatol 1986;4(2):208–12.

[146] Baer RL. Poison ivy dermatitis. Cutis 1990;46(1):34–6.

[147] Fisher AA. Poison ivy/oak/sumac. Part II: specific features. Cutis 1996;58(1):22–4.

[148] Gladman AC. Toxicodendron dermatitis: poison ivy, oak, and sumac. Wilderness Environ Med 2006;17(2):120–8.

[149] Corbett MD, Billets S. Characterization of poison oak urushiol. J Pharm Sci 1975;64(10): 1715–8.

[150] Craig JC, Waller CW, Billets S, et al. New GLC analysis of urushiol congeners in different plant parts of poison ivy, Toxicodendron radicans. J Pharm Sci 1978;67(4):483–5.

[151] Murphy JC, Watson ES, Harland EC. Toxicological evaluation of poison oak urushiol and its esterified derivative. Toxicology 1983;26(2):135–42.

[152] Guin JD. The black spot test for recognizing poison ivy and related species. J Am Acad Dermatol 1980;2(4):332–3.

[153] Hershko K, Weinberg I, Ingber A. Exploring the mango-poison ivy connection: the riddle of discriminative plant dermatitis. Contact Dermatitis 2005;52(1):3–5.

[154] Knight TE, Boll P, Epstein WL, et al. Resorcinols and catechols: a clinical study of cross-sensitivity. Am J Contact Dermat 1996;7(3):138–45.

[155] Pahwa R, Chatterjee VC. The toxicity of yellow oleander (*Thevetia neriifolia juss*) seed kernels to rats. Vet Hum Toxicol 1990;32(6):561–4.

[156] Peate WE. Occupational skin disease. Am Fam Physician 2002;66(6):1025–32.

[157] Guin JD, Gillis WT, Beaman JH. Recognizing the Toxicodendrons (poison ivy, poison oak, and poison sumac). J Am Acad Dermatol 1981;4(1):99–114.

[158] Lee NP, Arriola ER. Poison ivy, oak, and sumac dermatitis. West J Med 1999;171(5–6): 354–5.

[159] McGovern TW, LaWarre SR, Brunette C. Is it, or isn't it? Poison ivy look-a-likes. Am J Contact Dermat 2000;11(2):104–10.

[160] Allen PLJ. Leaves of three, let them be: if it were only that easy! [Erratum in: Pediatr Nurs 2004 May–Jun;30(3):249]. Pediatr Nurs 2004;30(2):129–35.

[161] Godfrey HP, Baer H, Watkins RC. Delayed hypersensitivity to catechols. V. Absorption and distribution of substances related to poison ivy extracts and their relation to the induction of sensitization and tolerance. J Immunol 1971;106(1):91–102.

[162] Byers VS, Castagnoli N Jr, Epstein WL. In vitro studies of poison oak immunity. II. Effect of urushiol analogues on the human in vitro response. J Clin Invest 1979;64(5):1449–56.

[163] Byers VS, Epstein WL, Castagnoli N, et al. In vitro studies of poison oak immunity. I. In vitro reaction of human lymphocytes to urushiol. J Clin Invest 1979;64(5):1437–48.

[164] Lepoittevin JP, Benezra C. Saturated analogues of poison ivy allergens. Synthesis of trans, trans- and cis, trans-3-alkyl-1,2-cyclohexanediols and sensitizing properties in allergic contact dermatitis. J Med Chem 1986;29(2):287–91.

[165] Dunn IS, Liberato DJ, Castagnoli N Jr, et al. Influence of chemical reactivity of urushiol-type haptens on sensitization and the induction of tolerance. Cell Immunol 1986;97(1): 189–96.

[166] Kalergis AM, Lopez CB, Becker MI, et al. Modulation of fatty acid oxidation alters contact hypersensitivity to urushiols: role of aliphatic chain beta-oxidation in processing and activation of urushiols. J Invest Dermatol 1997;108(1):57–61.

[167] Baer H, Watkins RC, Kurtz AP, et al. Delayed contact sensitivity to catechols. II. Cutaneous toxicity of catechols chemically related to the active principles of poison ivy. J Immunol 1967;99(2):365–9.

[168] Kalish RS, Morimoto C. Urushiol (poison ivy)-triggered suppressor T cell clone generated from peripheral blood. J Clin Invest 1988;82(3):825–32.

[169] Kalish RS, Morimoto C. Quantitation and cloning of human urushiol specific peripheral blood T-cells: isolation of urushiol triggered suppressor T-cells. J Invest Dermatol 1989; 92(1):46–52.

[170] Kalish RS, Johnson KL. Enrichment and function of urushiol (poison ivy)-specific T lymphocytes in lesions of allergic contact dermatitis to urushiol. J Immunol 1990;145(11): 3706–13.

[171] Kalish RS. Recent developments in the pathogenesis of allergic contact dermatitis. Arch Dermatol 1991;127(10):1558–63.

[172] Kalish RS, Wood JA, LaPorte A. Processing of urushiol (poison ivy) hapten by both endogenous and exogenous pathways for presentation to T cells in vitro. J Clin Invest 1994;93(5):2039–47.

[173] Kalish RS, Wood JA. Induction of hapten-specific tolerance of human CD8+ urushiol (poison ivy)-reactive T lymphocytes. J Invest Dermatol 1997;108(3):253–7.

[174] Enk AH, Katz SI. Early molecular events in the induction phase of contact sensitivity. Proc Natl Acad Sci U S A 1992;89(4):1398–402.

[175] Grabbe S, Schwarz T. Immunoregulatory mechanisms involved in elicitation of allergic contact hypersensitivity. Am J Contact Dermat 1996;7(4):238–46.

[176] Grabbe S, Schwarz T. Immunoregulatory mechanisms involved in elicitation of allergic contact hypersensitivity [see comment]. Immunol Today 1998;19(1):37–44.

[177] Wakabayashi T, Hu D-L, Tagawa Y-I, et al. IFN-gamma and TNF-alpha are involved in urushiol-induced contact hypersensitivity in mice. Immunol Cell Biol 2005;83(1):18–24.

[178] Kollef MH. Adult respiratory distress syndrome after smoke inhalation from burning poison ivy. JAMA 1995;274(4):358–9.

[179] Parker GF, Logan PC. Poison ivy (Rhus) dermatitis. Am Fam Physician 1972;6(1):62–6.

[180] Guin JD. Treatment of toxicodendron dermatitis (poison ivy and poison oak). Skin Therapy Lett 2001;6(7):3–5.

[181] Zafren K. Poison oak dermatitis. Wilderness Environ Med 2001;12(1):39–40.

[182] Kurlan JG, Lucky AW. Black spot poison ivy: a report of 5 cases and a review of the literature. J Am Acad Dermatol 2001;45(2):246–9.

[183] Mallory SB, Miller OFd, Tyler WB. Toxicodendron radicans dermatitis with black lacquer deposit on the skin. J Am Acad Dermatol 1982;6(3):363–8.

[184] Hurwitz RM, Rivera HP, Guin JD. Black-spot poison ivy dermatitis. An acute irritant contact dermatitis superimposed upon an allergic contact dermatitis. Am J Dermatopathol 1984;6(4):319–22.

[185] Cohen LM, Cohen JL. Erythema multiforme associated with contact dermatitis to poison ivy: three cases and a review of the literature. Cutis 1998;62(3):139–42.

[186] Schwartz RS, Downham TF 2nd. Erythema multiforme associated with Rhus contact dermatitis. Cutis 1981;27(1):85–6.

[187] Werchniak AE, Schwarzenberger K. Poison ivy: an underreported cause of erythema multiforme [Erratum in: J Am Acad Dermatol 2004 Dec;51(6):1040]. J Am Acad Dermatol 2004;51(5 Suppl):S159–60.

[188] Devich KB, Lee JC, Epstein WL, et al. Renal lesions accompanying poison oak dermatitis. Clin Nephrol 1975;3(3):106–13.

[189] Brook I. Secondary bacterial infections complicating skin lesions. J Med Microbiol 2002;51(10):808–12.

[190] Brook I, Frazier EH, Yeager JK. Microbiology of infected poison ivy dermatitis. Br J Dermatol 2000;142(5):943–6.

[191] Oh S-H, Haw C-R, Lee M-H. Clinical and immunologic features of systemic contact dermatitis from ingestion of Rhus (Toxicodendron). Contact Dermatitis 2003;48(5):251–4.

[192] Park SD, Lee SW, Chun JH, et al. Clinical features of 31 patients with systemic contact dermatitis due to the ingestion of Rhus (lacquer). Br J Dermatol 2000;142(5):937–42.

[193] Rietschel RL. Contact dermatitis and diagnostic techniques. Allergy Proc 1989;10(6):403–11.

[194] Rosenstreich DL. Evaluation of delayed hypersensitivity: from PPD to poison ivy. Allergy Proc 1993;14(6):395–400.

[195] Fisher AA. Poison ivy/oak dermatitis. Part I: prevention–soap and water, topical barriers, hyposensitization. Cutis 1996;57(6):384–6.

[195a] Anderson BE, Marks JG Jr, Mauger DT. Efficacy of tacrolimus ointment in the prevention and treatment of contact dermatitis. Dermatitis 2004;15:158–9.

[196] Epstein WL, Baer H, Dawson CR, et al. Poison oak hyposensitization. Evaluation of purified urushiol. Arch Dermatol 1974;109(3):356–60.

[197] Epstein WL, Byers VS, Frankart W. Induction of antigen specific hyposensitization to poison oak in sensitized adults. Arch Dermatol 1982;118(9):630–3.

[198] Marks JG Jr, Trautlein JJ, Epstein WL, et al. Oral hyposensitization to poison ivy and poison oak. Arch Dermatol 1987;123(4):476–8.

[199] Grevelink SA, Murrell DF, Olsen EA. Effectiveness of various barrier preparations in preventing and/or ameliorating experimentally produced Toxicodendron dermatitis. J Am Acad Dermatol 1992;27(2 Pt 1):182–8.

[200] Marks JG Jr, Fowler JF Jr, Sheretz EF, et al. Prevention of poison ivy and poison oak allergic contact dermatitis by quaternium-18 bentonite. J Am Acad Dermatol 1995;33 (2 Pt 1):212–6.

[201] Knight TE. Philodendron-induced dermatitis: report of cases and review of the literature. Cutis 1991;48(5):375–8.

[202] Arditti J, Rodriguez E. Dieffenbachia: uses, abuses and toxic constituents: a review. J Ethnopharmacol 1982;5(3):293–302.

[203] Rauber A. Observations on the idioblasts of Dieffenbachia. J Toxicol Clin Toxicol 1985; 23(2–3):79–90.

[204] Cumpston KL, Vogel SN, Leikin JB, et al. Acute airway compromise after brief exposure to a Dieffenbachia plant. J Emerg Med 2003;25(4):391–7.

[205] Hesse A, Siener R, Heynck H, et al. The influence of dietary factors on the risk of urinary stone formation. Scanning Microsc 1993;7(3):1119–27 [discussion: 27–8].

[206] Massey LK. Dietary influences on urinary oxalate and risk of kidney stones. Front Biosci 2003;8:s584–94.

[207] Massey LK, Roman-Smith H, Sutton RA. Effect of dietary oxalate and calcium on urinary oxalate and risk of formation of calcium oxalate kidney stones. J Am Diet Assoc 1993;93(8): 901–6.

[208] Mrvos R, Dean BS, Krenzelok EP. Philodendron/dieffenbachia ingestions: are they a problem? J Toxicol Clin Toxicol 1991;29(4):485–91.

[209] Gardner DG. Injury to the oral mucous membranes caused by the common houseplant, dieffenbachia. A review. Oral Surg Oral Med Oral Pathol 1994;78(5):631–3.

[210] Watson JT, Jones RC, Siston AM, et al. Outbreak of food-borne illness associated with plant material containing raphides. Clin Toxicol (Phila) 2005;43(1):17–21.

[211] Salinas ML, Ogura T, Soffchi L. Irritant contact dermatitis caused by needle-like calcium oxalate crystals, raphides, in Agave tequilana among workers in tequila distilleries and agave plantations. Contact Dermatitis 2001;44(2):94–6.

[212] Chiou AG, Cadez R, Bohnke M. Diagnosis of Dieffenbachia induced corneal injury by confocal microscopy. Br J Ophthalmol 1997;81(2):168–9.

[213] Robb H. Death from rhubarb leaves due to oxalic acid poisoning. JAMA 1919;73:627–8.

[214] Jacobziner H, Raybin HW. Rhubarb poisoning. N Y State J Med 1962;62:1676–8.

[215] McIntire MS, Guest JR, Porterfield JF. Philodendron—an infant death. J Toxicol Clin Toxicol 1990;28(2):177–83.

[216] Snajdauf J, Mixa V, Rygl M, et al. Aortoesophageal fistula—an unusual complication of esophagitis caused by Dieffenbachia ingestion. J Pediatr Surg 2005;40(6):e29–31.

ELSEVIER
SAUNDERS

EMERGENCY
MEDICINE
CLINICS OF
NORTH AMERICA

Emerg Med Clin N Am 25 (2007) 435–457

Herbal Drugs of Abuse: An Emerging Problem

William H. Richardson III, MD[a,b,*], Cheryl M. Slone, MD[a], Jill E. Michels, PharmD[b]

[a]Department of Emergency Medicine, Palmetto Health Richland,
3 Medical Park, Columbia, SC 29203, USA
[b]Palmetto Poison Center, South Carolina College of Pharmacy,
University of South Carolina, Columbia, SC 29208, USA

An herb is defined as a plant grown for culinary, medicinal, or in some cases spiritual value. In botanic terms, an herb is a plant not producing a woody stem [1]. There are many recognized, and some probably not-yet-identified, plants and herbs with hallucinogenic properties containing various psychoactive chemicals. Recreational abuse of certain plants can produce a spectrum of clinical effects often overlapping between psychedelic, stimulant, sedative, euphoric, and anticholinergic symptoms. Health care professionals need to be familiar with the emerging recreational use of certain plants and herbal supplements and recognize the potential toxicity and abuse potential of many of these products (Table 1).

It is difficult to quantify the extent of herbal recreational abuse in the United States. Statistical analysis of illegal drug abuse and herbal supplement use may provide a perspective of the problem. An estimated 19.1 million Americans (aged 12 and older) report using an illicit drug during the previous month as reported by the 2004 National Survey on Drug Use and Health. This represents a 7.9% overall rate of current illicit drug use by Americans in 2004 [2]. The Drug Abuse Warning Network reports that almost 2 million emergency department (ED) visits, from an estimated 106 million total ED visits in the United States in 2004, were drug related. Drug misuse or abuse of illicit drugs and pharmaceutics was responsible for 1.3 million of these cases [3].

* Corresponding author. Palmetto Poison Center, South Carolina College of Pharmacy, University of South Carolina, Columbia, SC 29208.
E-mail address: whrichardson@sc.rr.com (W.H. Richardson).

0733-8627/07/$ - see front matter © 2007 Elsevier Inc. All rights reserved.
doi:10.1016/j.emc.2007.02.009
emed.theclinics.com

Table 1
Herbal drugs of abuse

Common name	Active ingredient	Primary abuse potential
Salvia divinorum	Salvinorin A	Hallucinogen
Morning glory	LSA (lysergic acid hydroxyethylamide)	Hallucinogen
Hawaiian baby woodrose	LSA	Hallucinogen
Nutmeg	Myristicin, elemicin	Hallucinogen
Peyote	Mescaline	Hallucinogen
Ayahuasca	DMT (N,N-dimethyltryptamine)	Hallucinogen
Jimsonweed	Atropine, scopolamine, hyoscyamine	Hallucinogen, anticholinergic
Ma-huang	Ephedra alkaloids	Stimulant
Khat	Cathinone, cathine	Stimulant
Betel nut	Arecoline	Stimulant
Yohimbe	Yohimbine	Stimulant, hallucinogen
Guarana	Caffeine, xanthine alkaloids	Stimulant
Absinthe	Thujone	Euphoric, hallucinogen
Kava	Kavalactones	Anxiolytic
Cloves	Eugenol, nicotine	Analgesic, stimulant

Herbal dietary supplement use has increased dramatically in the United States during the last decade. Previously, the Federal Food, Drug, and Cosmetic (FD&C) Act of 1938 formed the legal basis for the US Food and Drug Administration (FDA) to have authority over food and food ingredients and defined requirements for truthful labeling of ingredients. The Food Additives Amendment to the FD&C Act passed in 1958 requiring FDA approval for the use of a food additive, including dietary supplements. The amendment additionally required a manufacturer to prove an additive's safety for its recommended use. The Dietary Supplement Health and Education Act passed in 1994 served to reduce the FDA oversight and premarket safety evaluation of dietary supplements [4]. As a result, food supplements of the herbal industry have become largely unregulated. Herbal supplement use in adults was reported to increase from 2.5% in 1993 to 12.1% in 1997 [5]. A survey of 1898 high-school adolescents in New York reported that 28.6% of students used herbal products at some point in their lifetime [6]. Increased on-line marketing and subsequent availability have culminated in a steady growth of herbal supplement sales. Sales of herbal dietary agents in the United States have grown from approximately $2 billion annually in 1994 to more than $4.4 billion in 2005 [7]. With this growth and popularity, recreational abuse of certain herbal dietary supplements has emerged as a serious problem, especially among adolescents and young adults. The legality and lack of regulation of herbal products, many with psychotropic, stimulant, and euphoric effects, has resulted in teenagers seeking an alternative "legal high" to illicit drugs of abuse. Internet advertising and on-line sales have become profitable techniques for marketing and distribution of many herbal drugs of abuse. In one study identifying 28 Web sites marketing dietary supplements for recreational use, 47% of dietary supplements on these sites appealed to the recreational drug user by comparing the effects of the herbal products to marijuana, ecstasy, lysergic acid diethylamide, cocaine, speed, and mushrooms. Seventy-nine percent of products were advertised claiming to be hallucinogens, stimulants, euphoria-producing, or sedatives. Most on-line suppliers were United States–based Web sites; however, all foreign Web sites included statements verifying shipping to the United States [8]. Some Web sites even continue to market ephedra-containing products despite the April 2004 FDA prohibition of the sale of dietary supplements containing ephedrine alkaloids [9].

Another consideration for many plant and herbal drug abusers is the perception that these legal alternatives are safer. Ephedra, marketed as a safe herbal weight-loss stimulant, was associated with significant adverse effects, including cerebrovascular accidents, seizures, cardiac arrhythmias, myocardial infarction, and death before its 2004 prohibition by the FDA [10,11]. Adverse effects were reported in the setting of manufacturer-recommended dosages, interaction with other medications, and abuse. There is little information assessing safety of manufacturer-recommended dosing of most herbal supplements, and significant safety concerns should exist with recreational use of these substances. Much of the medical literature describing abuse of herbal supplements is anecdotal, and the short- and long-term effects of abuse may be largely unrecognized.

Appealing to many users is the knowledge that most plant and herbal drugs of abuse are not detected on routine urine drug screens. The National Institute of Drug Abuse 5 includes the five most commonly tested-for drugs and those recommended for drug screening of federal employees: amphetamines, cannabinoids, cocaine, opiates, and phencyclidine. Other immunoassays may detect benzodiazepines, barbiturates, methadone, and propoxyphene. Certain amphetamine-like sympathomimetics, such as ephedrine-containing ma huang and cathinone-containing khat, could be detected on an amphetamine screen (dependent on immunoassay sensitivity and timing of use) but not specifically identified without additional qualitative testing. Most herbal supplements, however, are not detected with routine drug screening. Also, claims of common false positive immunoassay test results following use of common herbal supplements have not been validated [12,13].

Hallucinogens

Salvia divinorum

Salvia is a genus of more than 900 plants used for folk medicine, culinary purposes, and decorative foliage [14]. *Salvia divinorum*, a perennial herb from the mint family (*Lamiaceae*), was historically used for ceremonial purposes by the Mazatec Indians in Oaxaca, Mexico [15]. The plant grows to more than 3 feet tall with hollow square stems and large green leaves.

S divinorum is native to the Sierra Mazateca region of Mexico but is now grown domestically in the United States and imported from Central and South America. The plant has gained popularity since the mid-1990s as a recreational hallucinogen with various on-line botanic companies advertising it as a legal high. *S divinorum*, sometimes referred to as "Magic Mint," "Shepherdess's Herb," "Ska Maria Pastora," or "Sally-D," is widely available on the Internet and in certain tobacco shops, head shops, and herbal remedy stores. Marketing and promotion of *Salvia* as a legal alternative on Internet sites has increased the popularity and encouraged experimentation. On-line shoppers can purchase dried leaves, extract, seeds, or whole plants with prices, depending on concentration, ranging from $20 to $50 per gram. Smoking a concentrated extract is a preferred route of administration with users describing an intense, 15-minute, short-lived period of modified perception of external reality at doses of 200 to 500 μg [16]. Oral absorption following ingestion of the leaves or seeds of the plant produces a longer but less intense effect. The active ingredient, salvinorin-A, is a psychotropic neoclerodane diterpene and potent kappa opioid receptor agonist [17]. Kappa receptors are a subset of opioid receptors responsible for spinal and supraspinal analgesia, miosis, and psychotomimetic effects. Unlike many psychoactive drugs, salvinorin-A does not have $5\text{-}HT_{2A}$ serotoninergic activity [18]. Users, most commonly adolescents and young adults, describe profound hallucinogenic experiences similar to those induced by psilocybin, mescaline, and ketamine. Although monitored for emerging abuse potential, the US Drug Enforcement Administration (DEA) does not list this plant or its active ingredient in the Controlled Substances Act of scheduled chemicals [19]. The primary cause of morbidity associated with the use or abuse of *S divinorum* occurs from contaminated preparations or settings in which the intoxicating effects lead to accidents and injury [15]. Routine urine drug screening does not detect the use of this plant. Patients who develop mild anxiety may benefit from calm reassurance in a quiet environment. More severe reactions or agitation can be treated with benzodiazepines.

Lysergamide-containing plants

Lysergamides are a class of hallucinogens including LSD (D-lysergic acid diethylamide) and LSA (lysergic acid hydroxyethylamide). With LSD, a potent psychoactive chemical, a dose of 25 μg is capable of producing effects. LSD is not found in nature, but LSA, an analogue that is one-tenth as potent, exists naturally. LSA is a tryptamine found in the seeds of *Ipomoea violacea* (morning glory) and *Argyreia nervosa* (Hawaiian baby woodrose). $5\text{-}HT_{2A}$ receptor agonism likely contributes to hallucinogenic effects, but a complete neurochemical understanding of these psychedelic substances has not been elucidated.

Morning glory seeds, known as tlitlitzin, were traditionally used in Aztec rituals in ancient Mexico. In the 1960s, popularity increased when the seeds were used as a substitute for LSD. Seeds are taken orally, and doses may consist of pulverized seeds or an extract of the psychoactive alkaloids. A seed coat prevents drug absorption so the seeds must be chewed or pulverized before ingestion. Threshold effects are noted with ingestion of 25 to 50 seeds. Visual imagery and hallucinations are prominent following ingestion of 150 to 200 seeds (3–6 g), whereas dosages of 200 to 500 seeds produce intense hallucinations in addition to nausea, vomiting, and abdominal pain [20]. When taken on an empty gastrointestinal tract, hallucinogenic effects may occur within 1 hour of ingestion and can last for 6 to 10 hours. Although LSA is included as a schedule III substance by the DEA, morning glory seeds and plants are sold in most nurseries and botanic supply stores. Although possession of seeds for horticultural intent is legal, possession of extracts of lysergic acid or of pulverized morning glory seeds is illegal. Commercial morning glory seed producers treat the seeds with emetic agents in an attempt to discourage recreational ingestion [20].

Hawaiian baby woodrose is a perennial vine native to India and has derived its name because it grows prolifically in Hawaii where it has been historically used by Polynesians as a hallucinogen. The filtrate of these seeds was also used in religious and healing ceremonies by the Aztecs and later Native Americans but was recreationally used around 1965 when the seeds became available for purchase in head shops [21]. The plant contains LSA in large seeds surrounded by pods. These seeds are widely and legally available on the Internet with prices ranging from $5 to $20 for 100 seeds, although many Web sites mention that seeds are not for human consumption. By comparison, *A nervosa* contains 0.14% of LSA by dry weight of seeds versus 0.02% in *I violacea* seeds [22,23].

After being soaked in water, the seeds can be crushed, eaten whole, germinated, or consumed as an extract. Ingesting 5 to 10 seeds produces psychedelic effects similar to morning glory seeds, with effects beginning within 60 minutes and lasting 5 to 8 hours. Hallucinogenic effects occur with doses of 2 to 5 mg of LSA [15]. Sympathomimetic effects, such as tachycardia, hypertension, and mydriasis, are reported [21]. Primary treatment includes protection, reassurance, and sensory isolation, with use of benzodiazepines to blunt hallucinogenic-related agitation and sympathomimetic effects [24]. Routine urine drug immunoassays do not detect LSD or LSA. High-performance liquid chromatography or gas chromatography can confirm exposure, but these are rarely used in the acute clinical setting.

Nutmeg

Nutmeg is a product of the evergreen tree *Myristica fragrans* indigenous to the Spice Islands. The fruits of the tree look like peaches or apricots but when split open yield a single brown kernel, the nutmeg. The covering of the nutmeg, the net-like red aril, is used to produce mace. Nutmeg was used for centuries in Europe as a snuff [25]. Its various unproven clinical uses include treatment of gastrointestinal disorders, musculoskeletal problems, and psychiatric conditions. Although nutmeg has a long history of abuse, today it is imported into the United States where it is primarily used to spice baked goods and Christmas drinks. Large ingestions and periodic misuse are seen in adolescents or young adults in an attempt to achieve a euphoric or nutmeg narcosis effect. Still, nutmeg abuse is uncommon, likely a result of the unpalatable and undesirable emetic effects from doses needed to achieve the intended mental state [26]. Although nutmeg has a high incidence of unpleasant side effects, it is preferred by some users in search of a legal and easily obtainable euphoric drug with hallucinogenic effects. Presently, nutmeg is legal to buy, possess, and sell in the United States. A recent case series of 17 exposures involving nutmeg ingestion called to Texas poison centers from 1998 to 2004 reported more than 64% of these cases involved intentional abuse. No major effects were reported in this case series and most patients were managed outside of a health care facility [27]. Significant adverse effects and even death have been reported, however [28].

The psychotomimetic effects of nutmeg are caused by alkyl benzene derivatives (myristicin, elemicin, and safrole) and terpenes. The exact mechanism of central nervous system effects is not completely understood, but myristicin, a component of nutmeg oil with weak monoamine oxidase–inhibiting properties, was initially believed to be the active ingredient. A dose of myristicin twice that of a 20-g dose of nutmeg was shown to produce only mild clinical effects, however [29]. Myristicin and elemicin may be metabolized to amphetamine-like compounds similar to methoxymethylene-dioxyamphetamine (MMDA) and trimethoxyamphetamine, respectively. These and other active components (eugenol, borneol, and linalol) likely combine to produce psychotropic and sympathomimetic effects [26,30].

Ground nutmeg is ingested in 5- to 20-g doses (approximately 2 tablespoons of powder), either alone or in a paste with other ingredients designed to make the dose more palatable. Consuming large quantities of nutmeg may be difficult but can produce severe clinical and psychologic effects. Most users develop nausea and vomiting within an hour of ingestion, followed by central nervous system (CNS) intoxication and hallucinations 3 to 8 hours after ingestion. Undesirable effects include blurred vision, dizziness, drowsiness, xerostomia, flushing, palpitations, paresthesias, numbness, hypotension, and tachycardia. Desired effects may include euphoria, giddiness, and hallucinations (visual, auditory, and tactile) [26]. The primary effects of nutmeg are long lasting (up to 24 hours) and secondary effects can continue for 72 hours. One Internet blogger describes a "two day hangover" with lingering drowsiness, myalgias, depression, and headaches following nutmeg abuse [31].

There is no specific antidote for nutmeg poisoning. Symptomatic and supportive care is required to treat nausea and vomiting, agitation, hallucinations, and to address any sympathomimetic effects. Anticholinergic toxicity is occasionally suspected on initial presentation; however, physostigmine is not indicated, and most patients recover uneventfully. Myristicin is not detected on routine drug-of-abuse screens, but amphetamine-like metabolites of nutmeg's active components could theoretically cross-react in an immunoassay.

Peyote

Peyote (*Lophophora williamsii*) is a spineless cactus that grows on dry rocky slopes of the southwestern United States and northern Mexico. Archeological evidence suggests that peyote has been used by North American tribes for thousands of years. From a planted seed, 2 or more years are usually required for the plant to mature and flower. A peyote button is the 1- to 4-inch diameter top portion of the cactus that is harvested and dried. The buttons can be harvested repeatedly, and new ones will subsequently sprout. The buttons may be eaten fresh or dried, steeped, or ground into a powder [15]. Because of the acrid taste, some users disguise the powder in a gelatin capsule, use the tea as an enema, or smoke the powder with other substances [32]. A typical dose is 6 to 12 buttons taken orally, with each button containing approximately 1% to 6%, or 45 mg, mescaline. Larger doses can produce more sympathomimetic effects [33].

Mescaline (trimethoxyphenethylamine) is the primary psychoactive alkaloid responsible for the hallucinogenic properties of peyote. Central serotonergic and dopaminergic agonist effects are believed to be the physiologic cause of psychoactive and sympathomimetic stimulation, but the exact mechanism of action of mescaline is unclear. Mescaline is well absorbed in the gastrointestinal tract and within 1 hour of ingestion causes nausea, vomiting, abdominal cramps, dizziness, sweating, restlessness, and palpitations. Subsequently, a second phase within 1 to 3 hours of ingestion occurs, including the psychoactive effects of visual imagery, altered perceptions, and psychologic insight. Clinical effects commonly last 6 to 12 hours, and severe toxicity from peyote ingestion is rare. Symptomatic and supportive care is all that is generally required, and patients should be observed in a monitored setting until they are asymptomatic. Quantitative levels of mescaline are not routinely available, and blood levels do not always correlate with clinical effects. Routine urine drug screening does not detect mescaline.

Peyote and mescaline are considered schedule I substances under the Controlled Substance Act with one exemption [34]. Peyote can be used legally in the United States and Canada by the 300,000 members of the Native American Church for ceremonial or religious purposes or to promote physical and mental well-being. Only licensed representatives of the Native American Church may harvest peyote cactus [35,36]. There are other mescaline-containing cacti, *Trichocereus pachanoi* (San Pedro) and *Trichocereus peruvianus* (Peruvian torch), but these typically contain less mescaline by weight and are not indigenous to the United States.

DMT-containing plants

N,N-dimethyltryptamine (DMT) is an indole hallucinogen that shares its chemical structure with 5-MeO-DMT, bufotenine, psilocybin, and other hallucinogens. DMT is present naturally in many botanic sources in South and North America (eg, *Acacia* spp, *Mimosaceae* [*Piptadenia peregrina*], yopo tree [*Anadenanthera peregrina*], reed canary grass [*Phalaris arundinacea*]) and is most commonly used in ayahuasca tea (*Psychotria viridis*), traditionally prominent in shamanism of Amazonian tribes. Some plant preparations, such as ayahuasca, also naturally contain reversible monoamine oxidase–inhibiting beta-carboline alkaloids (harmine, harmaline, and tetrahydroharmine) that inhibit monoamine oxidase enzymes in the gastrointestinal tract and liver so that DMT is orally active [15]. Although popularized in its synthetic form in the 1960s, DMT is now more likely to be ingested in its natural forms, such as ayahuasca. A synthetic form is a white powder most often smoked or rarely injected. DMT is a $5\text{-HT}_{1A/1C/2A}$ receptor agonist and has cholinergic properties. The synthetic formulation is not active when taken orally because it is metabolized by monoamine oxidases in the gut and liver—thus the advantage of ayahuasca. When taken with monoamine oxidase inhibitors, the first pass metabolism of synthetic DMT is prevented, and it is able to enter the systemic circulation and central nervous system [37]. Peak effects occur within 3 minutes if smoked or injected but are delayed with oral ingestion. Clinical effects are described as intense, with vivid hallucinations, dissociation, and shifts in mood and perception. Other untoward adverse effects include mydriasis, hyperthermia, tachycardia, hypertension, and anxiety. Care is supportive because no specific antidote exists. Short-lived symptoms and clinical effects require observation until the patient is asymptomatic, and benzodiazepines should be administered for agitation. There is no proven benefit from gastrointestinal decontamination when DMT-containing plants are ingested, and there is no role for enhanced elimination [38]. DMT is a schedule I controlled substance but is not detected on routine urine drug screens. Detection by gas chromatography with surface ionization is possible, but this technique is not rapidly available in the acute setting [39].

Anticholinergics

Included in the *Solanaceae* family, the *Datura* genus contains a group of plants with tropane belladonna anticholinergic alkaloids, including atropine, scopolamine, and hyoscyamine [40,41]. Jimsonweed (*Datura stramonium*) grows in the wild throughout North America and can be found in open fields and blooming throughout the summer. The plant grows to approximately 1.5 m tall and has a solitary white, trumpet-shaped flower. In autumn, a spiny capsular fruit is produced that contains up to 50 small black seeds. Although all parts of the plant are toxic, the seeds contain the highest concentration of atropine [41–43]. One hundred seeds can contain up to 6 mg of atropine.

Jimsonweed is known by many local names, including thorn apple, locoweed, devil's trumpet, stink weed, and Jamestown weed [42,43]. Historically, jimsonweed was used by Native Americans for medicinal and religious purposes and has been used therapeutically to treat asthma [42]. Adolescents today most commonly use jimsonweed recreationally by ingesting, smoking, or brewing a tea from the seeds [40,41]. Other *Solanaceae* known to contain belladonna alkaloids include *Datura inoxia, Datura aurea, Datura sanguinea,* and *Brugmansia arborea.* Several other plants—deadly nightshade (*Atropa belladonna*), henbane (*Hyoscyamus niger*), and mandrake (*Mandragora officinarum*)—contain hyoscyamine and scopolamine alkaloids that are recreationally abused for their anticholinergic properties.

Although these plants are abused for their hallucinogenic and euphoric effects, anticholinergic intoxication can result in classic antimuscarinic symptoms because of competitive blockade of acetylcholine at the central and peripheral muscarinic receptor sites [40]. The mnemonic "hot as hare, blind as a bat, dry as a bone, red as a beet, and mad as a hatter" is commonly used to describe anticholinergic poisoning–related symptoms. Following ingestion, effects generally develop within 1 to 4 hours. Consumption of a tea prepared from the seeds or smoking the seeds results in a more rapid onset of symptoms. Patients initially develop xerostomia, blurred vision, and pupillary dilation. Dry skin, erythema, flushing, tachycardia, mild hyperthermia, and hypertension are common. The patient can develop confusion, disorientation, restlessness, and sometimes agitation later in the intoxication [44]. Hallucinations are often described as grasping or picking at imaginary objects [40,45], and amnesia of events after ingestion is common [44]. Anticholinergic intoxication can rarely result in seizures, coma, or death [40,41], but mortality is more commonly related to trauma and not direct toxic effects.

The duration of clinical effect is dose dependent but can last from a few hours to several days. Treatment remains primarily symptomatic. If ingested recently, activated charcoal may be beneficial for gastrointestinal decontamination, but this is unproven. Agitation should be treated with benzodiazepines while avoiding neuroleptics [40]. The patient should be kept in a nonthreatening and nonstimulating environment [44]. Other necessary supportive care may include treatment of hyperthermia, hypertension, urinary retention, and dehydration [40]. Patients who have mild symptoms that have resolved after 4 to 6 hours of observation can be discharged, but otherwise patients need admission until symptoms resolve.

Physostigmine, a short-acting acetylcholinesterase inhibitor, has been used as an antidote for severe anticholinergic poisonings [42,45–47]. Although controversy exists regarding its necessity because of safety concerns in overdose, case reports and retrospective studies have shown physostigmine to be effective in treating delirium and agitation attributable to anticholinergic substances [43,45–48]. Repeated doses may be required because of a shorter duration of effect than anticholinergic alkaloids, and the patient should be observed carefully for any signs of excessive secretions and bradycardia indicating cholinergic excess.

Sympathomimetics

Most plant or herbal recreational drugs touted as stimulants have sympathomimetic properties. Sympathomimetics are naturally-occurring and synthetically-produced chemicals that either increase the activity of the adrenergic nervous system or mimic its effect. Included in this class are direct-acting and indirect-acting agents. Direct-acting agents bind and stimulate α- or β-adrenergic receptors. Indirect-acting agents, such as amphetamines, cause increased presynaptic release and concentration of synaptic neurotransmitters, such as norepinephrine. Some substances cause both direct- and indirect-acting adrenergic effects, and certain herbal stimulants have sympathomimetic effects in combination with psychoactive and euphoric properties.

Plant-derived sympathomimetic toxicity is managed similarly to poisoning from synthetic stimulants. Begin with airway control, cardiac monitoring, and liberal use of benzodiazepines to treat agitation, hyperthermia, hypertension, tachycardia, and seizures. Passive or active cooling measures may be necessary for hyperthermia management. Life-threatening complications, such as myocardial infarction, cardiac dysrhythmias, intracranial hemorrhage, severe hyperthermia, coagulopathy, rhabdomyolysis, and acute renal failure, must be recognized and aggressively treated. There is no specific antidote for plant- and herbal-related stimulant toxicity, but benzodiazepines and intensive supportive care remain fundamental aspects of treatment.

Ephedra alkaloids

The *Ephedra* plant is a leafless shrub with a horsetail appearance that grows throughout the desert regions of Asia and North America. Plants belonging to the *Ephedra* genus, such as ma huang, have been used in Chinese medicine for thousands of years in the treatment of asthma. Mormons have historically been avid consumers of the ephedra-containing beverage "Mormon tea," which affords them the stimulatory effects of coffee or tea without the caffeine. More recent use in the United States has been in the form of dietary supplements for the purposes of increased energy and alertness, enhanced athletic performance, or weight loss. Estimates include approximately 12 million users and more than 3 billion servings sold of dietary supplements containing ephedra alkaloids in 1999 [10]. Plant preparations can contain 1% ephedrine but commercially sold products may contain 4% to 8% in combination with other stimulants, such as caffeine [49].

Ma-huang, containing the dried stems of *Ephedra equisetina*, contains the psychoactive alkaloids ephedrine, norephedrine, pseudoephedrine, and norpseudoephedrine. Ephedrine alkaloids are structurally related to amphetamines and act as direct-acting sympathomimetics with nonspecific α- and β-adrenergic agonist activity. Although ephedrine is closely related in structure to methamphetamine and is a commonly used precursor for the manufacture of methamphetamine, the CNS actions of ephedra alkaloids are significantly less potent.

Common stimulatory effects include insomnia, tachycardia, palpitations, nervousness, anxiety, restlessness, bronchodilation, headache, appetite suppression, mania, and psychosis. Ephedrine has been associated with significant adverse effects, including hepatotoxicity, hypertension, hemorrhagic stroke, ischemic stroke, seizures, cardiac arrhythmias, myocardial infarction, myocarditis, congestive heart failure, cardiomyopathy, and death [10]. Treatment of ephedra-related toxicity is similar to other CNS stimulants, with close attention paid to addressing the central sympathomimetic stimulation, cardiovascular toxicity, and secondary complications as a result of the heightened adrenergic state. Qualitative urine drug screening for amphetamines is available, but false-positive and false-negative results can occur. Ephedrine may cross-react with available urine immunoassays, but a true positive result only indicates usage during the last several days. Management of ephedra-related toxicity therefore must be based on the history of exposure and clinical manifestations.

Once classified as a food supplement under the 1994 Dietary Supplement Health and Education Act, there was no premarketing safety evaluation and regulation of ephedra-containing products by the FDA, and the actual content of active ingredients in herbal dietary supplements could vary greatly. Reported adverse effects of ephedra ultimately led the FDA to ban ephedra-containing products effective April 12, 2004 [9]. Despite the ban on ephedra alkaloids, these products continue to be available. One study of Internet sites advertising herbal dietary supplements reported 47% of Web sites continued to market ephedra products despite its illegality [8]. Most of the on-line marketing is targeted at teenagers and young adults. Ma huang herbal products are often advertised as "herbal ecstasy," "ultimate xphoria," "go," and "cloud 9," and are described as legal, inexpensive "natural highs." Ephedra alkaloids continue to be available and represent a serious health hazard alone or in combination with other stimulants.

Khat

Khat, *Catha edulis*, is a shrub grown in East Africa and the Arabian Peninsula where it is widely used as a stimulant. Fresh khat is typically consumed within 2 days because the active ingredient is degraded when the leaves age, and much of the potency is lost within a week. Users chew on the leaves, twigs, and young stems to produce alertness and appetite suppression with a potency reportedly ranging from caffeine to amphetamines. Leaves are chewed for several minutes and then placed into the cheek as the juice is slowly swallowed. Khat has increasingly been introduced to the United States and other countries by immigrants and is often found for sale in small, ethnic grocery stores [50]. The leaves are bundled and illegally imported into the United States and are now being used by other populations. Khat leaves are presently legal in Great Britain, although a growing movement has resulted in consideration of banning the product there [51]. Although khat is legal in East Africa and many European countries, cathinone, the active ingredient, is considered a schedule I substance by the DEA of the United States, and use of khat is illegal.

The plant contains two active components: cathinone (α-aminopropiophenone) and cathine (norpseudoephedrine). The primary active ingredient, cathinone, causes amphetamine-like sympathomimetic effects by stimulating a release of dopamine and other neurotransmitters from presynaptic neuronal storage. As the leaves dry, cathinone is converted to cathine, a less potent stimulant. Khat users describe the effects of increased energy, improved alertness, and euphoria. Other physiologic effects include increased blood pressure, tachycardia, bronchodilation, mydriasis, hyperthermia, and anxiety. Cathinone is physically and psychologically addictive. Withdrawal symptoms include irritability, fatigue, and rhinorrhea. Psychologic dependence leads many users to spend large portions of their household incomes on khat [52].

Khat is recommended by some herbalists as treatment of depression, obesity, fatigue, and gastric ulcers. But like other abused sympathomimetics, toxicity can develop to include rhabdomyolysis, cardiac dysrhythmias, stroke, altered sensorium, and convulsions. Adrenergic complications are less common than those associated with amphetamine abuse, however [53]. In the setting of overdose, khat can cause a psychosis with visual hallucinations and mania [54]. Reported long-term complications of khat use include oral carcinomas, hepatitis, ischemic cardiomyopathy, and cerebrovascular accidents [55–57].

Betel nut

Betel nut is the fourth most commonly abused substance worldwide, trailing only caffeine, alcohol, and nicotine [58]. The areca palm tree (*Areca catechu*) produces the egg-shaped betel nut. It is cultivated in India, East Africa, Southeast Asia, and the Asian Pacific, where it is chewed for its relatively mild stimulant effect. The betel nut is chewed alone or in a mixture known as betel quid, which also includes betel pepper leaf (*Piper betle*), lime (calcium hydroxide), spices, and often tobacco. The quid is tucked into the cheek for 15 to 20 minutes where it is absorbed by the oral and gastric mucosa [59]. Betel quid has been brought to the United States by immigrants, and although it has yet to establish mainstream use, its ingredients can be conveniently purchased in ethnic groceries and on the Internet.

The pharmacologic effect of betel nut is largely attributable to the alkaloid arecoline, which acts as a cholinomimetic agonist at nicotinic and muscarinic receptors and as an acetylcholinesterase inhibitor [60]. Users report a sense of well-being, heightened alertness, and increased capacity for work from the stimulant properties of the hydrolyzed arecoline combined with the essential oils of the betel pepper [61]. In a review of cases reported to the Taiwan Poison Control Center from January 1988 to June 1998, the most commonly reported manifestations were tachycardia, palpitations, hypotension, dyspnea, diaphoresis, vomiting, dizziness, and chest discomfort. Most cases recovered within 24 hours of ingestion, except one patient who developed lethal ventricular fibrillation suspected to be secondary to myocardial infarction. The amount ingested in most of these reports was 1 to 6 nuts, but the authors reported 66 nuts were chewed in one case and another ingested the extract of 100 nuts [62]. Autonomic symptoms may develop rapidly within 2 minutes, with peak effects at 4 to 6 minutes and mean symptom duration of approximately 17 minutes [63]. Symptoms of dizziness, vomiting, and flushing are more pronounced in first-time users [59]. Stimulation of glandular secretions, pupillary constriction, and bradycardia may follow. Adverse events include asthmatic exacerbation, cardiac arrhythmias, acute psychosis, dystonias, and seizures. The calcium hydroxide component of the betel quid can be responsible for causing milk-alkali syndrome and an increased risk for nephrolithiasis [64].

Betel nut has a strong addictive potential. A withdrawal syndrome is reported in infants of betel nut–abusing mothers [65]. The International Agency for Research on Cancer includes betel quid as a known human carcinogen even without combined tobacco use [66]. Chronic use causes characteristic red staining of the teeth and gums and increases the risk for oral leukoplakia, oral squamous cell carcinomas, and submucous fibrosis [67].

Most cases of acute toxicity are mild. The primary treatment is symptomatic and supportive care because no specific antidote exists. Serious adverse effects can occur, however, with reported cases of pulmonary edema, bronchospasm, and death [59]. Cholinergic crisis can result with first-time use or following large ingestions. In severe cases, atropine may be of benefit to antagonize arecoline at the muscarinic receptors. Betel nut and its active components are not detected with routine urine immunoassay, and use is not controlled in the United States.

Yohimbe

Yohimbine is an alkaloid stimulant derived from the bark of *Corynanthe yohimbe* and *Pausinystalia yohimbe* plants that grow in West Africa and the Congo. Yohimbine is marketed to the general public as a supplement for body-building and sexual enhancement and is consumed for its aphrodisiac and hallucinogenic properties. It is sold primarily in tablet form but can be purchased as a powder or tea. It is also available by prescription for the

treatment of erectile dysfunction, despite limited evidence regarding its efficacy [68–71].

Similar to reserpine, yohimbine has been used in research settings to
characterize the α2-adrenergic receptor [72]. Yohimbine is a selective α2-
adrenergic receptor antagonist and increases release of norepinephrine
that stimulates sympathetic outflow. Its effects are opposite of clonidine
and it has reportedly been used as an antidote for clonidine toxicity [73]. Autonomic changes include tachycardia, hypertension, mydriasis, nausea, diaphoresis, and vasodilatory-induced flushing. CNS excitation is prominent,
with symptoms of anxiety, hallucinations, and dissociation. Oral yohimbine
may produce maximal effects in 1 to 2 hours with total duration of effects
lasting 3 to 4 hours.

One case report describes a 16-year-old girl who took 250 mg of yohimbine powder and experienced an acute dissociative reaction. Within 20 minutes of ingestion, she experienced weakness, paresthesias, and loss of
coordination. At initial presentation she had tachycardia, hypertension,
and tachypnea. Over a 6-hour course she developed substernal chest pressure, severe headache, dizziness, tremors, anxiety, diaphoresis, and palpitations. She underwent observation and cardiac monitoring, with resolution
of symptoms at 36 hours following ingestion [74]. Another case report of
yohimbine toxicity in a 62-year-old man revealed a similarly benign, self-
limited course despite a large ingestion [75]. There are reports of significant
drug interactions with yohimbine use. Some authors recommend additional
caution when yohimbine is coingested with selective serotonin reuptake
inhibitor and monoamine oxygenase inhibitor preparations or in patients
taking tricyclic antidepressants [76,77].

Acute management is largely supportive. Although no specific antidote
exists, clonidine has been recommended for reversal of yohimbine toxicity
in adolescent and adult patients. β-adrenergic antagonists have been discouraged because of the theoretic possibility of worsening hypertension secondary to unopposed α-adrenergic stimulation [74]. Benzodiazepines may
provide safe, adequate management of severe symptoms associated with
yohimbine toxicity: agitation, seizures, hypertension, and tachycardia.

Yohimbine metabolites can be detected in the urine using high-
performance or thin-layer chromatography but are not detected in routine
urine drug screens. Serum norepinephrine will be elevated within 15 minutes
of ingestion [78], but no specific toxic blood concentration has been established for yohimbine. Yohimbine has limited regulation in the United States
by the FDA when used as a prescription drug. Otherwise, it is available as
a health food supplement without a prescription.

Caffeine-containing products

Following the FDA ban of the herbal weight-loss agent ephedra, many of
the top-selling weight-loss products switched to other stimulants, such as

guarana and yerba maté, that contain large amounts of caffeine. Guarana (*Paullinia cupana*) is a rainforest shrub containing significant quantities of caffeine and other xanthine alkaloids. A typical 2-teaspoon oral dose is most commonly used from a powder of the ground seeds of the plant. The seeds contain 2.5% to 7% caffeine by weight in comparison with 1% to 2% caffeine in coffee. A cup of coffee typically ranges from 50 to 150 mg of caffeine, whereas a serving of guarana can contain 200 mg of caffeine per dose [79]. Caffeine-related toxicity results from adenosine antagonism, phosphodiesterase inhibition, and endogenous release of norepinephrine with subsequent β-adrenergic receptor agonism. Clinical effects can range from a syndrome of caffeinism to cardiac dysrhythmias, seizures, and death. Caffeinism is characterized by restlessness, anxiety, diuresis, gastrointestinal disturbance, tachycardia, palpitations, headache, and insomnia. Laboratory abnormalities associated with caffeine intoxication can include transient hypokalemia from β-adrenergic agonism, hyperglycemia, lactic acidosis, and leukocytosis. One death from ventricular fibrillation is reported in a 25-year-old female, who had preexisting mitral valve prolapse, following ingestion of a Race 2005 Energy Blast drink containing guarana and ginseng [80]. Dennehy and colleagues [8] report that 10% of on-line herbal products contained guarana following a study of Web sites marketing supplements for recreational use.

Maté is a stimulant beverage prepared from the leaves of the South American holly *Ilex paraguariensis*. In addition to caffeine, it contains theobromine and theophylline and is most commonly consumed in South America. Adverse effects are similar to other teas or beverages containing large quantities of caffeine.

Analgesics/euphorics

Absinthe

Wormwood (*Artemisia absinthium*) is a woody herb that is native to Europe and has been naturalized in the United States [81–83]. Historically, oil of wormwood was used as an antihelminthic, and a bitter taken to stimulate digestion [81]. Absinthe, a liqueur derived from the wormwood plant, was first formulated in the late eighteenth century in Switzerland [84,85] and reached heightened popularity in the late nineteenth and early twentieth centuries primarily in France [81,82,85]. Known for its distinct green color, the "green fairy" was a favorite of the Bohemian life style of the late 1800s, and historically many famous artists and writers have been users: Oscar Wilde, Henri Toulouse-Lautrec, and Vincent van Gogh [81,83,85]. Because of its bitter taste, traditional preparation involved pouring cold water over a sugar cube atop a slotted spoon and into a glass containing absinthe liqueur. This also diluted the liqueur's high alcohol concentration by approximately 75% [82,84]. Thujone, a terpene found in oil of wormwood with α and β isomers, is the suspected source of hallucinations and psychosis from absinthe use [86]. Thujone has been shown to antagonize the γ-aminobutyric acid (GABA) receptor, and this may explain absinthe's excitatory and seizure-producing effects.

Acute effects of absinthe ingestion produce euphoria, confusion, delirium, and hallucinations, and it has also been described as an aphrodisiac [82–84]. Chronic use of absinthe, a syndrome referred to as absinthism, is reported to cause gastrointestinal disorders, sleeplessness, tremors, convulsions, auditory and visual hallucinations, brain damage, and death [82,85,87]. Because of acute and chronic effects, absinthe was banned in some countries in the early twentieth century, including the United States in 1912 [81,85]. There continues to be debate over the cause of absinthism: high alcohol content leading to alcoholism, natural components in wormwood oil, or adulteration [88].

The recent resurgence of absinthe has been fueled by its availability on the Internet and in European countries [8,88]. In the late 1980s, the European Union reinstated thujone as a food additive with a maximum concentration of 35 mg/kg for bitter spirits. It is believed that historic absinthe had concentrations as high as 260 mg/kg. Switzerland has since repealed absinthe prohibition, and it is expected that products with increased concentrations of thujone will be available [88]. In addition to euphoric effects, intentionally misleading advertisements often compare the clinical effects of absinthe to those of marijuana. Although there are structural similarities between thujone and tetrahydrocannabinol, studies have shown a low affinity of thujone for the cannabinoid receptor sites [83,88].

Treatment of ingestion is symptomatic and supportive because no specific antidote exists. One case report involving ingestion of 10 mL of essential oil of wormwood purchased from the Internet and mistaken for the liqueur describes seizures, rhabdomyolysis, and subsequent acute renal failure. The patient's symptoms resolved with supportive care [85].

Kava

Kava (*Piper methysticum*) has been used for centuries in tropical Pacific island communities for ceremonial purposes [89]. The roots and rhizomes of the pepper plant are crushed into an aqueous beverage and taken for its anxiolytic and psychotropic effects [90,91]. The aqueous emulsion causes a local anesthetic effect in the mouth and produces a general calming effect [92]. Weakness, numbness, and sedation may follow. One case report describes a 37-year-old man presenting with depressed mental status and ataxia similar to ethanol intoxication following several cups of kava tea. A urine toxicology screen and serum blood ethanol results were negative, and the symptoms resolved over 4 hours [93].

The anxiolytic actions of kava are the result of kavalactones (dihydrokawain, methysticin, dihydromethysticin, and kawain) that are believed to be

GABA-receptor agonists [90]. Long-term effects of kava use have included dermopathy, ataxia, anorexia, and hepatotoxicity [91,94]. Most of these effects are reported to be reversible on discontinuation [90,91,95,96]. Although uncommon, kava-induced hepatotoxicity is described, and the FDA released a consumer advisory in March 2002 regarding the use of kava and hepatic injury, including hepatitis, cirrhosis, and liver failure [97]. Several hypotheses for the cause of kava-induced hepatotoxicity have been explored: extraction process for commercial use involving alcohol or acetone extraction, genetic variations in metabolism, and coingestion of other herbs [89]. Because of increased popularity in Europe and North America and reports of hepatotoxicity, many countries, including Canada, have banned kava for consumer use [95,98]. Kava is an unregulated, unscheduled dietary health supplement in the United States and marketed by many herbal manufacturers as a treatment of insomnia, anxiety, and stress [90,98].

Most patients only require observation until clinical symptoms have resolved following acute intoxication. Other long-term toxic effects can occur after days or years of use at recommended doses, however. Discontinuation of the product and supportive care are the primary treatments, and there is no specific antidote. In 2002, the Centers for Disease Control and Prevention reported 10 cases in the United States, Germany, and Switzerland that required liver transplantation following hepatic failure associated with the ingestion of kava-containing supplements [98]. Although most patients recover with supportive care, clinical evidence of hepatic failure would warrant evaluation for liver transplant. Similar to other causes of toxin-induced hepatic injury, N-acetylcysteine (NAC), as a glutathione precursor and substitute, theoretically could serve as an adjunctive treatment of hepatotoxicity. One study suggested the formation of two novel electrophilic metabolites of kava in hepatic microsomes in vitro as a potential contributor to kava-induced hepatotoxicity [99]. Although unproven for hepatic injury secondary to kava, NAC has been proposed as a treatment of several hepatic toxins associated with reactive metabolite toxicity.

Cloves

Clove cigarettes, kreteks, are imported to the United States from Indonesia. Containing a mixture of approximately 30% ground or shredded cloves (*Syzygium aromaticum*) with 70% tobacco, clove cigarettes deliver twice as much tar, nicotine, and carbon monoxide as the average American cigarette [100,101]. On inhalation, eugenol, an ingredient in cloves, has a topical anesthetic effect and causes numbness in the throat. In the United States, deep inhalation and increased retention of the smoke, or toking, is the most common technique in which these cigarettes are smoked in an effort to enhance effects. There is concern that clove cigarettes may be a gateway drug for adolescents [100]. A national survey reported that 2.0% of middle school students and 2.7% of high school students currently smoke clove cigarettes [102]. Case reports of severe illness have been reported with clove cigarette use, including bronchospasm, hemoptysis, and pulmonary edema [101]. Treatment of any related toxicity is supportive.

Summary

Certain plants and herbal products, sold as dietary supplements, are emerging as popular drugs for recreational abuse. Like many synthetic drugs, plant and herbal supplements used recreationally can have a spectrum of clinical effects overlapping between euphoric, stimulant, and hallucinogenic experiences. Although some users may abuse a specific substance primarily to obtain an analgesic or euphoric effect, other individuals may be in search of the hallucinogenic effects from the same agent. Variations in individual response to certain drugs exist, and escalating doses may enhance some clinical effects while potentially decreasing others. Although attempts can be made to categorize herbal drugs of abuse based on the most commonly desired effects, it is clear that some of these substances have a spectrum of clinical effects and are used for various reasons.

With marketing focused at teenagers and young adults, these products are advertised to provide a "safe, natural high." Like many food supplements, however, these substances are largely unregulated and lack safety studies. Unfortunately, safety concerns are not often a deterrent for teenagers experimenting with an herbal supplement billed as "all natural" and often undetectable in routine urine immunoassays. Laws regarding these herbal supplements and plants vary by country and product, but several of these agents are scheduled substances by the United States DEA. Online purchasing by way of foreign-based Internet Web sites continues to make these products readily available and affordable. Despite the potential for abuse, addiction, and serious adverse effects, there may be a false perception that these products are all safe, legal, and organic. Often, patients do not consider herbal products as medications or worthy of mention to their caregivers, and many significant herbal–drug interactions exist. It should be expected that many recreational users may avoid reporting misuse even if the dietary supplement is legal. One complementary alternative medicine survey of patients presenting to an urban emergency department reported that only 67% of patients would inform their physician about herbal medication use, and 16% believed herbal remedies were all safe [103]. These perceptions and the ease of accessibility to herbal products could result in greater potential for recreational abuse and subsequent complications presenting to emergency departments. Health care professionals must be cognizant of this emerging problem because increased media coverage and Internet marketing have made these products accessible and recognizable to many young adults and teenagers.

References

[1] Available at: http://en.wikipedia.org/wiki/Herb. Accessed August 16, 2006.

[2] Substance Abuse and Mental Health Services Administration. Results from the 2004 National Survey on Drug Use and Health: National Findings (Office of Applied Studies, NSDUH Series H-28, DHHS Publication No. SMA 05–4062). Rockville (MD).

[3] Substance Abuse and Mental Health Services Administration. DAWN, 2004: National Estimates of Drug-Related Emergency Department Visits (Office of Applied Studies, DAWN Series D-28, DHHS Publication No. SMA 06-4143). Rockville (MD).

[4] Center for Food Safety and Applied Nutrition. Dietary Supplement Health and Education Act of 1994. U.S. Food and Drug Administration. Available at: http://www.cfsan.fda.gov/~dms/dietsupp.html. Accessed August 4, 2006.

[5] Eisenberg DM, Davis RB, Ettner SL, et al. Trends in alternative medicine use in the United States, 1990–1997: results of a follow-up national survey. JAMA 1998;280:1569–75.

[6] Yussman SM, Wilson KM, Klein JD. Herbal products and their association with substance use in adolescents. J Adolesc Health 2006;38:395–400.

[7] Ferrier GKL, Thwaites LA. US consumer herbal and herbal botanical supplement sales. Nutrition Business Journal; 2006. Available at: http://www.nutritionbusiness.com.

[8] Dennehy CE, Tsourounis C, Miller AE. Evaluation of herbal dietary supplements marketed on the Internet for recreational use. Ann Pharmacother 2005;39:1634–9.

[9] US Food and Drug Administration. FDA announces rule prohibiting sale of dietary supplements containing ephedrine alkaloids effective April 12. Department of Health and Human Services FDA Statement. Available at: http://www.fda.gov/bbs/topics/news/2004/NEW01050.html. Accessed August 4, 2006.

[10] Haller CA, Benowitz NL. Adverse cardiovascular and central nervous system events associated with dietary supplements containing ephedra alkaloids. N Engl J Med 2000;343:1833–8.

[11] Shekelle PG, Hardy ML, Morton SC, et al. Efficacy and safety of ephedra and ephedrine for weight loss and athletic performance: a meta-analysis. JAMA 2003;289:1537–45.

[12] Winek CL, Elzein EO, Wahba WW, et al. Interference of herbal drinks with urinalysis for drugs of abuse. J Anal Toxicol 1993;17:246–7.

[13] Markowitz JS, Donovan JL, DeVane CL, et al. Common herbal supplements did not produce false-positive results on urine drug screens analyzed by enzyme immunoassay. J Anal Toxicol 2004;28:272–3.

[14] Imanshahidi M, Hosseinzadeh H. The pharmacological effects of Salvia species on the central nervous system. Phytother Res 2006;20:427–37.

[15] Halpern JH. Hallucinogens and dissociative agents naturally growing in the United States. Pharmacol Ther 2004;102:131–8.

[16] Gonzalez D, Riba J, Bouso J, et al. Pattern of use and subjective effects of Salvia divinorum among recreational users. Drug Alcohol Depend 2006;85:157–62.

[17] Lee DY, Ma Z, Liu-Chen LY, et al. New neoclerodane diterpenoids isolated from the leaves of Salvia divinorum and their binding affinities for human kappa opioid receptors. Bioorg Med Chem 2005;13:5635–9.

[18] Roth BL, Banner K, Westkaemper R, et al. Salvinorin A: a potent naturally occurring nonnitrogenous kappa opioid selective agonist. Proc Natl Acad Sci USA 2002;99:11934–9.

[19] Available at: http://www.dea.gov/pubs/scheduling.html. Accessed August 30, 2006.

[20] Gahlinger PM. Chapter 7–Just say know (morning glory). In: Illegal drugs: a complete guide to their history, chemistry, use, and abuse. Salt Lake City (UT): Sagebrush Press; 2004. p. 163–93.

[21] Al-Assmar SE. The seeds of the Hawaiian baby woodrose are a powerful hallucinogen. Arch Intern Med 1999;159:2090.

[22] Chao JM, Der Marderosian AH. Ergoline alkaloidal constituents of Hawaiian baby woodrose, Argyreia nervosa (Burm. f.) Bojer. J Pharm Sci 1973;62:588–91.

[23] Miller MD. Isolation and identification of lysergic acid amide and isolysergic acid amide as the principle ergoline alkaloids in Argyreia nervosa, a tropical wood rose. Journal of the Association of Official Agricultural Chemists 1970;53:123–7.

[24] Shawcross WE. Recreational use of ergoline alkaloid from *Argyreia nervosa*. J Psychoactive Drugs 1983;15:251–9.

[25] Gahlinger PM. Chapter 7–Just say know (nutmeg). In: Illegal drugs: a complete guide to their history, chemistry, use, and abuse. Salt Lake City (UT): Sagebrush Press; 2004. p. 163–93.

[26] Sangalli BC, Chiang W. Toxicology of nutmeg abuse. J Toxicol Clin Toxicol 2000;38: 671–8.

[27] Forrester MB. Nutmeg intoxication in Texas, 1998–2004. Hum Exp Toxicol 2005;24:563–5.

[28] Stein U, Greyer H, Hentschel H. Nutmeg (myristicin) poisoning—report on a fatal case and a series of cases recorded by a poison information centre. Forensic Sci Int 2001;118: 87–90.

[29] Schultes RE, Hofmann A. Plants of hallucinogenic use. In: The botany and chemistry of hallucinogens. 2nd edition. Springfield (IL): Thomas; 1980. p. 121.

[30] Hung OL, Lewin NA, Howland MA. Herbal preparations. In: Goldfrank LR, Flomenbaum NE, Lewin NA, editors. Goldfrank's toxicologic emergencies. 7th edition. New York: McGraw-Hill Companies, Inc.; 2002. p. 1129–49.

[31] Available at: http://www.erowid.org/plants/nutmeg/. Accessed August 30, 2006.

[32] Gahlinger PM. Peyote and mescaline. In: Illegal drugs: a complete guide to their history, chemistry, use, and abuse. Salt Lake City (UT): Sagebrush Press; 2004. p. 393–412.

[33] Dart RC. Plants. In: Dart RC, Caravati EM, McGiugan MA, editors. Medical toxicology, 3rd edition. Philadelphia: Lippincott Williams & Wilkins; 2004. p. 1665–713.

[34] American Indian Religious Freedom Act Amendments of 1994 (1994):108 Statute 3124 Public Law103-344.42 USC.

[35] Halpern JH, Sherwood AR, Hudson JI, et al. Psychological and cognitive effects of long-term peyote use in Native Americans. Biol Psychiatry 2005;58:624–31.

[36] Calabrese JD. Spiritual healing and human development in the Native American Church: toward a cultural psychiatry of peyote. Psychoanal Rev 1997;84:237–55.

[37] Riba J, Valle M, Urbano G, et al. Human pharmacology of ayahuasca: subjective and cardiovascular effects, monoamine metabolite excretion, and pharmacokinetics. J Pharmacol Exp Ther 2003;306:73–83.

[38] Caravati EM. Hallucinogenic drugs. In: Dart RC, Caravati EM, McGiugan MA, editors. Medical toxicology, 3rd edition. Philadelphia: Lippincott Williams & Wilkins; 2004. p. 1103–11.

[39] Ishii A, Seno H, Suzuki O, et al. A simple and sensitive quantitation of N,N-dimethyltryptamine by gas chromatography with surface ionization detection. J Anal Toxicol 1997;21: 36–40.

[40] DeFrates LJ, Hoehns JD, Sakornbut EL, et al. Antimuscarinic intoxication resulting from the ingestion of moonflower seeds. Ann Pharmacother 2005;39:173–6.

[41] Coresman P, Lambrecht G, Schepens P, et al. Anticholinergic intoxication with commercially available thorn apple tea. Clin Toxicol 1994;32:589–94.

[42] Salen P, Shih R, Sierzenski P, et al. Effect of physostigmine and gastric lavage in datura stramonium-induced anticholinergic poisoning epidemic. Am J Emerg Med 2003;21:316–7.

[43] Epidemiologic notes and reports jimson weed poisoning—Texas, New York, and California, 1994. MMWR Morb Mortal Wkly Rep 1995;44:41–4.

[44] Vanderhoff BT, Mosser KH. Jimson weed toxicity: management of anticholinergic plant ingestion. Am Fam Physician 1992;46:526–30.

[45] Richardson WH, Williams SR, Carstairs SD. A picturesque reversal of antimuscarinic delirium. J Emerg Med 2004;26:463.

[46] Burns MJ, Linden CH, Graudins A, et al. A comparison of physostigmine and benzodiazepines for the treatment of anticholinergic poisoning. Ann Emerg Med 2000;35:374–81.

[47] Beaver KM, Gavin TJ. Treatment of acute anticholinergic poisoning with physostigmine. Am J Emerg Med 1998;16:505–7.

[48] Schneir AB, Offerman SR, Ly BT, et al. Complications of diagnostic physostigmine administration in emergency department patients. Ann Emerg Med 2003;42:14–9.

[49] Lynton RC, Albertson TE. Amphetamines and designer drugs. In: Dart RC, Caravati EM, McGiugan MA, editors. Medical toxicology, 3rd edition. Philadelphia: Lippincott Williams & Wilkins; 2004. p. 1071–83.

[50] Stefan J, Mathew B. Khat chewing: an emerging drug concern in Australia? Aust N Z J Psychiatry 2005;39:842–3.

[51] Available at: http://www.guardian.co.uk/uk_news/story/0,3604,1652424,00.html. Accessed August 16, 2006.

[52] Aden A, Dimba EA, Ndolo UM. Socio-economic effects of khat chewing in north eastern Kenya. East Afr Med J 2006;83:69–73.

[53] Chiang WK. Amphetamines. In: Goldfrank LR, Flomenbaum NE, Lewin NA, editors. Goldfrank's toxicologic emergencies, 7th edition. New York: McGraw-Hill Companies, Inc.; 2002. p. 1020–33.

[54] Giannini AJ, Castellani S. A manic-like psychosis due to khat. J Toxicol Clin Toxicol 1982; 19:455–9.

[55] Brostoff JM, Plymen C, Birns J. Khat—a novel cause of drug-induced hepatitis. Eur J Intern Med 2006;17:383.

[56] Saha S, Dollery C. Severe ischaemic cardiomyopathy associated with khat chewing. J R Soc Med 2006;99:316–8.

[57] Vanwalleghem IE, Vanwalleghem PW, De Bleecker JL. Khat chewing can cause stroke. Cerebrovasc Dis 2006;22:198–200.

[58] Gupta PC, Ray CS. Epidemiology of betel quid usage. Ann Acad Med Singap 2004;33(4 Suppl):31–6.

[59] Nelson BS, Heischober B. Betel nut: a common drug used by naturalized citizens from India, Far East Asia, and the South Pacific Islands. Ann Emerg Med 1999;34:238–43.

[60] Gilani AH, Ghayur MN, Saify ZS, et al. Presence of cholinomimetic and acetylcholinesterase inhibitory constituents in betel nut. Life Sci 2004;75:2377–89.

[61] Burton-Bradley BG. Arecaidinism: betel chewing in transcultural perspective. Can J Psychiatry 1979;24:481–8.

[62] Deng JF, Ger J, Tsai WJ, et al. Acute toxicities of betel nut: rare but probably overlooked events. J Toxicol Clin Toxicol 2001;39:355–60.

[63] Chu NS. Neurological aspects of areca and betel chewing. Addict Biol 2002;7:111–4.

[64] Allen SE, Singh S, Robertson WG. The increased risk of urinary stone disease in betel quid chewers. Urol Res 2006;34:239–43.

[65] Lopez-Vilchez MA, Seidel V, Farre M, et al. Areca-nut abuse and neonatal withdrawal syndrome. Pediatrics 2006;117:129–31.

[66] Available at: http://monographs.iarc.fr/ENG/Monographs/vol85/volume85.pdf. Accessed August 22, 2006.

[67] Norton SA. Betel: consumption and consequences. J Am Acad Dermatol 1998;38:81–8.

[68] Kunelius P, Hakkinen J, Lukkarinen O. Is high-dose yohimbine hydrochloride effective in the treatment of mixed-type impotence? A prospective, randomized, controlled double-blind crossover study. Urology 1997;49:441–4.

[69] Morales A, Condra M, Owen JA, et al. Is yohimbine effective in the treatment of organic impotence? Results of a controlled trial. J Urol 1987;137:1168–72.

[70] Reid K, Surridge DH, Morales A, et al. Double-blind trial of yohimbine in treatment of psychogenic impotence. Lancet 1987;2:421–3.

[71] Susset JG, Tessier CD, Wincze J, et al. Effect of yohimbine hydrochloride on erectile impotence: a double-blind study. J Urol 1989;141:1360–3.

[72] Goldberg MR, Roberson D. Yohimbine: a pharmacological probe for study of the alpha-2 adrenoreceptor. Pharmacol Rev 1983;35:143–80.

[73] Roberge RJ, McGuire SP, Krenzelok EP. Yohimbine as an antidote for clonidine overdose. Am J Emerg Med 1996;14:678–80.

[74] Linden CH, Vellman WP, Rumack B. Yohimbine: a new street drug. Ann Emerg Med 1985; 14:1002–4.

[75] Friesen K, Palatnick W, Tenenbein M. Benign course after massive ingestion of yohimbine. J Emerg Med 1993;11:287–8.

[76] Fugh-Berman A. Herb-drug interactions. Lancet 2000;355:134–8.

[77] De Smet PA, Smeets OS. Potential risks of health food products containing yohimbe extracts. BMJ 1994;309:958.

[78] Hedner T, Edgar B, Edvinsson L. Yohimbine pharmacokinetics and interaction with the sympathetic nervous system in normal volunteers. Eur J Clin Pharmacol 1992;43:651–6.

[79] Hess AM, Sullivan DL. Potential for toxicity with use of bitter orange and guarana for weight loss. Ann Pharmacother 2005;39:574–5.

[80] Cannon ME, Cooks CT, McCarthy JS. Caffeine-induced cardiac arrhythmia: an unrecognized danger of healthfood products. Med J Aust 2001;174:520–5.

[81] Gambelunghe C, Melai P. Absinthe: enjoying a new popularity among young people? Forensic Sci Int 2002;130:183–6.

[82] Holstege CP, Baylor MR, Rusyniak DE. Absinthe: return of the green fairy. Semin Neurol 2002;22:89–93.

[83] Olsen RW. Commentary: Absinthe and γ-aminobutyric acid receptors. Proc Natl Acad Sci USA 2000;97:4417–8.

[84] Strang J, Arnold WN, Peters T. Absinthe: what's your poison? BMJ 1999;319:1590–2.

[85] Weisbord SD, Soule JB, Kimmel PL. Poison on line—acute renal failure caused by oil of wormwood purchased through the Internet. N Engl J Med 1997;337:825–7.

[86] Hold KM, Sirisoma NS, Ikeda T, et al. α-Thujone (the active component of absinthe): γ-aminobutyric acid type A receptor modulation and metabolic detoxification. Proc Natl Acad Sci USA 2002;97:3826–31.

[87] Padosch SA, Lachenmeier DW, Kroner LU. Absinthism: a fictitious 19th century syndrome with present impact. Subst Abuse Treat Prev Policy 2006;1:1–14.

[88] Lachenmeier DW, Emmert J, Kuballa T, et al. Thujone—cause for absinthism? Forensic Sci Int 2006;158:1–8.

[89] Moulds RF, Malani J. Kava: herbal panacea or liver poison? Med J Aust 2003;178:451–3.

[90] Stickel F, Baumüller HM, Karlheinz S, et al. Hepatitis induced by kava (piper methysticum rhizome). J Hepatol 2003;39:62–7.

[91] Clough AR, Bailie RS, Currie B. Liver function test abnormalities in users of aqueous kava extracts. Clin Toxicol 2003;41:821–9.

[92] Kava. Lancet 1988;2(8605):258–9.

[93] Perez J, Holmes JF. Altered mental status and ataxia secondary to acute kava ingestion. J Emerg Med 2005;28:49–51.

[94] Wooltorton E. Herbal kava: reports of liver toxicity. CMAJ 2002;166:777.

[95] Russman S, Lauterberg BH, Helbling A. Kava hepatoxocity [letter]. Ann Intern Med 2001; 135:68–9.

[96] Grace R. Kava-induced urticaria [letter]. J Am Acad Dermatol 2005;53:906.

[97] Center for Food Safety and Applied Nutrition, USFDA. Consumer advisory: Kava-containing dietary supplements may be associated with severe liver injury, March 25, 2002. Available at: http://www.cfsan.fda.gov/~dms/addskava.html. Accessed August 29, 2006.

[98] Centers for Disease Control and Prevention. Hepatic toxicity possibly associated with kava-containing products—United States, Germany, and Switzerland, 1999–2002. MMWR 2002;51:1065–6.

[99] Johnson BM, Qiu SX, Khang S, et al. Identification of novel electrophilic metabolites of Piper methysticum Forst. (Kava). Chem Res Toxicol 2003;16:733–40.

[100] American Academy of Pediatrics Committee on Substance Abuse. Hazards of clove cigarettes. Pediatrics 1991;88:395–6.

[101] Centers for Disease Control and Prevention. Epidemiologic notes and reports illnesses possibly associated with smoking clove cigarettes. MMWR 1985;34:297–9.

[102] Centers for Disease Control and Prevention. Youth tobacco surveillance—United States, 2001–2002. MMWR Surveill Summ 2006;55(SS03):1–56.

[103] Weiss SJ, Takakuwa KM, Ernst AA. Use, understanding, and beliefs about complementary and alternative medicines among emergency department patients. Acad Emerg Med 2001;8: 41–7.

ELSEVIER
SAUNDERS

EMERGENCY
MEDICINE
CLINICS OF
NORTH AMERICA

Emerg Med Clin N Am 25 (2007) 459–476

Updates on the Evaluation
and Management of Caustic Exposures

Matthew Salzman, MD*, Rika N. O'Malley, MD

*Department of Emergency Medicine, Albert Einstein Medical Center, 5501 Old York Road,
Korman Building B-6, Philadelphia, PA 19141-3098, USA*

A caustic, also referred to as a *corrosive*, is a chemical capable of causing injury upon tissue contact. Generally, strong acids, with a pH of less than 3, and strong alkalis, with a pH of greater than 11, are of greatest concern in regard to human exposure. In 2004, the American Association of Poison Control Centers' Toxic Exposure Surveillance System documented over 200,000 exposures to caustic substances in both household and industrial products, including hydrochloric acid, potassium hydroxide, sodium hydroxide, sulfuric and phosphoric acids, as well as many others. Although the most commonly affected body areas are the face, eyes, and extremities, all reported fatalities were as a result of ingestion [1]. Little controversy exists in patient management following dermal or ocular caustic exposure. Immediate water irrigation of the site of exposure, followed by routine burn care with analgesia, fluid, and electrolyte replacement are the standards of care. In this manuscript, a thorough review of management of gastrointestinal caustic exposure is explored, not only because of the high rates of morbidity and mortality associated with these exposures, but also because there remains controversy regarding appropriate management of such exposures. Hydrofluoric acid (HF), a weak acid in its aqueous form, requires special consideration and specific antidotes, and as such, is addressed separately.

Caustic ingestion

Pathophysiology

The likelihood and severity of esophageal injury after caustic ingestion is related to several factors, including agent pH, titratable acid or alkaline

---

* Corresponding author.
E-mail address: salzmanm@einstein.edu (M. Salzman).

reserve, physical state (solid, liquid, or gel), and tissue contact time, as well as quantity and concentration of the substance ingested. The pH can be determined in the emergency department by litmus paper testing if there is product available, or by identifying the substance ingested and finding its material safety data sheet (www.msdsonline.com). The amount of acid or base required to titrate a chemical's pH to 8.00 may be a better predictor of esophageal injury than pH, especially after ingestion of near-neutral pH toxicants [2]; however, this information may not be as readily available as other chemical properties, such as pH and concentration. Tissue contact time may be influenced by the physical state of the toxicant, because ingested solids are more likely to adhere to mucous membranes of the gastrointestinal tract, resulting in prolonged contact. In a rat model, caustic soda (sodium hydroxide) has been shown to cause esophageal damage after 10 minutes of contact time, and esophageal perforation after 120 minutes of contact [3]. Further, in this animal study, solution concentration was determined to be the most important predictor of esophageal damage. Caustic soda concentrations of 1.83% were sufficient to cause epithelial necrosis, whereas concentrations of 7.33% induced submucosal damage, and concentrations of 14.33% resulted in muscle and adventitial damage [3].

Acids and alkalis are known to produce different types of tissue damage. Acids generally cause coagulation necrosis, with eschar formation that may limit substance penetration and injury depth [4]. Alkalis, in contrast, combine with tissue proteins and cause liquefactive necrosis and saponification, and are classically taught to penetrate deeper into tissues. Additionally, alkali absorption leads to thrombosis in blood vessels, impeding blood flow to already damaged tissue [5]. These mechanisms of injury suggest that alkali ingestion would lead to more serious injury and complications; however, this distinction is probably not clinically relevant in the setting of strong acid or base ingestion, because both are able to penetrate esophageal tissues rapidly, potentially leading to full-thickness damage to the esophageal wall [6]. In one study, strong acid ingestion was actually associated with longer hospital stays and increased incidence of systemic complications, such as renal failure, liver dysfunction, disseminated intravascular coagulation, and hemolysis, when compared with alkali ingestion [6].

Esophageal injury mechanisms may be more complicated than the chemical burns previously described. Reactive oxygen species generation with subsequent lipid peroxidation has been implicated as contributing to initial esophageal injury, and subsequent stricture formation seen commonly after caustic ingestion. Investigators have measured concentrations of malondialdehyde, a known end product of lipid peroxidation, as well as glutathione, a known endogenous free-radical scavenger, in esophageal tissue exposed to sodium hydroxide. The investigators found significantly higher malondialdehyde concentrations, indicating the presence of reactive oxygen species 24 hours postexposure. These concentrations remained high for 72 hours after exposure compared with noninjured controls. Furthermore, significantly lower glutathione concentrations in tissue exposed to sodium hydroxide were found in injured esophageal tissue compared with controls, further supporting the presence of reactive oxygen species and free-radical damage [7].

Esophageal injury may begin within minutes after corrosive ingestion, and may persist for hours thereafter [8]. Initially, tissue injury is marked by eosinophillic necrosis with swelling and hemorrhagic congestion [5]. Four to 7 days after ingestion, mucosal sloughing and bacterial invasion occur. This period is further marked by inflammation and the appearance of granulation tissue. During this time, ulcers become covered with a fibrinous layer. Perforation may occur during this time if ulceration exceeds the muscle plane. Fibroblasts appear at injury sites around day 4, and on day 5, roughly, an "esophageal mold" is formed, consisting of dead cells, secretions, and possibly food. On the 10th day after ingestion, esophageal repair begins. Finally, approximately 1 month after exposure, esophageal ulcerations begin to epithelialize [5].

Clinical assessment and studies

Patients who present for medical care following caustic ingestion may have varied signs and symptoms. Patients may be asymptomatic, but may also suffer from nausea, vomiting, dysphagia, odynophagia, drooling, abdominal pain, chest pain, or stridor. Attempts have been made to correlate symptomatology and physical findings with esophageal injury, but the literature is inconclusive. One study found that the presence of two or more signs or symptoms, including vomiting, drooling, or stridor, predicted serious esophageal injury [9]. A later study suggested that drooling and dysphagia alone correlated with esophageal injury [10]. A following study found that patients who have more than three signs or symptoms following corrosive ingestion had increased likelihood of esophageal injury [11]. Other studies [12,13], however, do not support these conclusions and suggest that clinical findings do not correlate with presence or severity of esophageal injury after corrosive ingestion. It has been demonstrated that absence of oropharyngeal injury does not exclude esophageal or gastric lesions [14], with one series finding a 12% incidence of grade II esophageal lesions in asymptomatic patients [12].

Investigators have attempted to correlate laboratory values with injury severity and outcome following caustic ingestion. One study found a white blood cell count greater than 20,000 cells/mm^3, as well as age, strong acid ingestion, and the presence of deep esophageal ulcers or necrosis, to be predictors of mortality [15]. A subsequent study found no correlation between C-reactive protein or leukocyte counts and esophageal injury or patient outcomes, and concluded that these are not useful predictive markers [11]. Despite these findings, hemolysis, disseminated intravascular coagulation, renal failure, and liver failure have all been reported following caustic ingestion [6], suggesting that laboratory studies may be useful in guiding patient management, but not in predicting morbidity or mortality.

Adult patients who have signs of perforated viscous, peritonitis, mediastinitis, or hemodynamic instability may require prompt surgical evaluation and intervention [16], including exploratory laparotomy or laparoscopy, necrotic tissue resection or esophagectomy with delayed colonic interposition. Patients presenting with abdominal pain and peritoneal findings should have chest and abdominal radiographs performed to determine the presence of intraperitoneal air or mediastinal air. Criteria for emergent surgery have been proposed, including presence of shock or disseminated intravascular coagulation, need for hemodialysis, acidosis, and degree of esophageal injury seen on endoscopy [17]. One study found that, following a caustic ingestion, an arterial pH less than 7.22 or a base excess lower than negative 12 indicate severe esophageal injury and the need for consideration of emergency surgery [18]. Some suggest that the presence of grade 3 lesions, described later, alone mandate immediate exploratory laparoscopy with removal of necrotic tissue, because this approach has been associated with improved outcomes and decreased mortality [4,19,20]. However, these criteria are reported in the adult patient literature only. In the pediatric population, these criteria have not been studied, and some authors recommend exhausting all resources to try to preserve the child's native esophagus [21].

Crucial in the initial evaluation of patients who have ingested corrosives is esophagogastroduodenoscopy (EGD). Initial endoscopes were rigid, and endoscopy was associated with increased incidence of esophageal perforation. However, flexible EGD has been established as a safe and reliable tool for assessing esophageal damage up to 96 hours after caustic ingestion [22], so long as gentle insufflation is used during the procedure. Only clinical or radiologic suspicion for perforated viscous is a contraindication for EGD [22]. Lesions are defined in Table 1.

Classifying burn degree is important for patient prognosis and management. Generally, patients who have grade 0 and 1 lesions do not develop

Table 1
Esophageal injury grading scale

Grade	Endoscopic findings
0	Normal esophagus
1	Mucosal edema and hyperemia
2a	Friability, hemorrhages, erosions, blisters, whitish membranes, exudates, and superficial ulcerations
2b	Deep or circumferential ulceration, in addition to 2a lesions
3a	Small and scattered areas of necrosis
3b	Extensive necrosis

Data from Zargar SA, Kochhar R, Mehta S, et al. The role of fiberoptic endoscopy in the management of corrosive ingestion and modified endoscopic classification of burns. Gastrointest Endosc 1991;37(2):165–9.

delayed sequelae, such as stricture or gastric outlet obstruction. These patients can be safely discharged to home after complete resolution of symptoms and their ability to tolerate ingestion of solids and liquids. As lesion severity increases, stricture formation incidence increases. Following a grade 2b burn, stricture incidence may be as high as 71% [22], and after a grade 3 burn, as high as 100% [23]. Additionally, the degree of esophageal injury visualized by endoscopy has been shown to be an accurate predictor of systemic complications and death, with each increased injury grade correlating with a ninefold increase in morbidity and mortality [6].

Attempts have been made to determine which patients should undergo EGD after corrosive ingestion. Some authors [14,16,24] recommend all patients who have ingested a corrosive undergo EGD, in light of the fact that studies have shown that patients who are asymptomatic may still have significant esophageal or gastric injury. One retrospective study, however, found that asymptomatic patients who had unintentionally ingested a corrosive were unlikely to have clinically significant esophageal injury [25]. Additionally, a retrospective review of children who had ingested hair relaxer, which often contains sodium or lithium hydroxide and may have a pH greater than 11, found that, despite the presence of lip and oropharyngeal injury, of the patients who underwent EGD, none had greater than grade 1 esophageal or gastric injury, and none had an adverse clinical outcome [26]. These data suggest that the need for endoscopy should be made on a clinical case-by-case basis. Typical indications for which EGD should be strongly considered include visible posterior pharyngeal burns, stridor, vomiting, chest or abdominal pain, or the inability or refusal to drink. Perhaps most notably, patients who have ingested corrosives as a suicide attempt should undergo EGD, because these patients often consume larger volumes of more corrosive agents as compared with those who have unintentionally ingested corrosives, and, as such, are at increased risk for esophageal or gastric injury.

In addition to EGD, other diagnostic modalities have been investigated to determine esophageal injury following caustic ingestion. High-resolution ultrasonography (endoscopic ultrasonography [EUS]) can be performed concomitantly with EGD, using a 20-MHz ultrasound miniprobe, which is smaller than a traditional transesophageal echocardiogram probe. EUS is better able to define deeper esophageal tissue layers and predict late complications, such as stricture formation. Early investigators [27] have proposed an injury grading system based on ultrasound findings, with grade 0 showing intact muscle layers; grade I demonstrating well-defined, but thickened layers; grade II demonstrating indistinct muscle layers; and grade III showing completely indistinguishable muscle layers. The authors further subdivide grade II and III lesions into a and b, with grade a showing noncircumferential injury and grade b showing full-circumference injury. A subsequent study confirmed that EUS was able to identify deeper tissue injury than conventional EGD [28]. However, the authors also concluded that this procedure does not add prognostic value over EGD alone. Despite their findings, the authors recognize that experience with EUS is limited and may warrant further investigation. An additional diagnostic tool for determining esophageal injury is the Technitium 99m sucralfate swallowing study. This tool was found to be useful in detecting esophageal injury in humans when performed within 24 hours of ingestion, as well as being useful in documenting healing on repeat studies [29].

Treatment

Initial treatment of patients after caustic ingestion includes hemodynamic stabilization and airway assessment, with possible endotracheal or nasotracheal intubation, or surgical airway management if there is evidence of upper airway compromise. Although activated charcoal administration is common after toxicant ingestion, this practice is contraindicated after caustic ingestion, because activated charcoal does not adsorb caustics and interferes with endoscopic evaluation.

A potential early intervention might include pH neutralization, with a patient consuming either a weak acid or base. This practice is generally not recommended for fear of compounding injury by inducing an exothermic reaction. This concern, however, is not borne out in animal studies, which demonstrate that intraluminal temperatures do not rise dangerously with neutralization therapy, and that there is no additive damage from an exothermic reaction [30,31]. Furthermore, Homan and colleagues [32] demonstrated that early neutralization therapy decreases esophageal injury on a histopathologic level in a rat model, and that delayed neutralization therapy results in increased esophageal damage. There is, however, no data to support this practice in humans and is currently not routinely recommended.

In addition to pH neutralization, dilution has been suggested as a possible technique for mediating esophageal injury after caustic ingestion. One study investigated dilution with milk and water after exposing rat esophagi to 50% sodium hydroxide. The investigators concluded that early dilution with milk or water decreased esophageal injury from alkali exposure [33]. No human clinical data exist to support this practice, and, as such, it is currently not recommended routinely because of concerns over potential for emesis, obscuring EGD evaluation and increasing luminal pressure and subsequent perforation.

Other treatments that have been suggested immediately following corrosive ingestions include enteral or parenteral proton-pump inhibitors and H-2 blockers. These agents are used to suppress reflux of gastric contents back into the esophagus, thereby minimizing esophageal injury [16]. However, one study found increased gastric injury when H-2 blockers were administered immediately following corrosive ingestion [5]. The authors postulated that this increase in gastric injury was a result of stomach acid suppression and decreased caustic neutralization, leading them to recommend starting this treatment 24 hours after caustic ingestion. To date, however, human clinical studies demonstrating efficacy are lacking.

The most concerning chronic complications after caustic ingestions include stricture formation and esophageal malignant transformation. Although strictures may develop in 26% to 55% of patients who ingest caustic substances [19,34], early interventions are aimed at preventing or minimizing this complication. The most common, and perhaps most controversial, treatments used to prevent stricture formation are parenteral corticosteroids and antibiotics. Corticosteroids are believed to attenuate inflammation and granulation and fibrous tissue formation [35]. One prospective study found no benefit from systemic steroid administration in children who had ingested caustic substances and that the development of strictures was related only to severity of esophageal injury [36]. A subsequent study found that high doses of methylprednisolone were beneficial in patients who had grade 2b esophageal lesions, with a decreased incidence of stricture formation and decreased need for bougienage after stricture formation [37]. However, some animal studies have demonstrated increased morbidity and mortality associated with corticosteroid use [38]. In addition, a meta-analysis of studies published between 1991 and 2004 ultimately found that corticosteroids are of no benefit and do not significantly decrease the incidence of strictures after corrosive ingestion [39], and recommends the abandonment of this practice. Other investigators have supported this conclusion, finding that systemic steroid treatment has no beneficial effect on esophageal wound healing following caustic esophageal burns [40]. There have been no prospective clinical trials evaluating the utility of antibiotics alone, and their value in the setting of caustic ingestion without signs of concomitant infection, such as peritonitis or mediastinitis, is unknown. Despite the 1000-times greater incidence of esophageal cancer in patients who have ingested caustics over the general population [41], routine screening is not currently recommended [16].

There are some potential new treatment modalities for stricture formation prevention. Because of the reactive oxygen species generated after caustic ingestion, investigators have been focusing on antioxidant treatment to prevent esophageal strictures. In a rat model, treatment with vitamin E caused decreased collagen synthesis and stricture formation [42]. Additionally, ketotifen, an H-1 blocker and mast-cell stabilizer, when given either orally or intraperitoneally to rats, decreased stricture formation and fibrosis after caustic ingestion [43]. Further, phosphatidylcholine, which stimulates collegenase activity and prevents excessive collagen accumulation, when given to rats after caustic ingestion, prevented stricture formation as well [44]. Data in humans are lacking, but these treatments may represent options worthy of further investigation.

Other treatment modalities exist for the prevention and treatment of strictures, including bougienage, esophageal stent placement, intralesional corticosteroid injection, and endoscopic dilatation after stricture formation. Instrumentation of the esophagus can lead to perforation, especially during days 7 to 21 after ingestion, at which time the burn area is weakest, as necrotic tissue begins to slough [16]. Despite this, Tiryaki and colleagues [34] found early, prophylactic dilatation with bougienage to be safe as well as effective at reducing time for stricture resolution. Esophageal stents have also been shown to reduce the incidence of stricture formation [45–47].

Once strictures have formed, patients often require endoscopic balloon dilatation, or bougienage. Multiple dilatations may be required long term for strictures to resolve; however, stable patients may be able to perform this task at home, eliminating the need for frequent hospital admissions [48]. In addition, some authors advocate intralesional corticosteroid injections as augmentation to stricture dilation and have found that using this technique, although technically difficult, reduces the number or dilatations required for stricture resolution [49]. Surgical intervention may be necessary if these treatments fail, or in the presence of malignant transformation or lengthy or tight strictures [50]. Surgical options include colonic or small bowel interposition and gastric transposition [46]. Although these procedures are often highly invasive, a minimally invasive technique has been described, using thoracoscopic and laparscopic technique [50].

Caustic enemas

Although less common than caustic ingestion, caustic enema use and abuse has been reported, at times with devastating consequences. Caustic enemas have been used in suicide and homicide attempts, as abortifacients, as tribal therapeutics, or by accident [51]. Patients who have underlying psychiatric disorders reportedly have used alkali enemas in a misguided attempt to purge parasites from their intestines [52]. Caustics that have been rectally administered include car battery acid (sulphuric acid), potash, muriatic acid, acetic acid, hydrofluoric acid, and ammonia (Haroz, personal communication, 2006) [51,53,54]. Corrosive enemas may be more damaging than corrosive ingestion, because the agent has increased tissue contact time in the lower gastrointestinal tract than in the upper [53]. Despite the potentially devastating consequences associated with caustic enemas, less is known about treatment and prognosis.

Patients presenting after rectal caustic administration may have varied symptoms, including ano-rectal pain, abdominal pain or colic, and tenesmus. In one report, a 5-year-old boy who had received an acetic acid enema presented with lethargy and cyanosis [53]. Clinical findings may include hematochezia, hypotension, hypogastric tenderness, flank tenderness, and a hyper- or hypotonic anal sphincter [51,53]. Frank peritonitis has never been reported immediately following rectal caustic administration.

Patients who present following caustic enemas may require hemodynamic stabilization and should be assessed for potential intestinal bleeding and the need for emergent transfusion. Chest and abdominal radiographs may need to be obtained to determine the presence of free air. In the absence of peritoneal findings, lower endoscopy, such as sigmoidoscopy or colonoscopy, should be considered to determine the extent and depth of injury. However, some authors suggest that this may be of little help and may increase risk of perforation [51]. There is no injury grading system for corrosive enema injuries as described for corrosive esophagitis. Injury may range from none, to friable mucosa, to extensive, full thickness necrosis, extending as far proximally as the terminal ileum. Surgical management with exploration and resection of bowel may be necessary if there is evidence of necrotic tissue, peritonitis, or pneumoperitoneum. However, postoperative mortality rates have been reported as greater than 50% [51].

Similar to patients who have corrosive esophagitis, patients who have corrosive colitis are at risk for significant morbidity and mortalitiy, including strictures, bowel perforation, peritonitis, renal and hepatic dysfunction, and disseminated intravascular coagulation [53]. Early interventions to alleviate pain and minimize sequelae include mesalamine enema, beclamethasone enema [55], and parenteral steroids and antibiotics. To date, no clinical studies have been done to evaluate the efficacy of these treatments. Supportive care remains the mainstay of treatment, with early surgical and gastroenterology consultation for endoscopic evaluation and possible surgical intervention. Patients may also require prolonged observation or close follow-up, because delayed viscous perforation has been reported, and patients who have strictures may require dilatation, as well as possible surgical resection, should dilatation fail [51].

Hydrofluoric acid

HF is marketed in several formulations for both industrial and commercial use. It is available as an anhydrous acid in concentrations greater than 99%, as well as in aqueous solution in concentrations up to 70% [56]. In its anhydrous form, it is considered a strong acid, but in aqueous solution, it is considered a weak acid. Even in its aqueous form as a weak acid, HF exposure may have devastating consequences. Industrial uses include the manufacturing of refrigerants, herbicides, pesticides, pharmaceutics, high-octane gasoline, aluminum, plastics, electrical components, and light bulbs. It can also be found in commercial products for rust removal, brass and crystal cleaning, and enamel etching [57]. Ammonium bifluoride is also available in over-the-counter products, especially in car wheel cleaners, and exposure to it should be treated in a similar manner to an exposure to HF.

Mechanism of action

HF, in its aqueous form, is a weak acid that slowly dissociates into hydrogen and fluoride ions, resulting in tissue penetration by way of a nonionic diffusion gradient potentially causing extensive liquefaction necrosis, behaving more like an alkali than an acid [58]. Additionally, fluoride ions penetrate tissues and form insoluble salts with positively charged ions such as calcium and magnesium, causing tissue injury, hypocalcemia, hypomagnesemia, and pain that is often out of proportion to visible tissue injury [59].

Clinical manifestations and initial assessment

Dermal contact with HF is the most common route of exposure, especially injuries to the hands with the use of low-concentration rust remover and aluminum cleaning products [60]. After HF skin contact, symptoms may be immediate or delayed. HF concentrations greater than 50% may cause immediate, severe, and throbbing pain and a whitish discoloration of the skin. Concentrations of 20% to 50% generally produce pain and swelling on the exposed areas that may be delayed up to 8 hours. HF solutions less than 20% may cause no immediate symptoms on skin contact, but may cause serious injury that may be delayed 12 to 24 hours [61].

Aqueous HF solutions are highly volatile and produce vapors that are lighter than ambient air, often resulting in concomitant inhalational and dermal injury, especially with head and neck exposures [58]. Pulmonary effects include upper airway irritation, narrowing, swelling, and obstruction of the upper airway that may be immediate or delayed up to 36 hours [61]. Physical findings may include stridor, wheezing, or rhonchi, as well as erythema and ulceration of the upper respiratory tract [62]. High concentration HF inhalation may result in rapid onset of noncardiogenic pulmonary edema and death [63].

Ocular exposure to HF may be the result of aqueous or HF vapor contact. Eye contact may result in pain, corneal sloughing, revascularization, corneal opacification, and occasionally keratoconjunctivitis sicca as a long-term complication [64].

HF ingestion can cause gastritis while sparing the remainder of the gastrointestinal tract. After ingestion, patients may present with nausea, vomiting, or abdominal pain. Systemic absorption is rapid and usually fatal within the first 30 minutes after ingestion, but potentially as long as 7 hours after ingestion [59].

Death following HF exposure is often a result of cardiac dysrhythmias, most notably ventricular fibrillation [64]. These cardiac dysrhythmias are most likely multifactoral, secondary to electrolyte abnormalities, acidosis, or hypoxia [60]. Hypocalcemia alone is probably insufficient to explain the dysrhythmias, because rats exposed to sodium fluoride still died of cardiovascular failure despite calcium replacement [65]. Some authors postulate that hyperkalemia precipitates cardiac toxicity, because fluoride ions increase intracellular calcium concentration, subsequently causing potassium efflux and systemic hyperkalemia [66].

Because of concerns for both upper and lower airway edema, close inspection of the patient's airway is paramount. Evidence of oropharyngeal edema may prompt early endotracheal or nasotracheal intubation, or surgical airway management. Intravenous access may need to be obtained to monitor serum electrolyte levels, such as calcium, potassium, magnesium, and sodium, as well as to administer analgesia, intravenous fluids, and electrolytes. An increase in ionized serum fluoride and decrease in total and ionized serum calcium, hyponatremia, and hyperkalemia can occur following moderate HF exposure [67]; however, because there is little correlation between clinical outcomes and serum fluoride levels, monitoring serum fluoride is of little value [68].

Cardiac monitoring and serial electrocardiography (ECG) may demonstrate electrolyte abnormalities before serum studies are available, although the sensitivity of ECG is unclear [59]. The ECG may show sinus tachycardia, nonspecific ST segment abnormalities, QTc prolongation, QRS widening, or ventricular fibrillation. Patients manifesting pulmonary symptoms such as cough or dyspnea may require chest radiography evaluation.

Decontamination and topical treatments

All patients suffering HF exposure require immediate decontamination, with emergency personnel taking care not to contaminate themselves [69]. All areas that have been in contact with HF should be promptly irrigated with copious amounts of water. Contaminated clothing should be removed and stored in sealed plastic bags to avoid secondary exposure to care providers.

Topical treatments are aimed at decreasing pain, skin injury, and systemic absorption of fluoride ions. Quaternary ammonium compounds, such as benzalkonium chloride, have been used to decontaminate and irrigate HF burns. These compounds are purported to inactivate fluoride ions on the skin. Exposed skin can be soaked in a 0.13% benzalkonium chloride water solution or dressed in benzalkonium chloride–soaked compression dressings to be changed every 2 to 4 minutes. These compounds are useful in mild burns, but less useful in deeper burns [58]. These compounds should not be used in the eye.

Calcium-containing gels can also be applied topically to low-concentration (less then 20%) HF burns. A 2.5% calcium gel can be prepared by mixing 3.5 g of calcium gluconate powder with 5 ounces of a water-soluble lubricant, such as K-Y jelly, or mixing 25 mL of 10% calcium gluconate with 75 mL of a water-soluble lubricant [60,69]. The gel should be left in place for 15 minutes, rinsed, and reapplied as often as necessary until pain is relieved [58]. Topical magnesium has also been proposed as a treatment for HF burns, but its efficacy is uncertain. Some studies report effectiveness similar to topical calcium [70,71], whereas others report little evidence to support the routine use of magnesium to treat low-concentration dermal HF exposure [69].

Hexafluorine is a hypertonic agent that has been used for many years in Europe to decontaminate skin and ocular HF burns. It is believed to chelate both hydrogen and fluoride ions, thereby decreasing systemic absorption. Despite case reports describing successful HF burn treatment with Hexafluorine [72,73], animal studies of HF-induced dermal injury treated with Hexafluorine showed no difference in electrolyte disturbances in the Hexafluorine treated animals compared with those decontaminated with water. Further, animals decontaminated with Hexafluorine had more severe skin burns compared with those treated with water or calcium gluconate gel [74].

Regional and systemic treatments

Intradermal calcium injection has been recommended when application of topical calcium gel fails to relieve the pain within the first few minutes following HF exposure or following skin exposure to HF of greater than 20% concentration. Recommendations suggest using a 27- or 30-gauge needle; no more than 0.5 mL/cm^2 of 10% calcium gluconate is injected into the subcutaneous tissue surrounding the exposed areas [61]. Calcium chloride should not be used because it can cause further tissue damage. Despite reported successful treatment of HF exposure with local calcium injection, there are several concerns with this technique, and its routine use is discouraged. First, patients may experience more pain from multiple injections. Second, the volume that can be infiltrated into digits is limited, and vascular compromise can occur if too much fluid volume is infiltrated into a closed finite space such as fingertips. Further, there is concern that digital calcium injection may extend the burn into the subungal area. Finally, local hyperosmolality and tissue toxicity of calcium may cause more damage than the HF itself [56,60,75].

Following inhalational exposure to HF, nebulized calcium gluconate may attenuate local and systemic toxicity. Calcium gluconate 2.5% (2.5 g or 25 mL of calcium gluconate in 100 mL of water) can be nebulized by way of conventional means to treat serious HF inhalation with systemic hypocalcemia [58,61,69,76,77]. However, this treatment has never been formally studied, and evidence to support its routine use is lacking.

Parenteral calcium can be administered both through standard peripheral intravenous means, as well in combination with a Bier block. Peripheral intravenous calcium administration of calcium gluconate, which contains 0.45 mEq/mL of calcium, should be limited to 0.1 to 0.2 mL/kg pushed slowly over 5 minutes. Calcium chloride, which contains 1.36 mEq/mL of calcium, should be administered through central venous access slowly, because it is an irritant and can cause tissue injury and necrosis should it extravasate.

The Bier block was originally intended for regional anesthesia of the distal extremities. Its use in the treatment of HF burns was first reported in 1992 [78]. This technique involves achieving intravenous access in the hand or foot of the affected extremity. A tourniquet, such as a blood pressure cuff, is then applied to the proximal portion of the limb and inflated to 50 mm Hg above the patient's systolic blood pressure. The cuff or tourniquet should not be applied on the forearm or lower leg because adequate arterial compression cannot be obtained. The block is more effective if the extremity is exsanguinated before the tourniquet is inflated. This can be done by tightly wrapping the distal part of the extremity with an Esmarch rubber bandage. It is also acceptable to simply elevate the extremity for 20 to 30 seconds while applying firm digital pressure on the brachial or femoral artery [79]. A volume of 25 mL of 2.5% calcium gluconate is then infused slowly while the cuff remains inflated. After 25 minutes, the cuff pressure is decreased gradually over 5 minutes. This technique should not be used for patients who have poor peripheral vascular circulation. Additionally, gradual cuff deflation is important so as not to cause systemic hypercalcemia.

Magnesium sulfate has been proposed as a treatment for HF burns, but its efficacy has not been firmly established. One rat study showed that high-dose intravenous magnesium sulfate infusion decreased mortality [80]. However, a subsequent study of intravenous magnesium sulfate failed to demonstrate decreased fluoride bioavailabilty or risk of death after HF exposure [81].

Intra-arterial calcium infusion is an additional treatment option, if the HF burn involves a large part of an extremity or is a high-concentration exposure to the hands. An arterial line should be placed ipsilaterally and proximally to the affected area. A solution of 10 mL of 10% calcium gluconate in 40 mL of normal saline or D5W is run through the line over 4 hours. The infusion can be repeated every 4 to 8 hours, with pain relief considered the indication for therapy cessation [61,75]. The arterial pressure waveform should be monitored continuously after the infusion is completed for as long as the artery is cannulated. Complications of this therapy include ulnar, radial, and median nerve palsy; hematoma formation; and inflammation of the puncture site. One case series of patients suffering HF extremity injuries described a slight decrease in serum magnesium levels requiring correction and clinically insignificant hypercalcemia with this technique [82]. Further, an increased incidence of microperforation of blood vessels with higher-concentration calcium gluconate solutions was described in a rat model of intra-arterial calcium infusion [83]. High-concentration intra-arterial calcium chloride infusion has been described, but the potential for vessel injury and tissue necrosis from extravasation mandates extreme caution. When canulating a major artery, such as the brachial artery, consultation with a surgeon or interventional radiologist may be warranted.

Hemodialysis and burn excision are other modalities available for treating patients who have HF burns. One case report describes a patient who suffered a 7% body surface area burn with 71% HF. The patient developed fluoride-induced cardiotoxicity and ventricular fibrillation, which was treated successfully with hemodialysis. Utility of hemodialysis for the management of high-concentration HF exposure is otherwise unproven [84]. Additionally, one case report describes a favorable outcome for a patient treated with aggressive surgical resection of hydrofluoric acid burns [85]. Further, a recent rabbit study showed a decrease in the serum fluoride and in the degree of hypocalcemia and mortality in a group treated with excision of the exposed area 30 minutes after the injury was induced, compared with groups treated conservatively and with calcium gluconate infusion [86]. In most HF exposures, however, surgical treatment should be limited to debridement of blisters and necrotic tissues to enhance the efficacy of medical treatment [58].

Ocular exposure

Ocular exposure to HF in the form of a liquid splash or vapor requires vigorous irrigation with water, normal saline, or lactated Ringers solution. Copious irrigation with nonmineral containing solutions is the only widely accepted therapy for HF exposure to the eyes. Generally accepted treatment for HF skin exposure, such as calcium or magnesium application, may not be appropriate for ocular burn [87]. Urgent ophthalmology consultation is appropriate once the patient is stabilized. Commercially available calcium gluconate containing solutions are available [88]; however, an animal study of 1% calcium gluconate irrigation did not show any significant advantage over saline irrigation [89]. Another animal study suggests possible benefit with magnesium chloride solution irrigation [87], and there are case reports of successful treatment of ocular HF exposure with calcium gluconate eye drops [90,91]. However, these therapies should only be instituted after emergent consultation with an opthalmologist.

Summary

Patients who have ingested caustic substances have great potential for morbidity and mortality. Close evaluation of the patient's airway, with aggressive supportive care, remains paramount. Currently, there is little evidence to support the use of parenteral corticosteroids or systemic antibiotics without concomitant signs of infection following caustic ingestion. Early consultation with a gastroenterologist, otolaryngologist, or surgeon should be considered, because the patient may warrant EGD or surgical intervention. Patients exposed to hydrofluoric acid by any route require decontamination as well as specialized treatments, including topical, regional, and systemic treatments to reduce burns, pain, and systemic complications. These patients may also require early consultation with a surgeon or interventional radiologist, should there be a need for surgical debridement or intra-arterial therapies.

References

[1] Watson WA, Litovitz TL, Rodgers GC Jr, et al. 2004 Annual report of the American Association of Poison Control Centers Toxic Exposure Surveillance System. Am J Emerg Med 2005;23(5):589–666.

[2] Hoffman RS, Howland MA, Kamerow HN, et al. Comparison of titratable acid/alkaline reserve and pH in potentially caustic household products. J Toxicol Clin Toxicol 1989; 27(4–5):241–6.

[3] Mattos GM, Lopes DD, Mamede RC, et al. Effects of time of contact and concentration of caustic agent on generation of injuries. Laryngoscope 2006;116(3):456–60.

[4] Havanond C. Is there a difference between the management of grade 2b and 3 corrosive gastric injuries? J Med Assoc Thai 2002;85(3):340–4.

[5] Mamede RC, de Mello Filho FV. Ingestion of caustic substances and its complications. Sao Paulo Med J 2001;119(1):10–5.

[6] Poley JW, Steyerberg EW, Kuipers EJ, et al. Ingestion of acid and alkaline agents: outcome and prognostic value of early upper endoscopy. Gastrointest Endosc 2004;60(3): 372–7.

[7] Gunel E, Caglayan F, Caglayan O, et al. Reactive oxygen radical levels in caustic esophageal burns. J Pediatr Surg 1999;34(3):405–7.

[8] Satar S, Topal M, Kozaci N. Ingestion of caustic substances by adults. Am J Ther 2004;11(4): 258–61.

[9] Crain EF, Gershel JC, Mezey AP. Caustic ingestions. Symptoms as predictors of esophageal injury. Am J Dis Child 1984;138(9):863–5.

[10] Nuutinen M, Uhari M, Karvali T, et al. Consequences of caustic ingestions in children. Acta Paediatr 1994;83(11):1200–5.

[11] Chen TY, Ko SF, Chuang JH, et al. Predictors of esophageal stricture in children with unintentional ingestion of caustic agents. Chang Gung Med J 2003;26(4):233–9.

[12] Gaudreault P, Parent M, McGuigan MA, et al. Predictability of esophageal injury from signs and symptoms: a study of caustic ingestion in 378 children. Pediatrics 1983;71(5):767–70.

[13] Gorman RL, Khin-Maung-Gyi MT, Klein-Schwartz W, et al. Initial symptoms as predictors of esophageal injury in alkaline corrosive ingestions. Am J Emerg Med 1992; 10(3):189–94.

[14] Previtera C, Giusti F, Guglielmi M. Predictive value of visible lesions (cheeks, lips, oropharynx) in suspected caustic ingestion: may endoscopy reasonably be omitted in completely negative pediatric patients? Pediatr Emerg Care 1990;6(3):176–8.

[15] Rigo GP, Camellini L, Azzolini F, et al. What is the utility of selected clinical and endoscopic parameters in predicting the risk of death after caustic ingestion? Endoscopy 2002;34(4): 304–10.

[16] Katzka DA. Caustic injury to the esophagus. Curr Treat Options Gastroenterol 2001;4(1): 59–66.

[17] Brun JG, Celerier M, Koskas F, et al. Blunt thorax oesophageal stripping: an emergency procedure for caustic ingestion. Br J Surg 1984;71(9):698–700.

[18] Cheng YJ, Kao EL. Arterial blood gas analysis in acute caustic ingestion injuries. Surg Today 2003;33(7):483–5.

[19] Estrera A, Taylor W, Mills LJ, et al. Corrosive burns of the esophagus and stomach: a recommendation for an aggressive surgical approach. Ann Thorac Surg 1986;41(3):276–83.

[20] Cattan P, Munoz-Bongrand N, Berney T, et al. Extensive abdominal surgery after caustic ingestion. Ann Surg 2000;231(4):519–23.

[21] Erdogan E, Eroglu E, Tekant G, et al. Management of esophagogastric corrosive injuries in children. Eur J Pediatr Surg 2003;13(5):289–93.

[22] Zargar SA, Kochhar R, Mehta S, et al. The role of fiberoptic endoscopy in the management of corrosive ingestion and modified endoscopic classification of burns. Gastrointest Endosc 1991;37(2):165–9.

[23] Baskin D, Urganci N, Abbasoglu L, et al. A standardised protocol for the acute management of corrosive ingestion in children. Pediatr Surg Int 2004;20(11–12):824–8.

[24] Squires RH Jr, Colletti RB. Indications for pediatric gastrointestinal endoscopy: a medical position statement of the North American Society for Pediatric Gastroenterology and Nutrition. J Pediatr Gastroenterol Nutr 1996;23(2):107–10.

[25] Gupta SK, Croffie JM, Fitzgerald JF. Is esophagogastroduodenoscopy necessary in all caustic ingestions? J Pediatr Gastroenterol Nutr 2001;32(1):50–3.

[26] Aronow SP, Aronow HD, Blanchard T, et al. Hair relaxers: a benign caustic ingestion? J Pediatr Gastroenterol Nutr 2003;36(1):120–5.

[27] Kamijo Y, Kondo I, Kokuto M, et al. Miniprobe ultrasonography for determining prognosis in corrosive esophagitis. Am J Gastroenterol 2004;99(5):851–4.

[28] Chiu HM, Lin JT, Huang SP, et al. Prediction of bleeding and stricture formation after corrosive ingestion by EUS concurrent with upper endoscopy. Gastrointest Endosc 2004;60(5): 827–33.

[29] Millar AJ, Numanoglu A, Mann M, et al. Detection of caustic oesophageal injury with technetium 99m-labelled sucralfate. J Pediatr Surg 2001;36(2):262–5.

[30] Homan CS, Singer AJ, Henry MC, et al. Thermal effects of neutralization therapy and water dilution for acute alkali exposure in canines. Acad Emerg Med 1997;4(1):27–32.

[31] Homan CS, Singer AJ, Thomajan C, et al. Thermal characteristics of neutralization therapy and water dilution for strong acid ingestion: an in-vivo canine model. Acad Emerg Med 1998;5(4):286–92.

[32] Homan CS, Maitra SR, Lane BP, et al. Histopathologic evaluation of the therapeutic efficacy of water and milk dilution for esophageal acid injury. Acad Emerg Med 1995;2(7): 587–91.

[33] Homan CS, Maitra SR, Lane BP, et al. Therapeutic effects of water and milk for acute alkali injury of the esophagus. Ann Emerg Med 1994;24(1):14–20.

[34] Tiryaki T, Livanelioglu Z, Atayurt H. Early bougienage for relief of stricture formation following caustic esophageal burns. Pediatr Surg Int 2005;21(2):78–80.

[35] Jain AL, Robertson GJ, Rudis MI. Surgical issues in the poisoned patient. Emerg Med Clin North Am 2003;21(4):1117–44.

[36] Anderson KD, Rouse TM, Randolph JG. A controlled trial of corticosteroids in children with corrosive injury of the esophagus. N Engl J Med 1990;323(10):637–40.

[37] Boukthir S, Fetni I, Mrad SM, et al. High doses of steroids in the management of caustic esophageal burns in children [abstract]. Arch Pediatr 2004;11(1):13–7 [in French].

[38] Rosenberg N, Kunderman PJ, Vroman L, et al. Prevention of experimental esophageal stricture by cortisone. II. Control of suppurative complications by penicillin. AMA Arch Surg 1953;66(5):593–8.

[39] Pelclova D, Navratil T. Do corticosteroids prevent oesophageal stricture after corrosive ingestion? Toxicol Rev 2005;24(2):125–9.

[40] Ulman I, Mutaf O. A critique of systemic steroids in the management of caustic esophageal burns in children. Eur J Pediatr Surg 1998;8(2):71–4.

[41] Zwischenberger JB, Savage C, Bidani A. Surgical aspects of esophageal disease: perforation and caustic injury. Am J Respir Crit Care Med 2002;165(8):1037–40.

[42] Gunel E, Caglayan F, Caglayan O, et al. Effect of antioxidant therapy on collagen synthesis in corrosive esophageal burns. Pediatr Surg Int 2002;18(1):24–7.

[43] Yukselen V, Karaoglu AO, Ozutemiz O, et al. Ketotifen ameliorates development of fibrosis in alkali burns of the esophagus. Pediatr Surg Int 2004;20(6):429–33.

[44] Demirbilek S, Aydin G, Yucesan S, et al. Polyunsaturated phosphatidylcholine lowers collagen deposition in a rat model of corrosive esophageal burn. Eur J Pediatr Surg 2002;12(1): 8–12.

[45] Berkovits RN, Bos CE, Wijburg FA, et al. Caustic injury of the oesophagus. Sixteen years experience, and introduction of a new model oesophageal stent. J Laryngol Otol 1996; 110(11):1041–5.

[46] Zhou JH, Jiang YG, Wang RW, et al. Management of corrosive esophageal burns in 149 cases. J Thorac Cardiovasc Surg 2005;130(2):449–55.

[47] Wang RW, Zhou JH, Jiang YG, et al. Prevention of stricture with intraluminal stenting through laparotomy after corrosive esophageal burns. Eur J Cardiothorac Surg 2006; 30(2):207–11.

[48] Bapat RD, Bakhshi GD, Kantharia CV, et al. Self-bougienage: long-term relief of corrosive esophageal strictures. Indian J Gastroenterol 2001;20(5):180–2.

[49] Kochhar R, Ray JD, Sriram PV, et al. Intralesional steroids augment the effects of endoscopic dilation in corrosive esophageal strictures. Gastrointest Endosc 1999;49(4 Pt 1): 509–13.

[50] Nwomeh BC, Luketich JD, Kane TD. Minimally invasive esophagectomy for caustic esophageal stricture in children. J Pediatr Surg 2004;39(7):e1–6.

[51] Diarra B, Roudie J, Ehua Somian F, et al. Caustic burns of rectum and colon in emergencies. Am J Surg 2004;187(6):785–9.

[52] da Fonseca J, Brito MJ, Freitas J, et al. Acute colitis caused by caustic products. Am J Gastroenterol 1998;93(12):2601–2.

[53] Kawamata M, Fujita S, Mayumi T, et al. Acetic acid intoxication by rectal administration. J Toxicol Clin Toxicol 1994;32(3):333–6.

[54] Cappell MS, Simon T. Fulminant acute colitis following a self-administered hydrofluoric acid enema. Am J Gastroenterol 1993;88(1):122–6.

[55] Michopoulos S, Bouzakis H, Sotiropoulou M, et al. Colitis due to accidental alcohol enema: clinicopathological presentation and outcome. Dig Dis Sci 2000;45(6):1188–91.

[56] Burd A. Hydrofluoric acid-revisited. Burns 2004;30(7):720–2.

[57] CDC chemical emergencies, facts about hydrogen fluoride. Available at: http://www.bt.cdc.gov/agent/hydrofluoricacid/basics/facts.asp. Accessed October 8, 2006.

[58] Kirkpatrick JJ, Enion DS, Burd DA. Hydrofluoric acid burns: a review. Burns 1995;21(7): 483–93.

[59] Kao WF, Dart RC, Kuffner E, et al. Ingestion of low-concentration hydrofluoric acid: an insidious and potentially fatal poisoning. Ann Emerg Med 1999;34(1):35–41.

[60] Caravati EM. Acute hydrofluoric acid exposure. Am J Emerg Med 1988;6(2):143–50.

[61] Agency for toxic substances and diseases registry: medical management guideline for hydrogen fluoride. Available at: http://www.atsdr.cdc.gov/MHMI/mmg11.htm. Accessed October 8, 2006.

[62] Wing JS, Brender JD, Sanderson LM, et al. Acute health effects in a community after a release of hydrofluoric acid. Arch Environ Health 1991;46(3):155–60.

[63] Dote T, Kono K, Usuda K, et al. Lethal inhalation exposure during maintenance operation of a hydrogen fluoride liquefying tank. Toxicol Ind Health 2003;19(2–6):51–4.

[64] Rao RB, Hoffman RS. Caustics and batteries. In: Goldfrank LR, NF, Lewis NA, editors. Goldfrank's toxicologic emergencies. 7th edition. New York: McGraw-Hill; 2002. p. 1323–45.

[65] Strubelt O, Iven H, Younes M. The pathophysiological profile of the acute cardiovascular toxicity of sodium fluoride. Toxicology 1982;24(3–4):313–23.

[66] Cummings CC, McIvor ME. Fluoride-induced hyperkalemia: the role of Ca2+-dependent K+ channels. Am J Emerg Med 1988;6(1):1–3.

[67] Murano M. Studies of the treatment of hydrofluoric acid burn. Bull Osaka Med Coll 1989;5: 39–48.

[68] Saady JJ, Rose CS. A case of nonfatal sodium fluoride ingestion. J Anal Toxicol 1988;12(5): 270–1.

[69] Kirkpatrick JJ, Burd DA. An algorithmic approach to the treatment of hydrofluoric acid burns. Burns 1995;21(7):495–9.

[70] Burkhart KK, Brent J, Kirk MA, et al. Comparison of topical magnesium and calcium treatment for dermal hydrofluoric acid burns. Ann Emerg Med 1994;24(1):9–13.

[71] Dunn BJ, MacKinnon MA, Knowlden NF, et al. Topical treatments for hydrofluoric acid dermal burns. Further assessment of efficacy using an experimental piq model. J Occup Environ Med 1996;38(5):507–14.

[72] Soderberg K, Kuusinen P, Mathieu L, et al. An improved method for emergent decontamination of ocular and dermal hydrofluoric acid splashes. Vet Hum Toxicol 2004;46(4): 216–8.

[73] Mathieu L, Nehles J, Blomet J, et al. Efficacy of hexafluorine for emergent decontamination of hydrofluoric acid eye and skin splashes. Vet Hum Toxicol 2001;43(5):263–5.

[74] Hulten P, Hojer J, Ludwigs U, et al. Hexafluorine vs. standard decontamination to reduce systemic toxicity after dermal exposure to hydrofluoric acid. J Toxicol Clin Toxicol 2004; 42(4):355–61.

[75] Vance MV, Curry SC, Kunkel DB, et al. Digital hydrofluoric acid burns: treatment with intraarterial calcium infusion. Ann Emerg Med 1986;15(8):890–6.

[76] Schiettecatte D, Mullie G, Depoorter M. Treatment of hydrofluoric acid burns. Acta Chir Belg 2003;103(4):375–8.

[77] Kono K, Watanabe T, Dote T, et al. Successful treatments of lung injury and skin burn due to hydrofluoric acid exposure. Int Arch Occup Environ Health 2000;73(Suppl):S93–7.

[78] Henry JA, Hla KK. Intravenous regional calcium gluconate perfusion for hydrofluoric acid burns. J Toxicol Clin Toxicol 1992;30(2):203–7.

[79] Casey W. Intravenous regional anesthesia (Bier's block). Update in Anesthesia. Available at: http://www.nda.ox.ac.uk/wfsa/html/u01_003.htm. Accessed October 8, 2006.

[80] Williams JM, Hammad A, Cottington EC, et al. Intravenous magnesium in the treatment of hydrofluoric acid burns in rats. Ann Emerg Med 1994;23(3):464–9.

[81] Heard K, Hill RE, Cairns CB, et al. Calcium neutralizes fluoride bioavailability in a lethal model of fluoride poisoning. J Toxicol Clin Toxicol 2001;39(4):349–53.

[82] Siegel DC, Heard JM. Intra-arterial calcium infusion for hydrofluoric acid burns. Aviat Space Environ Med 1992;63(3):206–11.

[83] Dowbak G, Rose K, Rohrich RJ. A biochemical and histologic rationale for the treatment of hydrofluoric acid burns with calcium gluconate. J Burn Care Rehabil 1994;15(4):323–7.

[84] Bjornhagen V, Hojer J, Karlson-Stiber C, et al. Hydrofluoric acid-induced burns and life-threatening systemic poisoning–favorable outcome after hemodialysis. J Toxicol Clin Toxicol 2003;41(6):855–60.

[85] Buckingham FM. Surgery: a radical approach to severe hydrofluoric acid burns. A case report. J Occup Med 1988;30(11):873–4.

[86] Yang SJ, Zhang YH, Liu LP, et al. Comparison of various methods of early management of hydrofluoric acid burn in rabbits [abstract]. Zhonghua Shao Shang Za Zhi 2005;21(1):40–2 [in Chinese].

[87] McCully J. Ocular hydrofluoric acid burns: animal model. Trans Am Ophthalmol Soc 1990; 88:649–84.

[88] Recommended medical treatment for hydrofluoric acid exposure [pamphlet]. Honeywell International Inc.; 2006.

[89] Beiran I, Miller B, Bentur Y. The efficacy of calcium gluconate in ocular hydrofluoric acid burns. Hum Exp Toxicol 1997;16(4):223–8.

[90] Bentur Y, Tannenbaum S, Yaffe Y, et al. The role of calcium gluconate in the treatment of hydrofluoric acid eye burn. Ann Emerg Med 1993;22(9):1488–90.

[91] Rubinfeld RS, Silbert DI, Arentsen JJ, et al. Ocular hydrofluoric acid burns. Am J Ophthalmol 1992;114(4):420–3.

ELSEVIER
SAUNDERS

EMERGENCY
MEDICINE
CLINICS OF
NORTH AMERICA

Emerg Med Clin N Am 25 (2007) 477–497

Atypical Antipsychotics and Newer Antidepressants

Tracey H. Reilly, MD[a],*, Mark A. Kirk, MD[b]

[a]Division of Medical Toxicology, Department of Emergency Medicine, University of Virginia,
P.O. Box 800774, Charlottesville, VA 22908-0774, USA
[b]Blue Ridge Poison Center, Division of Medical Toxicology, Department of Emergency
Medicine, University of Virginia, P.O. Box 800744, Charlottesville, VA 22908-0774, USA

Atypical antipsychotics and antidepressants are two of the most commonly prescribed drug classes as well as two of the most commonly reported drug classes associated with human exposure reported to the American Association of Poison Control Centers. Of the 2,438,644 human exposures reported to the American Association of Poison Control Centers in 2004, antidepressants represented 103,155 exposures, and 129,855 exposures were from sedatives/hypnotics/antipsychotics [1]. These figures likely underrepresent the true number of exposures because they reflect only the exposures reported to United States poison centers. These two drug categories are the number two and number three leading causes of death from exposure to all substances as classified by the American Association of Poison Control Centers in 2004 [1]. The emergency medicine physician should be aware of the potential side effects of these commonly prescribed medications because they are frequently encountered in overdose, both therapeutic and intentional, and frequently occur in multiple-drug exposures.

Atypical antipsychotics

Traditional antipsychotics, introduced into clinical practice in the 1950s, were used in the treatment of the positive symptoms of schizophrenia (eg, hallucinations, delusions). However, they proved not useful for the treatment of the negative symptoms of schizophrenia (eg, poverty of thought, withdrawal, and poor motivation) and caused severe extrapyramidal side effects and tardive dyskinesia. Ultimately these drawbacks limited their clinical effectiveness because of the high noncompliance rate and eventual treatment failure.

---

* Corresponding author.
E-mail address: tr3p@virginia.edu (T.H. Reilly).

0733-8627/07/$ - see front matter © 2007 Elsevier Inc. All rights reserved.
doi:10.1016/j.emc.2007.02.003

In the late 1980s, the "atypical" antipsychotics were made available for clinical use. These second-generation antipsychotics include clozapine, risperidone, olanzapine, quetiapine, ziprasidone, and aripiprazole. These agents have a lower propensity to cause extrapyramidal symptoms and an increased ability to treat the negative as well as positive symptoms of schizophrenia.

The terms *neuroleptic* and *antipsychotic* are synonymous when referring to this class of pharmacologic agent. To be classified as an atypical neuroleptic, a drug has to have a lower affinity or propensity to bind to and antagonize D_2-dopaminergic receptors as compared with the traditional antipsychotics. Also, the agent must have a more selective antagonism of the D_2-dopaminergic receptor. Older neuroleptic agents antagonized not only D_2 receptors in the mesolimbic pathway, which treated the positive symptoms of psychosis, but also antagonized the D_2 receptors in the nigrostriatal pathway, which brought about unwanted extrapyramidal side effects and tardive dyskinesia. To be considered atypical, agents have to produce little or no extrapyramidal symptoms at therapeutic dosing and also have little or no propensity to cause tardive dyskinesia [2,3]. Also, the agent must be effective in treating the negative signs and symptoms of schizophrenia (eg, anhedonia, apathy, poverty of thought).

It is the D_2-receptor antagonism that likely causes the extrapyramidal effects seen with neuroleptic drug therapy. The atypical neuroleptics do antagonize the D_2 receptor but do so with more selectivity for mesolimbic versus nigrostriatal pathways in the brain and with less binding potency than the traditional agents. Also, the atypical neuroleptics avidly block serotonergic 5-HT_{1A} and 5-HT_{2A} receptors. Reduction in brain serotonergic activity has been associated with reduced extrapyramidal effects in animals given neuroleptics [3]. Atypical neuroleptic agents with a high serotonergic receptor blockade activity as compared with dopamine receptor blockade have improved efficacy to treat the negative signs and symptoms of schizophrenia, likely due to disinhibition of serotonin effect on the dopamine pathways in the prefrontal cortex. Adverse drug effects can occur with therapeutic dosing as well as supratherapeutic or overdosing. In general, exposure to the atypical neuroleptic drug class tends to cause less toxicity and rarely results in fatality when compared with the older more traditional antipsychotics. The following sections describe in detail the relevant drug effects of this drug class, clinical manifestations of toxicity including neuroleptic malignant syndrome and drug-induced heat stroke, and the management of the patient who has toxicity from atypical neuroleptics.

Drug effect in therapeutic dosing

Atypical neuroleptics demonstrate a wide range of antagonism at many different receptors in the central nervous system. This range of antagonism allows each neuroleptic to have a somewhat unique clinical profile.

Although all of the atypical neuroleptics have dopamine and serotonin receptor blockade activity, they do so with varying affinities.

Several agents interact with muscarinic receptors. An inverse relationship exists between muscarinic receptor blockade and occurrence of extrapyramidal side effects. In other words, when muscarinic receptor blockade is high, extrapyramidal side effects are low. This effect is seen clinically with clozapine and olanzapine, atypical agents with little or no known extrapyramidal side effects [3]. Clozapine causes sialorrhea as a side effect. This is counter intuitive because of its antimuscarinic effects, and this hypersalivation can be treated with a muscarinic receptor antagonist. Clozapine has been shown to be an agonist at specific muscarinic receptors in animal cell model experiments. Although the complete pharmacologic mechanism behind clozapine's ability to cause hypersalivation remains to be elucidated, this drug is an example of how complex and varied the receptor pharmacology of the atypical neuroleptics can be.

Many of the atypical neuroleptics are potent histamine H_1-receptor blocking agents. For example, olanzapine is the most potent antihistaminic agent of all the neuroleptics and may be the most potent H_1-receptor antagonist known [3].

The atypical neuroleptic agents can antagonize the alpha-adrenergic receptors as well. The overall pharmacodynamic effects of this drug class are best represented by receptor affinity. This is depicted in Table 1 [2,4–7]. A summary of the effects of blockade at the different receptors is shown in Box 1 [3,7,8].

Clinical picture in overdose

In general, exaggeration of the normal drug effects of atypical neuroleptics can be expected in overdose. Overdoses of the atypical neuroleptics are rarely fatal unless other coingestants are involved [2,4]. Frequently in polydrug ingestions, when one of the agents is an atypical neuroleptic, the most severe symptoms are likely not due to the atypical neuroleptic, but to one or more of the other coingestants. The most common clinical effects seen in patients who have neuroleptic overdose typically consists of central nervous

Table 1
Receptor affinity of the atypical neuroleptics

	Alpha-1 receptor	H-1 receptor	M-1 receptor	D-2 receptor	5-HT2A receptor
Clozapine	+	+	+	±	+
Olanzapine	+	+	±	+	+
Quetiapine	+	+	Ø	Ø	±
Risperidone	+	+	Ø	+	+
Aripiprazole	Ø	Ø	N/A	+	+
Ziprasidone	+	±	Ø	+	+

Ø, no clinically significant effect seen; ±, receptor affinity but likely clinically insignificant; +, clinically significant antagonistic effect seen.

Box 1. Signs and symptoms associated with receptor antagonism

α-adrenoreceptor (more potent effects seen with α1 blockade than α2)
Miosis, dizziness, hypotension, reflex tachycardia, nasal
   congestion

Histamine H1 receptor
Sedation, drowsiness, appetite stimulation

Muscarinic receptor
Blurred vision (may precipitate narrow-angle glaucoma), dry
   mucous membranes, sinus tachycardia, urinary retention,
   constipation

Serotonin receptor 5HT2A
Reduce anxiety, improve sleep, alleviate depression, and
   psychosis

Dopamine D2 receptor
Extrapyramidal symptoms, hyperprolactinemia

---

system depression, miosis, hypotension, and reflexive tachycardia [2]. The central nervous system depression can lead to profound sedation or a coma-like state that may require the treating physician to use advanced airway management if the patient is unable to protect their airway. This level of intensive care is usually not required for long periods of time because the depressive effects resolve fairly rapidly. The cardiovascular effects are easily treatable and also resolve fairly quickly. All of the atypical neuroleptics have been associated with prolongation of the duration of the cardiac action potential (QT interval). This topic is addressed in a later section of this article.

Treatment in overdose

The treatment of patients who have symptoms from atypical neuroleptic overdose is largely supportive because no specific antidote exists to reverse drug effects. Airway, breathing, and circulation should be quickly assessed. Patients should be placed on continuous cardiac monitoring and intravenous access obtained. Basic laboratories including electrolytes, acetaminophen, aspirin, and an electrocardiogram should be obtained on all patients who have both therapeutic and intentional overdose. A pregnancy screen should be done on all women of child-bearing years.

The hypotension and reflexive tachycardia that frequently occurs with overdose of atypical antipsychotics should initially be treated with intravenous crystalloid solutions. If the patient is still profoundly hypotensive after adequate fluid resuscitation, vasopressor therapy may be initiated. An agent with primarily peripheral alpha-1–receptor effect should be used, such as phenylephrine or norepinephrine [2].

Patients whose mental status does not improve after 4 to 6 hours of observation should be admitted to a monitored setting. Patients who experience serious symptoms such as seizure or cardiac dysrhythmias should be admitted to an intensive care unit [2].

Special considerations

Several of the atypical neuroleptics have been associated with fatal and nonfatal ketoacidosis, hyperglycemia, and diabetic ketoacidosis. Olanzapine, clozapine, and quetiapine all have been associated with new-onset diabetes and ketoacidosis [9–11]. In many reported cases, patients who discontinued treatment with the drug had significant improvement of glycemic control, and some of the patients returned to their baseline glycemic state with no further glycemic control required [9,12]. It is recommended that patients who are begun on an atypical neuroleptic have frequent serum glucose monitoring; however, there are no current evidence-based recommendations on how often this monitoring should occur [10,11].

The two newest atypical neuroleptics deserve additional discussion because their pharmacologic mechanism is somewhat unique.

Ziprasidone

Ziprasidone is one in the latest class of atypical antipsychotics known as dopamine system stabilizers. This agent not only antagonizes serotonin 5-HT_{2A} and dopamine D_2 receptors but can also act as an agonist at dopamine D_2 receptors and serotonin 5-HT_{1A} receptors. It also blocks the reuptake of norepinephrine and serotonin. This combination of receptor pharmacology has the effect of treating both the negative and positive symptoms of schizophrenia without causing extrapyramidal symptoms [13,14]. The dopamine agonism/antagonism effect works to modulate the level of dopamine in different parts of the brain. Where there is too much dopamine effect, it works as an antagonist, and where there is not enough dopamine effect, it works to increase dopamine activity [13]. Ziprasidone has some modest alpha-1–receptor antagonism that may manifest as mild orthostatic hypotension or dizziness [5]. A modest increase in QT interval has been published in clinical trial studies on ziprasidone [14]. What this means clinically is still to be determined, and no literature regarding significant cardiac toxicity caused by ziprasidone was found while researching this publication. A case report by Burton [15] described a ziprasidone overdose in an adult male who developed a corrected QT interval (QTc) of 490 milliseconds without any dysrhythmias. His QTc returned to normal without any adverse sequelae. However, it has been recommended that ziprasidone not be prescribed to patients who are already on medications that can prolong the QT interval or to patients who have a known history of QT prolongation or cardiac disease [14].

Aripiprazole

Aripiprazole is also a member of the dopamine system stabilizer class of atypical neuroleptics. In addition to its partial dopamine agonism and dopamine D_2-receptor antagonism, aripiprazole has low histamine H_1-receptor and alpha-1–adrenergic receptor blocking effects, which may cause sedation and mild hypotension, respectively [6]. Ataxia, somnolence, and vomiting have been reported in patients who have acute overdose of aripiprazole [6]. Aripiprazole has not been associated with prolongation of the QTc interval or ventricular dysrhythmias [6,13].

Dystonic reactions

Acute dystonic reactions are unpleasant extrapyramidal side effects seen most commonly with the use of dopamine blocking agents such as antipsychotic, antiemetic, and antidepressant drugs [16,17]. Ninety percent of dystonic reactions usually occur within the first few days to weeks of treatment initiation [18,19]. These reactions can be classified as sudden, involuntary tonic contractions of a muscle or group of muscles in a patient demonstrating normal mentation [16]. Muscle groups of the face, neck, and back are commonly affected. Dystonic reactions are one of the leading causes for noncompliance with drug treatment. Although disconcerting for the patient, dystonic reactions are rarely life-threatening. However, rare occurrences of laryngeal and esophageal dystonia are documented and may be responsible for some of the sudden death cases associated with antipsychotic drug use [20,21].

Acute dystonic reactions usually occur within the first few days of starting a causative medication or after a rapid increase in dose of the medication [17]. Risk factors include male sex, young age, use of cocaine, and a history of hypersensitivity to neuroleptic-induced side effects [17,21]. All of the traditional as well as the atypical neuroleptics can cause acute dystonic reactions [17,20,22].

Treatment of dystonia

The treatment of dystonic reactions can be gratifying for the clinician both in terms of abatement of the symptoms for the patient and confirmation that the diagnosis of dystonia was indeed correct. The differential diagnosis of dystonia includes not only adverse drug effect but also focal seizure disorder, stroke, meningitis or encephalitis, electrolyte imbalances, conversion reaction, tetanus, and strychnine poisoning [16,17].

Treatment usually consists of administration of one of various drugs with central anticholinergic activity. Treatment with dopamine blocking agents leads to an excessive effect of acetylcholine in the nigrostriatal pathway causing dystonia [16]. Suppression of acetylcholine effect with an anticholinergic agent brings the balance between acetylcholine and dopamine back into equilibrium. Intramuscular or parenteral administration of benztropine mesylate, diphenhydramine HCl, biperiden HCl, or trihexyphenidyl have all been found useful for the rapid relief of dystonic reactions [16,21].

The presentation of an alert patient who has acute respiratory distress and stridor with a history of neuroleptic therapy should alert the clinician to the possibility of laryngeal dystonia [21]. Although rare, this is a potentially life-threatening condition, and the patient should be placed in a monitored environment. Supplemental humidified oxygen should be delivered to the patient, and advanced airway management equipment and a cricothyroidotomy tray should be placed at the bedside. The patient should be given intravenous centrally acting anticholinergic agents such as diphenhydramine or benztropine mesylate. Additionally, parenteral administration of a benzodiazepine such as lorazepam should be considered for its muscle relaxant and anxiolytic effects [23].

Resolution of dystonic symptoms typically occur within 10 to 30 minutes of administration of the previously mentioned anticholinergic agents [23]. Oral anticholinergic therapy should continue for several days after the dystonic occurrence. Suggested duration of oral anticholinergic therapy ranges from 3 to 7 days and depends on the elimination half-life of the offending agent [16,20,23]. It is recommended that the patient be instructed to return if dystonic symptoms should redevelop and to follow-up promptly for re-evaluation by the physician who prescribed the offending agent to discuss the change to a less-potent dopamine blocking agent.

Drug-induced heat stroke

Temperatures above 41.6°C to 42°C can produce significant injury to humans over a short period of time [24]. Temperatures above 49°C can result in almost immediate cell death and tissue necrosis [24]. Heat stoke is defined by a triad of hyperpyrexia with core temperatures above 41.1°C, anhydrosis, and central nervous system disturbance [25]. Patients who have psychiatric illness are at increased risk of developing heat-related illnesses with high mortality. This may be because of underlying physiologic pathology associated with mental illness or because of the kinds of medications prescribed to patients who have psychiatric illness. However, drug-induced heat stroke is more often seen in the elderly population versus younger individuals [26]. Also, additional use of anticholinergic agents increases the risk of a drug-induced heat stroke [26].

Heat intolerance and heat stroke are well-recognized clinical phenomena in patients taking neuroleptic and anticholinergic medications. The pathophysiologic mechanisms responsible for these hyperpyrexic syndromes involve suppressed function of the thermoregulatory center in the anterior hypothalamus and loss of sweating ability to dissipate heat. The suppression of activity of the dopaminergic pathways in the thermoregulatory center can produce either hypothermia or hyperthermia, depending on the ambient temperature [27]. A third mechanism by which drugs can affect body temperature is by cutaneous vasoconstriction reducing the amount of heat dissipation by convection and radiation [25].

Even before the introduction of antipsychotic medications, psychiatric patients were at increased risk of dying during weather-related heat waves [28]. Patients who have schizophrenia have been shown to be less tolerant to heat stress when compared with a healthy population [29,30]. Their intolerance to heat may due to an inherent dysfunction of thermoregulation associated with schizophrenia in addition to an adverse drug effect from medications frequently prescribed for the schizophrenic condition [29]. Other risk factors include extremes of age, comorbid diseases, dehydration, alcoholism, prolonged exertion in or exposure to elevated environmental heat, wearing excessive clothing, and previous history of heat-related illness [31].

The clinical picture of drug-induced heat stroke usually includes sudden onset of hyperthermia, central nervous system disturbance, and anhydrosis in a patient who has the history of antipsychotic or anticholinergic drug therapy [25,26]. Sweating is usually absent in classic heat stroke but may be present in cases of exertional heat stroke [31]. Seizures can occur in drug-induced heat stroke [26].

In drug-induced heat stroke, excess heat is commonly derived from the ambient environment and its occurrence does have seasonal variation [32]. Ambient heat, humidity, and radiant stress from direct sunlight must all be considered when assessing environmental heat stress [24]. By far the most important variable is humidity. When the temperature of the ambient air is greater than 33°C, body heat is lost primarily through sweating [25]. High humidity can interfere with this sweating process, and a patient taking antipsychotic or anticholinergic medications could be at increased risk of heat-related illness because their ability to sweat may be compromised. Physicians should counsel their patients who take antipsychotic medications as well as patients who are poorly conditioned or not acclimated to high heat and humidity to avoid strenuous outdoor activity on warm days [24].

Treatment of drug-induced heat stroke

Early recognition of drug-induced heat stroke versus neuroleptic malignant syndrome is critical because heat stroke is a medical emergency. Rapid cooling is essential in the initial management of all patients who have heat stroke. Prolonged hyperthermia increases the risk for development of multisystem organ failure. Patients should be cooled to a core temperature of 38.5°C to 39°C [24]. Further cooling is not advised because it may lead to hypothermia [24]. Hypotension due to drug-induced heat stroke usually responds to cooling, which causes a decrease in peripheral perfusion. Unresponsive hypotension is an ominous sign [25]. Sympathomimetic vasopressors should be avoided because they impede cutaneous dissipation of heat [25]. Intravenous crystalloid fluids should be used to treat hypotension; however, their use should be monitored closely to avoid complications from fluid overload.

Neuroleptic malignant syndrome

Neuroleptic malignant syndrome (NMS) is an adverse, idiosyncratic drug reaction to neuroleptics with a mortality rate of 4% to 30% [31,33]. Initially called "akinetic hypertonic syndrome," neuroleptic malignant syndrome was first described by Delay in 1960 [34,35]. NMS encompasses a spectrum of clinical signs and symptoms; thus, no single set of criteria for its diagnosis has been accepted [34]. Generally, it can be characterized by hyperthermia, muscle rigidity, autonomic dysfunction, and an altered level of consciousness (Table 2) [34,36,37]. Associated features include akinesia, tremor, dystonias, dysphagia, dyspnea, diaphoresis, sialorrhea, incontinence, tachycardia, fluctuating blood pressure, flushing, and pallor [37]. It is postulated to be caused by a disruption of central dopamine neurotransmission in the nigrostriatal and hypothalamic dopamine pathways [26]. Other neurotransmitters such as epinephrine, serotonin, and acetylcholine may also be involved in the development of NMS because they are present in neuronal pathways involved in hypothalamic thermoregulation [26]. It may be distinguished from drug-induced heat stroke by the presence of muscle rigidity and sweating.

NMS is a rare occurrence, with an incidence estimated to be between 0.07% and 1% [37,38]. NMS has been most commonly associated with haloperidol and fluphenazine, but all of the atypical neuroleptics have been associated with its occurrence [38–42]. The duration of use of an antipsychotic medication has not been correlated with the development of NMS; hence, NMS can occur at anytime during treatment [26]. Also, NMS is not limited to just neuroleptic use in psychiatric patients. It has been documented to occur in patients who have Huntington's chorea and Parkinson's disease [36].

Two important laboratory findings are leucocytosis with white blood cell counts ranging from 10,000/μg/L to 40,000/μg/L with or without shift, and

Table 2
Clinical and laboratory features useful in the diagnosis of NMS

Fever/Hyperthermia	Tachypnea	Elevated Serum
Tachycardia	Diaphoresis	Creatine Phosphokinase
Muscle Rigidity	Incontinence	Leukocytosis
Altered Mental Status	Dyspnea	
Akinesia	Sialorrhea	

elevated serum creatine kinase levels [26,37]. The elevated white blood cell is thought to be due to stress response [37]. The elevated creatine kinase may be due to stress, agitation, and rhabdomyolysis secondary to muscular rigidity [26,37].

Treatment of neuroleptic malignant syndrome

Treatment of NMS should also be quickly initiated because it too can be a life-threatening condition. Rapid withdrawal of the offending neuroleptic agent, establishment of intravenous access, initiation of cooling measures, and implementation of aggressive critical care management are essential to success. Numerous case reports in the literature support the use of dantrolene and bromocriptine in the treatment of NMS [43]. However, high-quality, intensive, supportive care has also been shown to successfully treat NMS [44].

Aggressive supportive care should focus on hydration status, rapid cooling measures, and anticoagulation [37]. Low-dose heparin should be initiated as soon as possible to prevent thrombotic events in these critically ill patients [34]. Respiratory failure may develop due to chest wall muscle rigidity and autonomic instability and require advanced airway management [26]. Hydration status should be optimized with intravenous crystalloid solutions and renal function monitored closely especially if rhabdomyolysis is present. Renal failure is an important predictor of mortality in NMS [26]. Anticholinergic agents have been suggested to treat NMS. However, there is no strong support for this in the literature, and the interference with sweating and possible exacerbation of the hyperpyrexia point against the recommendation for the use of anticholinergic agents to treat NMS.

Dantrolene is a peripheral muscle relaxant that inhibits calcium release from the sarcoplasmic reticulum, which decreases the available calcium for ongoing muscle contraction [34]. Dantrolene is the drug of choice for the treatment of malignant hyperthermia, but its use in the treatment of NMS is not as well accepted. In one prospective study by Rosebush [45], the use of dantrolene to treat patients diagnosed with NMS did not improve outcome. A dose of intravenous dantrolene of 1 mg/kg can be given initially and may be increased 10 fold if necessary to control symptoms [46]. This dose may be repeated every 10 minutes up to a total dose of 10 mg/kg/day [34,36]. Hepatic toxicity has occurred with doses of greater than 10 mg/kg/day [34]. The major side effects to be expected are muscle weakness and nausea [46].

Bromocriptine mesylate is a dopamine agonist given to counter the dopamine blocking effects of neuroleptic agents. This agent is available in an oral formulation only. Doses have ranged from 2.5 to 10 mg four times per day [34]. In a study by Rosenberg [43] that compared treatment options for NMS, bromocriptine was shown to have a more rapid response and resolution of symptoms than compared with supportive care alone. Bromocriptine has been associated with worsening psychosis in patients being treated for NMS [37].

Intravenous administration of levodopa has been reported in the literature to successfully treat cases of NMS [47]. In this case series, treatment of NMS with dantrolene for several days had not resulted in improvement of symptoms. Initiation of intravenous levodopa therapy ranging from 50 mg/day to 100 mg/day resulted in rapid improvement in the patients' clinical status.

Benzodazepines should be considered in the treatment of NMS. In addition to treating muscular rigidity and agitation, they also reduce patient anxiety and the hyperadrenergic state that can contribute to the disorder [33].

Drug-induced heat stroke versus neuroleptic malignant syndrome

Distinguishing drug-induced heat stroke from NMS is important for proper clinical management (Table 3) [26,30–32,48]. The degree of elevation of body temperature and creatine kinase level may not dependably discriminate between drug-induced heat stroke and NMS [32]. These two hyperpyrexic conditions require slightly different management, and a delay in the treatment of heat stroke can have fatal consequences in up to 50% of cases [30].

In general, patients who have drug-induced heat stroke do not demonstrate extrapyramidal muscle rigidity or sweating [30,32]. Drug-induced heat stroke tends to cause a higher core body temperature [30,31]. Compared to NMS, onset of drug-induced heat stroke is abrupt, often with seizures, and frequently is associated with weather-related heat waves [32]. Patients who have drug-induced heat stroke frequently are dehydrated and may be hyponatremic. Although aggressive supportive treatment with rapid cooling is critical to effective care of both conditions, dopaminergic agents and benzodiazepines may be of additional benefit in the treatment of NMS [32].

Table 3
A comparison of clinical signs and symptoms

Drug-induced heat stroke	Neuroleptic malignant syndrome
Abrupt onset	Insidious onset
Absence of sweating	Sweating present
No muscle rigidity	Muscle rigidity
Decreased mental status	Decreased mental status
Seizures likely	No seizures
Rhabdomyolysis causing acute renal failure	Rhabdomyolysis causing acute renal failure
Mortality 20–50%	Mortality 10–20%
Core temperature greater than 40°C	Fever ranges from low grade to very high
Metabolic acidosis	Metabolic acidosis
Elevated creatine kinase possible	Elevated creatine kinase common
Leukocytosis possible	Leukocytosis common
Disseminated intravascular coagulopathy	Generalized autonomic dysfunction

Psychiatric patients should be counseled on avoiding situations that could put them at risk for developing a heat-related illness. They should be warned not to exercise heavily or perform highly exertional work when ambient temperatures are elevated above 30°C [25]. They should be encouraged to drink plenty of noncaffeinated, electrolyte-balanced beverages, wear loosely fitted light clothing, and stay in an air-conditioned environment as much as possible [28].

Newer antidepressants

Depression has plagued mankind for thousands of years. Possibly the first antidepressant was *Papaver somniforum* or poppy. Given to mankind by the goddess Ceres, it was used to relieve pain and sorrow [49]. Opium tincture, introduced by Emil Kraepelin, was the first-line agent in the treatment of depression from the 1920s to the mid-1950s [49,50].

The mechanistic theory of depression has evolved over the years. Initially postulated as a deficiency of cerebral monoamine neurotransmitters, the theory of the cause of depression now describes a complicated picture of receptor biochemistry and gene expression. As the theory of depression has evolved, so too has the research and development of pharmacology and pharmacologic agents necessary to treat the many symptoms of depression. Newer antidepressants with unique pharmacologic effects focusing on serotonin, norepinephrine, and dopamine modulation in the brain have largely replaced the traditional cyclic antidepressants and monoamine oxidase inhibitors. The following sections describe the actions of these newer agents with a focus on the management of acute poisonings and common adverse effects of these agents (Table 4).

Drug effect in therapeutic dosing

The selective serotonin reuptake inhibitors (SSRIs) were considered the first agents of the newer antidepressant agent drug class. SSRIs are designed to increase the amount of serotonin activity, either by inhibition of presynaptic reuptake of the neurotransmitter or by postsynaptic modulation of serotonin receptors to achieve an enhanced serotonin effect. As a class, SSRIs are part of the first line of therapy in the treatment of depression. Also, they have a much improved safety profile over the traditional cyclic antidepressants with an average 10 fold lower fatal toxicity index when compared with cyclic antidepressants [51]. Signs and symptoms associated with enhanced serotonin effect may be pronounced, such as dizziness, blurred vision, nausea, vomiting, diarrhea, and restlessness.

Additional agents with more selective pharmacology continue to be developed. Agents that selectively inhibit reuptake of one or more of the monoamine neurotransmitters are available for use in the United States. Additionally, there are agents that modulate presynaptic and postsynaptic

Table 4
Newer or atypical antidepressants

SSRI	NSSA[a]	SARI[b]	NRI	NDRI	SNRI
Prozac (fluoxetine)			Edronax (reboxetine)	Wellbutrin (bupropion)	Effexor (venlafaxine)
Zoloft (sertraline)					Cymbalta (duloxetine)
Paxil (paroxetine)					
Celexa (citalopram)	Remeron (mirtazapine)	Serzone (nefazodone)			
Lexapro (escitalopram)					
Luvox (fluvoxamine)		Desyrel (trazodone)			

Abbreviations: NDRI, norepinephrine and dopamine reuptake inhibitor; NRI, selective noradrenergic reuptake inhibitor; NSSA, noradrenergic and specific serotonergic antidepressant; SARI, serotonin 2A antagonist reuptake inhibitor; SNRI, serotonin and norepinephrine reuptake inhibitor.

[a] Additional mechanisms: blocks presynaptic alpha 2 receptors, serotonin receptors, and histamine receptors.

[b] Additional mechanisms: blocks serotonin reuptake and serotonin 5HT2A receptors, weak norepinephrine reuptake inhibition, and weak alpha 1 receptor blockade.

receptor function to achieve enhanced pharmacologic effect (see Table 4) [52]. All of these agents have unique receptor affinity profiles that allow for some additional clinical signs and symptoms appreciated best in overdose.

Clinical picture in overdose

In overdose, clinicians can expect to see signs and symptoms of excessive serotonergic stimulation: altered mentation or sedation, blurred vision, tremor, nausea, vomiting, hypotension, and tachycardia. Additional signs and symptoms such as seizures, cardiac conduction disturbances, priapism, and the syndrome of inappropriate antidiuretic hormone secretion occur more rarely and are unique to certain agents [53–55]. Deaths from overdose of any of the newer antidepressants, although rare, have occurred [56,57].

Treatment in overdose

In general, patients who have ingestions of serotonergic agents require minimal interventions and are frequently asymptomatic. If after an observation time of 6 to 8 hours from ingestion the patient who ingested the overdose demonstrates no signs of toxicity, clinicians should be able to determine their final dispositions for these patients. However, patients who have exposure to extended-release formulations, who demonstrate even mild toxicity, or who have coingestants should be observed in a monitored environment for at least 12 hours or until completely asymptomatic.

Management usually consists of supportive care with the use of intravenous fluids for hypotension and benzodiazepines for agitation.

For agents that cause seizures, benzodiazepines and barbiturates are first-line therapy. Conduction disturbances with prolongation of the QRS intervals should be treated with sodium bicarbonate. Torsade de pointes is a rare cardiac toxicity and should be treated with magnesium or overdrive pacing.

Most of the newer antidepressants have few serious or life-threatening side effects. Agents with more significant toxicity are described.

Venlafaxine

Venlafaxine is an atypical antidepressant that inhibits the reuptake of serotonin, norepinephrine, and dopamine. Most commonly available as an extended-release preparation, venlafaxine can also block cardiac sodium channels in a dose-dependent fashion [58,59]. In overdose, central nervous system depression, symptoms of serotonergic excess, seizures, sinus tachycardia, and cardiac conduction abnormalities with prolongation of the QRS and QTc intervals have been reported [60,61]. Seizures frequently occur earlier in ingestion, whereas cardiac toxicity presents later. Toxicity may be delayed many hours, especially if an extended-release formulation was ingested. Patients who have ingested an extended release formulation and are symptomatic can be at risk for seizures up to 15 hours after their ingestion [58,62]. Most recently, the US Food and Drug Administration has alerted physicians to an increased risk of fatal outcome with an overdose of venlafaxine as compared with other SSRIs (http://www.fda.gov/medwatch/index.html).

Citalopram

Citalopram is a selective serotonin reuptake inhibitor antidepressant. Seizures and prolongation of the QTc interval have been documented after overdose with citalopram. More commonly, seizures occur earlier in the ingestion, whereas QTc prolongation may be delayed [54,57,63,64]. Citalopram may cause toxicity more often than other SSRIs [64,65].

Bupropion

Bupropion (Wellbutrin) is a norepinephrine and dopamine reuptake inhibitor. Sinus tachycardia, lethargy, tremors, and seizures are the most commonly reported toxicities in bupropion overdose [66]. Onset of seizure activity may occur from minutes to as many as 8 hours postingestion and be delayed with exposure to extended-release formulations [66]. Fatalities are rare, but have been reported [67].

Serotonin syndrome

Serotonin is a neurotransmitter derived from dietary intake of tryptophan and is involved in the modulation of a wide variety of clinical states, such as sleep, appetite, anxiety and depression, platelet function, movement disorders, and emesis [52]. The development of serotonin syndrome (SS) is thought to result from the presence of excessive serotonin, which leads to overstimulation of serotonin 5-HT$_{1A}$ and 5-HT$_{2A}$ receptors in the peripheral and central nervous systems [68–70]. Classically, SS has been described as a triad of altered mental status, autonomic instability, and abnormal neuromuscular activity (Table 5) [68,70,71]. An established definition of the salient clinical features of SS has not been validated [68]. However, Dunkley [69] did a retrospective analysis of patients admitted for an overdose of a serotonergic agent and found that clonus, agitation, diaphoresis, tremor, and hyperreflexia were required clinical features necessary for diagnosis of serotonin toxicity by a toxicologist. Because SS can be life threatening and several deaths have been reported in the literature, hyperthermia and increased rigidity were also included in their criteria for diagnosing serotonin toxicity. The hyperreflexia and increased muscular rigidity is frequently more pronounced in the lower extremities [70].

The presence of excessive serotonin can develop from one of many pharmacologic actions and usually the consumption of more than one serotonergic agent. SS can develop due to decreased breakdown of the neurotransmitter or increased synthesis such as from increasing dietary tryptophan [72]. Decreased reuptake or increased release of the neurotransmitter can also precipitate SS. Agents that are capable of this include sympathomimetics (ie, cocaine or amphetamines), dextromethorphan, cyclic antidepressants, meperidine, and tramadol [71].

Treatment of serotonin syndrome

The management of patients who have SS is largely supportive with a focus on removing the offending agent, reducing hyperthermia with

Table 5
Clinical signs and symptoms associated with serotonin toxicity

	Altered mental status	Autonomic instability	Neuromuscular abnormalities
Mild			
	Confusion	Fever < 38°C	Hyperreflexia
	Restlessness	Tachycardia	Clonus
		Diarrhea	Ataxia
		Mydriasis	Akathisia
Moderate			
	Somnolence	Fever < 39.5°C	Myoclonus
	Agitation	Hyper/hypotension	Clonus
		Mydriasis	Ataxia
Severe			
	Coma	Fever > 39.6°C	Rigidity
	Seizures	Diaphoresis	
		Dyspnea	
		Tachycardia	

cooling measures, and reducing muscular rigidity and agitation with judicious use of benzodiazepines [68,70]. The onset of symptoms is usually rapid, frequently within hours to days of initiation of treatment or escalation of dose [71]. Rapid treatment usually results in rapid resolution of symptoms. Although supportive treatment is the mainstay for management of serotonin syndrome, there are published data on the use of 5-HT$_2$ blockers for the treatment of SS. Although no large randomized, double-blinded, controlled trials of these agents versus supported care alone have been published, agents such as cyproheptadine, risperidone, and chlorpromazine have been tried with mixed results [68]. Cyproheptadine may be one of the more commonly reported agents used in the treatment of SS [68,70]. Cyproheptadine is a 5-HT$_{1A}$ and 5-HT$_{2A}$ receptor antagonist with histamine H$_1$-receptor blocking and antimuscarinic activities [70]. Only available in on oral formulation, cyproheptadine has been administered in various dose concentrations and frequencies (eg, 4 to 16 mg; doses every 6 to 8 hours; duration of therapy 24 hours or greater) [68,70]. Kapur [73] suggests a single dose of 30 mg is needed to achieve adequate serotonin receptor blockade.

Cardiovascular effects of psychotropic drugs

There is a growing awareness by the public as well as clinicians of the potentially harmful cardiovascular side effects of the newer antidepressants and atypical neuroleptics. The wide range of chemical structure and unique receptor affinities make it difficult to categorically include all of the psychotropic agents as having cardiovascular effects. Rather, clinicians now have to be keenly aware of the novel effects of individual drugs and how each drug may potentially interact with already prescribed medications as they pertain to the physiologic uniqueness of their patients.

Alpha-1–adrenergic blockade

Many of the newer antidepressants and atypical neuroleptics can have peripheral effects on the cardiovascular system. Alpha-1–receptor blockade can lead to orthostatic hypotension, reflex tachycardia, and symptoms of dizziness and syncope. Clinicians who evaluate patients who have the complaint of dizziness or syncope should always review the patient's medication list for potential drug interactions or the presence of medications with significant peripheral cardiovascular effects. In many cases, the alpha-1–receptor blockade leads to tachyphylaxis, and the hypotensive effects of the medications decrease with continued use [74]. In certain populations, such as the elderly or patients who have cardiovascular disease, the peripheral effects may lead to significant morbidity with increased risk or occurrence of falls in the elderly and worsening angina symptoms in patients who have significant cardiovascular disease [74,75]. In overdose, alpha-1–adrenergic blockage can precipitate significant hypotension with reflexive tachycardia.

Usually transient and responsive to intravenous crystalloid fluids, hypotension due to alpha-1–receptor blockade can be refractory and may require treatment with a direct alpha agonist vasopressor such as phenylephrine.

Drug-induced QT prolongation

The QT interval encompasses the entire duration of the cardiac action potential from the onset of depolarization to the completion of repolarization [76,77]. Normal QT intervals are less than 440 milliseconds in men and less than 450 milliseconds in women. Prolongation of the QT interval is a common effect of many drug classes. A measured QT of greater than 500 milliseconds is considered abnormal and carries with it a potential risk of development of ventricular tachydysrhythmias and rarely torsade de pointes [14]. However, the degree of QT prolongation is not associated with increased risk of ventricular dysrhythmias [76,77].

Frequently, agents that have been demonstrated to cause torsade de pointes do not cause a high degree of QT prolongation, and agents that produce significant QT prolongation do not cause ventricular dysrhythmias or torsades [76]. A consistent association between the length of the QT interval and the risk for development of dysrhythmias or torsades has not been established [77]. The University of Arizona Center for Education and Research on Therapeutics has put together an informative website (www.torsades.org) on medications with varying degrees of risk for causing torsade de pointes.

In general, prolongation of the QT interval is caused by impedence of potassium efflux out of the cardiac cell. Likely the most physiologically relevant cause of drug-induced QT prolongation is by inhibition of I_{Kr}, known as the "rapid delayed rectifier" potassium current [77]. I_{Kr} is an outward potassium current through a potassium channel encoded by the human ether-á-go-go gene [76]. This channel allows efflux of potassium out of myocardial cells and rapid repolarization in phase 3 of the cardiac action potential [77]. An increase in the length of phase 3 prolongs the QT interval and increases the risk for an asynchronous electrical potential that could lead to an arrhythmia such as torsade de pointes [75].

Many factors exist that can contribute to the occurrence of torsade de pointes. An increase of the QT by 60 milliseconds or more from baseline during neuroleptic drug treatment mandates close monitoring of the patient for signs of ventricular dysrhythmias [75]. An increase in the QT dispersion of 100 milliseconds or more, or increases of more than 100% from baseline may put the patient at risk for the development of dysrhythmias or sudden death [77]. Additionally, genetic polymorphisms in ion channels, female gender, electrolyte abnormalities, congestive heart failure, ischemic heart disease, renal dysfunction, in addition to the use of one or more pharmacologic agents that prolong the QT interval may predispose the patient to serious dysrhythmias [75,77].

Clinicians should be aware of the cardiovascular side effects that medications they prescribe may cause in their patients. Also, obtain a baseline ECG before the initiation of any medication with the potential to cause QT prolongation or the addition of a medication that may prolong the QT to an existing drug regimen. Such additions may create conditions that amplify the effect of individual medications and make otherwise safe drug therapies potentially harmful or even life threatening.

Summary

Tens of thousands of adverse drug reactions occur each year due to exposure by therapeutic dosing or intentional overdosing of the atypical antipsychotics and newer antidepressants. Most often, patients will have little or no symptoms from their exposure. Less frequently, patients will be symptomatic and require an observation period with minimal supportive care only during a short hospital stay. Rarely, patients can develop significant toxicity that will require critical care intervention and intensive monitoring. It is for these patients that emergency medicine physicians need to be well informed about the pharmacology, toxicity, and management of atypical antipsychotic and newer antidepressant drug exposures.

References

[1] Watson WA. 2004 Annual report of the American Association of Poison Control Centers Toxic Exposure Surveillance System. Am J Emerg Med 2005;23(5):589–666.
[2] Burns M. The pharmacology and toxicology of atypical antipsychotic agents. J Toxicol Clin Toxicol 2001;39(1):1–14.
[3] Richelson E. Basic neuropharmacology of antidepressants relevant to the pharmacotherapy of depression. Clin Cornerstone 1999;1(4):17–30.
[4] Raggi MA. Atypical antipsychotics: pharmacokinetics, therapeutic drug monitoring and pharmacological interactions. Curr Med Chem 2004;11(3):279–96.
[5] Keck PE. Clinical pharmacodynamics and pharmacokinetics of antimanic and mood-stabilizing medications. J Clin Psychiatry 2002;63(4):3–11.
[6] Seifert SA. Aripiprazole (abilify) overdose in a child. Clinical Toxicology 2005;43(3):193–5.
[7] Richelson E. Receptor pharmacology of neuroleptics: relation to clinical effects. J Clin Psychiatry 1999;60(10):5–14.
[8] Richelson E, Souder T. Binding of antipsychotic drugs to human brain receptors: focus on newer generation compounds. Life Sci 2000;68(1):29–39.
[9] Wilson DR, Souza L, Sarkar N, et al. New-onset diabetes and ketoacidosis with atypical antipsychotics. Schizophr Res 2003;59(1):1–6.
[10] Torrey EF, Swalwell CI. Fatal olanzapine-induced ketoacidosis. Am J Psychiatry 2003; 160(12):2241.
[11] Ragucci KR, Wells BJ. Olanzapine-induced diabetic ketoacidosis. Ann Pharmacother 2001; 35(12):1556–8.
[12] Koller EA, Doraiswamy PM. Olanzapine-associated diabetes mellitus. Pharmacotherapy 2002;22(7):841–52.
[13] Launer M. Partial dopamine agonists in schizophrenia. Hosp Med 2005;66(5):300–3.
[14] Goodnick PJ. Ziprasidone: profile on safety. Expert Opin Pharmacother 2001;2(10): 1655–62.

[15] Burton S. Ziprasidone overdose. Am J Psychiatry 2000;157(5):835.
[16] Corre KA. Extended therapy for acute dystonic reactions. Ann Emerg Med 1984;13(3): 194–7.
[17] van H. Acute dystonia induced by drug treatment. BMJ 1999;319(7210):623–6.
[18] Burgyone K. The use of antiparkinsonian agents in the management of drug-induced extrapyramidal symptoms. Curr Pharm Des 2004;10(18):2239–48.
[19] Wirshing WC. Movement disorders associated with neuroleptic treatment. J Clin Psychiatry 2001;62(21):15–8.
[20] Christodoulou C, Kalaitzi C. Antipsychotic drug-induced acute laryngeal dystonia: two case reports and a mini review. J Psychopharmacol 2005;19(3):307–11.
[21] Koek RJ, Pi EH. Acute laryngeal dystonic reactions to neuroleptics. Psychosomatics 1989; 30(4):359–64.
[22] McCarthy RH. Esophageal dysfunction in two patients after clozapine treatment. J Clin Psychopharmacol 1994;14(4):281–3.
[23] Fines RE, Brady JWJ, Martin ML. Acute laryngeal dystonia related to neuroleptic agents. Am J Emerg Med 1999;17(3):319–20.
[24] Lugo A. Heat-related illness. Emerg Med Clin North Am 2004;22(2):315-viii.
[25] Stadnyk AN. Drug-induced heat stroke. Can Med Assoc J 1983;128(8):957–9.
[26] Bhanushali MJ. The evaluation and management of patients with neuroleptic malignant syndrome. Neurol Clin 2004;22(2):389–411.
[27] Forester D. Fatal drug-induced heat stroke. Journal of American College of Emergency Physicians 1978;7(6):243–4.
[28] Bark N. Deaths of psychiatric patients during heat waves. Psychiatr Serv 1998;49(8):1088–90.
[29] Hermesh H, Shiloh R, Epstein Y, et al. Heat intolerance in patients with chronic schizophrenia maintained with antipsychotic drugs. Am J Psychiatry 2000;157(8):1327–9.
[30] Kerwin RW. Heat stroke in schizophrenia during clozapine treatment: rapid recognition and management. J Psychopharmacol 2004;18(1):121–3.
[31] Kwok JSS, Chan TYK. Recurrent heat-related illnesses during antipsychotic treatment. Ann Pharmacother 2005;39(11):1940–2.
[32] Lazarus A. Differentiating neuroleptic-related heatstroke from neuroleptic malignant syndrome. Psychosomatics 1989;30(4):454–6.
[33] Rosebush P, Stewart T. A prospective analysis of 24 episodes of neuroleptic malignant syndrome. Am J Psychiatry 1989;146(6):717–25.
[34] Adnet P. Neuroleptic malignant syndrome. Br J Anaesth 2000;85(1):129–35.
[35] Delay J, Pichot P, Lemperiere T, et al. [A non-phenothiazine and non-reserpine major neuroleptic, haloperidol, in the treatment of psychoses] [in French]. Ann Med Psychol 1960;118(1):145–52.
[36] Levenson JL. Neuroleptic malignant syndrome. Am J Psychiatry 1985;142(10):1137–45.
[37] Susman VL. Clinical management of neuroleptic malignant syndrome. Psychiatr Q 2001; 72(4):325–36.
[38] Totten VY, Hirschenstein E, Hew P. Neuroleptic malignant syndrome presenting without initial fever: a case report. J Emerg Med 1994;12(1):43–7.
[39] Hasan S, Buckley P. Novel antipsychotics and the neuroleptic malignant syndrome: a review and critique. Am J Psychiatry 1998;155(8):1113–6.
[40] Solomons K. Quetiapine and neuroleptic malignant syndrome. Can J Psychiatry 2002;47(8): 791.
[41] Sing KJ, Ramaekers GMGI, Van Harten PN. Neuroleptic malignant syndrome and quetiapine. Am J Psychiatry 2002;159(1):149–50.
[42] Trosch RM. Neuroleptic-induced movement disorders: deconstructing extrapyramidal symptoms. J Am Geriatr Soc 2004;52(12):S266–71.
[43] Rosenberg MR. Neuroleptic malignant syndrome. Review of response to therapy. Arch Intern Med 1989;149(9):1927–31.
[44] Caroff SN. The neuroleptic malignant syndrome. J Clin Psychiatry 1980;41(3):79–83.

[45] Rosebush PI. The treatment of neuroleptic malignant syndrome. Are dantrolene and bromocriptine useful adjuncts to supportive care? [see comment] Br J Psychiatry 1991;159: 709–12.

[46] Paasuke RT. Drugs, heat stroke and dantrolene. Can Med Assoc J 1984;130(4):41–3.

[47] Nisijima K, Noguti M, Ishiguro T. Intravenous injection of levodopa is more effective than dantrolene as therapy for neuroleptic malignant syndrome. Biol Psychiatry 1997;41(8): 913–4.

[48] Lefkowitz D. Cerebellar syndrome following neuroleptic induced heat stroke. J Neurol Neurosurg Psychiatry 1983;46(2):183–5.

[49] Ban TA. Pharmacotherapy of depression: a historical analysis. J Neural Transm 2001; 108(6):707–16.

[50] Ban TA. Pharmacotherapy of mental illness—a historical analysis. Prog Neuropsychopharmacol Biol Psychiatry 2001;25(4):709–27.

[51] Sarko J. Antidepressants, old and new. A review of their adverse effects and toxicity in overdose. Emerg Med Clin North Am 2000;18(4):637–54.

[52] Stahl SM. Essential psychopharmacology: neuroscientific basis and practice applications. 2nd edition. New York: Cambridge University Press; 2000. p. 601.

[53] Kirchner V. Selective serotonin reuptake inhibitors and hyponatraemia: review and proposed mechanisms in the elderly. J Psychopharmacol 1998;12(4):396–400.

[54] Personne M. Citalopram overdose—review of cases treated in Swedish hospitals. J Toxicol Clin Toxicol 1997;35(3):237–40.

[55] Warner MD. Trazodone and priapism. J Clin Psychiatry 1987;48(6):244–5.

[56] Harris CR. Fatal bupropion overdose. J Toxicol Clin Toxicol 1997;35(3):321–4.

[57] Ostrom M, Eriksson A, Thorson J, et al. Fatal overdose with citalopram. Lancet 1996; 348(9023):339–40.

[58] Buckley NA. 'Atypical' antidepressants in overdose: clinical considerations with respect to safety. Drug Saf 2003;26(8):539–51.

[59] Khalifa M, Daleau P, Turgeon J. Mechanism of sodium channel block by venlafaxine in guinea pig ventricular myocytes. J Pharmacol Exp Ther 1999;291(1):280–4.

[60] Blythe D. Cardiovascular and neurological toxicity of venlafaxine. Hum Exp Toxicol 1999; 18(5):309–13.

[61] Oliver JJ. Venlafaxine poisoning complicated by a late rise in creatine kinase: two case reports. Hum Exp Toxicol 2002;21(8):463–6.

[62] Whyte IM, Dawson AH, Buckley NA. Relative toxicity of venlafaxine and selective serotonin reuptake inhibitors in overdose compared to tricyclic antidepressants. QJM 2003;96(5): 369–74.

[63] Personne M. Citalopram toxicity. Lancet 1997;350(9076):518–9.

[64] Kelly CA. Comparative toxicity of citalopram and the newer antidepressants after overdose. J Toxicol Clin Toxicol 2004;42(1):67–71.

[65] Isbister GK. Relative toxicity of selective serotonin reuptake inhibitors (SSRIs) in overdose. J Toxicol Clin Toxicol 2004;42(3):277–85.

[66] Spiller HA. Bupropion overdose: a 3-year multi-center retrospective analysis. Am J Emerg Med 1994;12(1):43–5.

[67] Bergmann F. Seizure and cardiac arrest during bupropion SR treatment. J Clin Psychopharmacol 2002;22(6):630–1.

[68] Gillman PK. The serotonin syndrome and its treatment. J Psychopharmacol 1999;13(1): 100–9.

[69] Dunkley EJC. The hunter serotonin toxicity criteria: simple and accurate diagnostic decision rules for serotonin toxicity. QJM 2003;96(9):635–42.

[70] Chan BSH. Serotonin syndrome resulting from drug interactions. Med J Aust 1998;169(10): 523–5.

[71] Rusyniak DE. Toxin-induced hyperthermic syndromes. Med Clin North Am 2005;89(6): 1277–96.

[72] Steiner W. Toxic reaction following the combined administration of fluoxetine and L-tryptophan: five case reports. Biol Psychiatry 1986;21(11):1067–71.

[73] Kapur S. Cyproheptadine: a potent in vivo serotonin antagonist. Am J Psychiatry 1997; 154(6):884.

[74] Buckley NA. Cardiovascular adverse effects of antipsychotic drugs. Drug Saf 2000;23(3): 215–28.

[75] Piepho RW. Cardiovascular effects of antipsychotics used in bipolar illness. J Clin Psychiatry 2002;63(4):20–3.

[76] Heist EK. Drug-induced proarrhythmia and use of QTc-prolonging agents: clues for clinicians. Heart Rhythm 2005;2(2):S1–8.

[77] Kao LW. Drug-induced q-T prolongation. Med Clin North Am 2005;89(6):1125-x.

ELSEVIER
SAUNDERS

EMERGENCY
MEDICINE
CLINICS OF
NORTH AMERICA

Emerg Med Clin N Am 25 (2007) 499–525

Criminal Poisoning: Drug-Facilitated Sexual Assault

Laura K. Bechtel, PhD[a],
Christopher P. Holstege, MD[b],*

[a]Blue Ridge Poison Center, University of Virginia Health System,
P.O. Box 800744, Charlottesville, VA 22908-0774, USA
[b]Division of Medical Toxicology, Department of Emergency Medicine,
University of Virginia, P.O. Box 800744, 1222 Jefferson Park Avenue,
4th Floor, Charlottesville, VA 22908-0774, USA

Sexual assault is defined as any undesired physical contact of a sexual nature perpetrated against another person. Sexual assault is much broader than the term rape, traditionally referred to as forced vaginal penetration of a woman by a male assailant [1]. In 2003 to 2004 an average of 204,370 sexual assaults were reported to law-enforcement agencies in the United States [2]. Because most sexual assaults are not reported, this national average is grossly underrepresented. The National Women's Study documented that 84% of women in their sample did not report their rapes to the police [3]. Among United States college students, approximately 25% of women reported experiencing completed or attempted rape [4]. In 2003, approximately 9% of high school students reported having been forced to have sexual intercourse [5]. Current estimates from available data indicate that 1 in 6 women will be the victim of a sexual assault at least once in her lifetime [6].

Drug-facilitated sexual assault (DFSA) is a complex and prevalent problem presenting to North American emergency departments (EDs) [7–10]. DFSA is defined as the use of a chemical agent to facilitate sexual assault. The reported prevalence of DFSA varies. The US Department of Justice estimates 44% of sexual assaults are perceived to occur under the influence of drugs or alcohol [2,11,12]. Often drugs and alcohol are used voluntarily by

---

* Corresponding author. Division of Medical Toxicology, Department of Emergency Medicine, University of Virginia, P.O. Box 800744, 1222 Jefferson Park Avenue, 4th Floor, Charlottesville, VA 22908-0774.

E-mail address: ch2xf@virginia.edu (C.P. Holstege).

0733-8627/07/$ - see front matter © 2007 Elsevier Inc. All rights reserved.
doi:10.1016/j.emc.2007.02.008
emed.theclinics.com

the victim and offender [11]. One multicenter study estimates 4.3% of the DFSAs examined were surreptitiously drugged victims and 35.4% of the DFSAs involved voluntarily use of illicit drugs [10]. Because of the absence of national scientific studies examining the prevalence of DFSAs in the United States, the exact number of alcohol and illicit drug–related sexual assaults is unknown. Yet an increasing number of independent testing programs are performing analyses on urine, blood, and hair samples collected from individuals who claim to have been sexually assaulted and believe that drugs were involved in the United Kingdom, France, and the United States [8,10,13,14]. These reports are attributable to an increased awareness of the problem and technological advances in rapid drug analyses.

Sexual assault victims and the emergency department

Identifying victims of DFSA and addressing specific medical and ultimately legal issues are essential roles of the emergency health care provider. When treating a victim of sexual assault, health care personnel have encountered numerous problems, such as not recognizing the urgency of medical attention, not treating the patient as a victim, and failing to document all available forensic evidence in a timely fashion. To help alleviate these problems, the Office for Victims of Crime (US Department of Justice) granted funding for implementing Sexual Assault Nurse Examiner (SANE) programs. A SANE is a registered nurse who works closely with medical staff and interacts with sexual assault crisis centers, law enforcement officers, prosecutors, judges, forensic laboratory staff, and child protective services workers to meet the multiple needs of victims and to hold offenders accountable for their crimes [15,16].

Physicians may encounter unique circumstances when treating DFSA victims because of potential delays when victims present for medical attention or not perceiving the patient as a sexual assault victim. The sedative-hypnotic and amnesic properties of the drugs used to facilitate a sexual assault can alter the victim's behavior, increase the victim's susceptibility to sexual assault, and diminish recollection of events surrounding the sexual assault. Often victims are reluctant to report incidents because of a sense of embarrassment, guilt, perceived responsibility, or acquaintance to their assaulter. Numerous reports have documented that the victims either do not seek medical attention or delay seeking medical treatment for 3 to 7 days after the assault [17–23]. Extended delays in collecting specimens from DFSAs may reduce the probability of detecting drugs potentially used to facilitate a sexual assault. Most of the drugs typically used in the facilitation of sexual assaults are rapidly absorbed and metabolized by the body, thereby rendering them difficult to detect in routine urine and blood drug screenings.

The most commonly reported symptoms from victims of DFSA are confusion, dizziness, drowsiness, impaired judgment, anterograde amnesia, lack of muscle control, loss of consciousness, reduced inhibitions, nausea,

> **Box 1. Common clinical effects reported by DFSA victims**
>
> Confusion
> Dizziness
> Anterograde amnesia
> Impaired judgment
> Reduced inhibitions
> Drowsiness
> Lack of muscle coordination
> Loss of consciousness
> Nausea
> Vomiting
> Hypotension
> Bradycardia

hypotension, and bradycardia (Box 1). Victims of sexual assault may present to the ED with physical injuries resulting from the assault or clinical effects of the drugs. For example, a victim may present to the ED with one or a combination of the following: contusions, lacerations, broken bones, altered metal status, or intoxication [24]. The health care team treats the urgent injuries but may not inquire about the possibility of sexual assault. They may mistake the clinical effects of the drug used on the victim for self-induced substance abuse. Physicians should be aware that symptoms mimicking alcohol toxicity may point to the possibility of a DFSA. SANEs are trained in investigative interview techniques that may help a patient recall specific events leading up to injuries caused by DFSA. Physicians must recognize the need to provide prophylaxis against sexually transmitted disease, assess female patients for pregnancy risk, or provide follow-up care for medical and emotional needs. In addition, the emergency medical staff must be aware of the necessity of collecting sensitive forensic evidence if the victim decides to report the assault.

Forensic laboratory analyses

All reported sexual assault cases are tested for the abuser's DNA using a "rape kit." Care must be taken to ensure chain of custody. Semen, blood, urine, vaginal secretions, saliva, vaginal epithelial cells, hair, and other biologic evidence may be identified and genetically typed by a crime laboratory [23,25]. The information derived from the analysis can often help determine whether sexual contact occurred, provide information regarding the circumstances of the incident, and be compared with reference samples collected from patients and suspects. The most common form of DNA analysis used in crime labs for identification is called polymerase chain reaction (PCR). PCR allows the analysis of evidence samples of limited quality and quantity by making millions of copies of very small amounts of DNA. Using an advanced form of PCR testing called short tandem repeats (STR), the laboratory is able to generate a DNA profile that can be compared with DNA from a suspect or a crime scene [25].

Sexual assault cases suspected of involving alcohol or drugs should have samples sent to the state Department of Forensics for toxicology testing. In addition to DNA testing, collection of urine and blood for forensic analysis at a state laboratory is typically performed to identify drugs used to facilitate sexual assault. Hair samples removed from the scalp may be requested for drug analysis when there is a significant delay in reporting a DFSA. Analysis of drugs present in hair can offer several advantages over urine and blood specimens in specific cases. The window of drug detection may be extended from days to weeks and even months because of the stability of the drug once it is deposited [26]. Analysis of sequential hair segments can provide a chronicle of drug use. Because the mechanisms by which drugs are deposited in hair are not well understood, prosecution of sexual abuse offenders based solely on results obtained from hair analysis is controversial [27]. Several factors are known to contribute to the deposition of drugs in hair: rate of hair growth, anatomic location of hair, thickness and color (melanin content) of hair, and environmental contamination. Drugs in hair are usually present in low concentrations (pg/mg to ng/mg); therefore, sensitive laboratory methods are required for detection [28–30].

Samples must be collected under strict chain-of-custody guidelines. A three-tier chain of testing may be used to analyze drugs used to facilitated sexual assault at many state forensic laboratories nationwide (Fig. 1). The first tier of testing quantitatively screens for ethanol from blood specimens using a gas chromatography with flame-ionization detection (GC-FID) or a gas chromatography linked to mass spectrometry detection (GC-MS). The second tier quantitates drugs of abuse, such as amphetamines, barbiturates, benzodiazepines, cannabinoids, cocaine, lysergic acid diethylamide, opioids, γ-hydroxybutyrate (GHB), chloral hydrate, and dextromethorphan, using immunoassays and fluorescent polarization assays. Confirmation assays are performed using GC-MS or high-pressure liquid chromatography linked to tandem mass spectroscopy (HPLC-MS/MS) analyses. The third tier of testing, focusing on basic amine drugs (BAD), uses an extremely sensitive and specific means of screening (HPLC-MS/MS) for analysis of a broad array of 300 to 400 amine-containing compounds, such as tricyclic antidepressants and benzodiazepines, that may not be detected using tier two methodologies. In many states, victims perceived to be under the influence of alcohol and having a blood alcohol concentration greater than 0.08 are not typically analyzed beyond the level of first tier ethanol testing without specific medical documentation suspecting symptoms of additional drug exposure. Many DFS cases (other than alcohol) may therefore be undetected under the current screening protocols performed at some state forensic laboratories. Several published reports

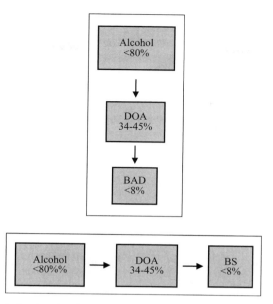

Fig. 1. Three-tier chain of testing for drug-facilitated sexual assault at state forensic laboratories. Recent publications indicate up to 80% of victims of sexual assaults are under the influence of alcohol; 34% to 45% of sexual assaults are under the influence of drugs of abuse; and less than 8% are under the influence of other basic amine drugs.

document 34% to 45% of victims of sexual assault are under the influence of drugs of abuse (DOA); 8% are under the influence of drugs not typically detected by standard DOA methods (eg, BAD) [7,8,10,21,31]. It is important for physicians and SANE teams to document suspicions of drugs in the patient's medical record, especially in cases of sexual assault. Documentation of these suspicions justifies drug-specific analyses by the state forensic laboratory. These analytic results are mandatory for the prosecution of sexual predators.

The Drug-Induced Rape Prevention and Punishment Act of 1996 (Public Law 104-305) modified 21 U.S.C. § 841 to provide penalties of up to 20 years' imprisonment and fines for people who intend to commit a crime of violence (including rape) by distributing a controlled substance to another individual without that individual's knowledge. This act provides specific definitions of controlled substances and crimes of violence that assist prosecutors in maximizing the penalties against sexual predators. Controlled substances are categorized as schedule I to V drugs by the US Drug Enforcement Administration (DEA) (Box 2). Extensive efforts have focused on documenting detection limits for common drugs used to facilitate sexual assault to aid in prosecution of sexual predators [10]. Without the extensive efforts of medical staff, forensic toxicologists, police, and judicial officials these penalties against sexual assault offenders cannot be implemented.

Box 2. Classification of scheduled drugs in the United States

Schedule I drugs
The substance has a high potential for abuse.
The substance has no currently accepted medical use in treatment in the United States.
There is a lack of accepted safety for use of the substance under medical supervision.
The drugs are not available by prescription and are deemed to have no medical use.

Schedule II drugs
The substance has a high potential for abuse.
The substance has a currently accepted medical use in treatment in the United States or a currently accepted medical use with severe restrictions.
Abuse of the substances may lead to severe psychologic or physical dependence.
The drugs or other substances are only available by prescription, and distribution is carefully controlled and monitored by the DEA.

Schedule III drugs
The substance has less potential for abuse than the drugs or other substances in schedules I/II.
The substance has a currently accepted medical use in treatment in the United States.
Abuse of the substance may lead to moderate or low physical dependence or high psychologic dependence.
The drugs or other substances are available only by prescription, although control of wholesale distribution is somewhat less stringent than schedule II drugs.

Schedule IV drugs
The drug or other substance has a low potential for abuse relative to the drugs or other substances in schedule III.
The drug or other substance has a currently accepted medical use in treatment in the United States.
Abuse of the drug or other substance may lead to limited physical dependence or psychologic dependence relative to the drugs or other substances in schedule III.
The drugs are available only by prescription, although control of wholesale distribution is somewhat less stringent than schedule III drugs.

Schedule V drugs

The drug or other substance has a low potential for abuse relative
to the drugs or other substances in schedule IV.
The drug or other substance has a currently accepted medical
use in treatment in the United States.
Abuse of the drug or other substance may lead to limited
physical dependence or psychologic dependence relative to
the drugs or other substances in schedule IV.
Schedule V drugs are sometimes available without
a prescription.

In addition to providing immediate, prophylactic, and follow-up medical care to the sexual assault victim, physicians need to implement resources necessary to maintain the integrity of physical evidence, document the victim's examination results/interpretation and interview history, and serve as an expert opinion during judicial proceedings. Integration of all these events is necessary to assist a victim of DFSA and support the prosecution of the sexual predator [11,32].

What drugs are used to facilitate sexual assault?

Most sexual assaults have been linked to the abuse of alcohol [7,9,31,33,34]. It is commonly accepted that there is a high degree of correlation between alcohol intoxication and the risk for being sexually assaulted [10]. In recent years, however, there has been increased attention in the literature to people using other drugs to render their victims unconscious or lower their level of resistance with the intent to sexually assault them [14,20,35,36]. In addition to alcohol, the drugs most often implicated in DFSAs are GHB, flunitrazepam, and ketamine, although others, including other benzodiazepines and sedative-hypnotics, are used also (Box 3). These drugs share similar characteristics for producing sedation, hypnosis, and anterograde amnesia. These effects often rapidly incapacitate victims and the effects can be intensified when they are willingly or involuntarily taken with alcohol. Because of the sedative and amnesic properties of these drugs, victims often have no memory of an assault, only an awareness or sense that they were violated.

Ethanol

The most common drug associated with DFSA is alcohol [7]. Because most sexual assault cases are not reported, the percent of alcohol-associated sexual assault cases varies greatly (30%–75%). Because of the prevalence of

---

Box 3. Drugs used to facilitate sexual assault

Ethanol
Chloral hydrate
Benzodiazepines
Nonbenzodiazepine sedative-hypnotics
GHB
Ketamine
Opioids
Dextromethorphan
Barbiturates
Anticholinergics
Antihistamines

---

alcohol consumption by college students, numerous institutions across the United States offer health information programs focused on increasing the awareness of alcohol-associated sexual assaults [37,38]. These programs heighten awareness that alcohol is a drug often used to facilitate sexual assault and they assist victims in finding medical and legal aid.

Clinical effects

The clinical effects of alcohol are dose and time dependent. Ethanol metabolism follows zero-order kinetics. Although the rate of metabolism varies from person to person, because of phenotypic differences in alcohol dehydrogenase and metabolic tolerance in chronic drinkers, the reported average rate of metabolism is found to be constant (about 15 mL/dL/h) [39,40]. The clinical effects of ethanol intoxication include impaired judgment, incoordination, behavioral changes, ataxia, cognitive slowing, memory impairment, nausea, vomiting, diplopia, and lethargy. Depending on a person's pre-existing tolerance, respiratory depression, coma, and death may occur at levels of 300 to 400 mg/dL. It takes little volume to intoxicate a person. For example, to achieve levels of intoxication of 200 mg/dL requires consumption of about 100 mL of absolute ethanol in a 70 kg adult. Many liquors contain 40% to 50% ethanol; therefore six to seven shots (30 mL per shot) of liquor in rapid succession may result in an ethanol level of 200 mg/dL [41]. Significantly lower concentrations of ethanol are required to incapacitate (or increase the susceptibility for sexual assault in) a smaller-framed victim or a person who voluntarily or unwillingly coingests drugs with sedative or psychotropic effects.

Laboratory monitoring

Analysis of ethanol levels from urine and blood specimens are commonly evaluated in many clinical laboratories, private laboratories, and state laboratories. Blood alcohol is determined using enzymatic analyses. Blood alcohol and urine analysis confirmation is performed using a GC-FID or gas GC-MS [42,43]. Although most clinical laboratories set the limit of detection at 10 mg/dL, published reports document the limits of detection for ethanol using GC-FID and GC-MS as low as 1 and 0.02 mg/dL, respectively [40,42]. These sensitive detection assays may therefore extend the time (12–24 hours) required for submitting specimens from sexual assault cases and enhance the possibility of prosecuting a perpetrator for a DFSA crime. Back-tracking calculations (15 mg/dL/h and one half-life every 4 h) are often performed to estimate the blood alcohol level at a given time before the actual time the blood sample was taken. Caution must be used with this method of reverse extrapolation, because chronic alcohol abusers and heavy drinkers metabolize alcohol faster than social or naïve drinkers [40].

Choral hydrate "Mickey Finn"

Anecdotal reports of combining drugs and alcohol to assault victims date back to the early nineteenth and twentieth centuries. An infamous example is Mickey Finn, the proprietor of Chicago's Lone Star Saloon in the late nineteenth and early twentieth centuries. He was alleged to have drugged his customers with the addition of chloral hydrate to their ethanol-based beverages and subsequently robbed them.

Chloral hydrate is classified as a nonbarbiturate hypnotic. It is an inexpensive transparent crystalline compound that can be easily dissolved in beverages. It was first synthesized in 1832 and was one of the original depressants developed for the specific purpose of inducing sleep. At therapeutic single doses, chloral hydrate has a rapid onset (30 minutes), produces minimal side effects, and is useful in alleviating sleeplessness caused by pain or insomnia in a relatively short time. The abuse and misuse of this drug and subsequent introduction of newer sedatives (barbiturates and benzodiazepines) led to its decline for medicinal purposes.

Clinical effects

The diagnosis of chloral hydrate can be difficult to differentiate from alcohol, benzodiazepine, and barbiturate intoxication, because all share similar clinical effects. Although the exact mechanism of action of chloral hydrate has not been determined, it is a general central nervous system (CNS) depressant having sedative effects with minimal analgesic effects when administered independently. At low doses (<20 mg/kg) symptoms may include relaxation, dizziness, slurred speech, confusion, disorientation, euphoria, irritability, and hypersensitivity rash. At higher doses (>50 mg/kg) chloral hydrate can cause hypotension, hypothermia, hypoventilation, tachydysrhythmia, nausea, vomiting, diarrhea, headache, and amnesia [44]. The elimination half-life ($t_{1/2}$) of chloral hydrate is 4 to 12 hours

[44,45]. If coingested with alcohol, chloral hydrate metabolism may be seriously impaired. Because ethanol and chloral hydrate are both metabolized by CYP2E1 and alcohol dehydrogenase, coingestion may not only exacerbate their clinical effects but also prolong their duration of action [45,46].

Laboratory monitoring

Chloral hydrate is not detected on routine, commercially available drug screens. Quantification of chloral hydrate and its metabolites trichloroethanol (TCE), TCE-glucuronide, and trichloroacetic acid can be detected in less than 1 mL plasma using HPLC-MS/MS and capillary gas chromatography with electron-capture detection (GC/ECD) [47–49]. Limit of detection for chloral hydrate is 5 ng/mL and 10 ng/mL for its metabolites using GC/ECD [49].

Benzodiazepines

Benzodiazepines are a large class of drugs that bind to specific receptor sites on γ-aminobutyric acid (GABA)-mediated receptor synapses in the brain. Benzodiazepines are believed to increase GABA-mediated chloride conduction into the postsynaptic neuron, prolonging hyperpolarization of the cell and diminishing synaptic transmission, thereby producing its sedative properties. Drugs within this class vary in their affinity and efficacy at their receptor. This variation results in differences in the degree of clinical effects, time of onset, and rate of metabolism. Ultimately, with a faster rate of onset there tends to be greater abuse potential [50]. Although national statistics are not available to estimate the prevalence of benzodiazepines used to facilitate sexual assault, recent publications estimate approximately 8% of sexual assault cases are positive for benzodiazepines [7,8,10,28]. Flunitrazepam (Rohypnol) is the most frequently reported (4% of sexual assault cases) date rape drug belonging to the benzodiazepine class [7]. The high incidence of flunitrazepam in DFSA is partially attributable to the development and implementation of specific toxicologic tests in response to increased public awareness resulting in a testing bias [7,9,32,51,52]. Other benzodiazepines that have been reported in sexual assault victims are diazepam, triazolam, temazepam, tetrazepam, and clonazepam [13,19,28,53,54].

Flunitrazepam is a fast-acting sedative-hypnotic and is categorized as a schedule I drug in the United States. Because it is still licensed for use in Europe, Asia, and Latin America for sedation and treatment of insomnia, sexual predators can acquire this drug through illegal trafficking [55]. On the street, flunitrazepam is known as Roofies, Forget pill, Rubies, Ruffies, Rope, Roopies, Ropies, Rib, R-2, Roaches, Papas, Mexican Valium and Circles. Sexual assault predators use flunitrazepam because it can be easily dissolved into a beverage, it is relatively tasteless and odorless, it quickly incapacitates victims, and routine drug screens do not detect its presence.

Clinical effects

Flunitrazepam is more potent than diazepam owing to its slower dissociation from the GABA receptor [56–58]. It is rapidly absorbed and distributed into tissues on oral administration. The onset of its sedative, amnesic, hypnotic, and disinhibitory effects can occur within 20 to 30 minutes [56]. Although the effects of flunitrazepam occur rapidly when used alone, it is often coingested with alcohol, which amplifies its effects [59,60]. Initial symptoms may consist of dizziness, disorientation, lack of coordination, and slurred speech, which mimic alcohol intoxication. Other unique effects are anterograde amnesia as early as 15 minutes after oral administration [20]. Rapid alternation of hot and cold flashes may precipitously be followed by loss of consciousness. Large doses (> 2 g) have produced aspiration, muscular hypotonia, hypotension, bradycardia, coma, and death [13,21,54,61]. The clinical diagnosis of flunitrazepam can be difficult to differentiate from alcohol intoxication.

Laboratory monitoring

Patients who have a complaint of sexual assault who seem intoxicated or have anterograde amnesia should be suspected of unknowingly ingesting a benzodiazepine. Commonly marketed drug screens turn positive for most benzodiazepines, but not all (ie, flunitrazepam; other benzodiazepines marketed outside the United States). Point of care testing is available for benzodiazepines in the ED, but clinical samples must be confirmed and documented under strict chain-of-custody procedures [62]. In addition to adhering to standard rape protocols, a urine or hair specimen should be analyzed for benzodiazepine and their metabolites by a state forensic laboratory using GC-MS or HPLC-MS/MS [30,61,63–65]. Flunitrazepam metabolites can be detected up to 60 hours in the urine using an automated immunoassay system (EMIT II), categorized as a general toxicologic screen that is available in many hospital laboratories. Flunitrazepam metabolites can be detected and as early as 7 days in hair samples (HPLC-MS/MS) [54].

Nonbenzodiazepine hypnotics

Zopiclone, eszopiclone, zolpidem, and zaleplon belong to a new generation of sedative-hypnotics that are structurally different from benzodiazepines (Fig. 2). Like benzodiazepines, these drugs modulate the GABA$_A$ receptor chloride channel by binding to the benzodiazepine (BZ) receptors, otherwise known as the omega (ω_1) receptors, in the brain [66] without binding to peripheral BZ receptors [67,68]. These drugs therefore have fewer muscle-relaxant properties [68]. The rapid-onset and amnesic properties of this class of drugs can result in disinhibition, passivity, and retrograde amnesia, making it a favored DFSA drug. These drugs require only a low dose

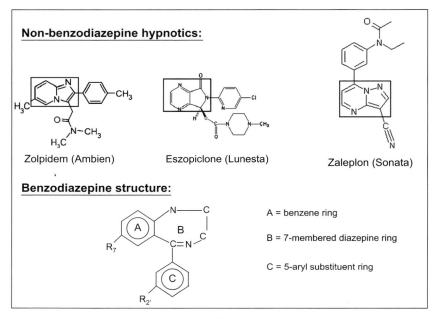

Fig. 2. Structural similarities between benzodiazepine and nonbenzodiazepine sedative-hyp-notics. The nonbenzodiazepine hypnotics share a common pyrimidine ring (*boxed*) structure containing various chemical side groups. Members of the benzodiazepine class share common structural features: (*A*) benzene ring; (*B*) 7-membered diazepine ring; (*C*) 5-aryl substituent ring.

to cause an effect and are rapidly metabolized. Because of the amnesic prop-erties of these drugs, victims are often confused following the event and may be delayed in reporting the sexual assault [7]. Commonly used drug screens do not test for these substances; therefore, suspected amnestic drug use must be documented to justify more elaborate drug testing by state agencies. All these characteristics make these drugs potential agents in DFSA.

Recognition of these new-generation sleep aids as potential agents used in facilitating sexual assault has only recently been reported in the United States, United Kingdom, and France [7,8,21,69,70]. Few published reports in the United States tested sexual assault victims for the presence of zolpi-dem, and unfortunately those that tested did not report its prevalence rate [61,71]. Because of the increased prevalence of short-acting nonbarbiturate use on college campuses and across the United States and minimal data es-timating the prevalence of these drugs used in sexual assault, there is a strong demand for national systematic studies to estimate the prevalence of non-barbiturate sleep aids in DFSA.

Most of the nonbenzodiazepine sleep aids are available through a pre-scription as a schedule IV drug and are readily available in North American social circles (ie, college campuses). These highly prescribed insomnia drugs are available in a tablet form that may be crushed and dissolved into a beverage or food of an unsuspecting victim. All may produce additive CNS-depressant effects when coadministered with other psychotropic medications, such as anticonvulsants, antihistamines, ethanol, and other drugs that themselves produce CNS depression.

Clinical effects and drug characteristics

Zolpidem

Zolpidem is available as an immediate- or extended-release tablet. An average oral dose of 10 to 15 mg has a rapid onset of clinical symptoms between 10 and 30 minutes. Clinical effects peak at approximately 1.5 hours for immediate release, duration lasts for about 6 to 8 hours for both immediate- and extended-release preparations, and the $t_{1/2}$ is approximately 2.5 hours [72]. Clinical effects may include dizziness, psychomotor, confusion, nervousness, amnesia, and hallucinations. There is evidence of minimal respiratory depression when used as a single agent, but zolpidem may produce additive CNS-depressive effects and death when coadministered with other sedatives [73].

Zaleplon

Zaleplon is available as an immediate-release tablet or capsule. An average oral dose of 10 to 15 mg has a rapid onset of clinical symptoms of approximately 10 to 30 minutes. Although the $t_{1/2}$ for zaleplon is about 1 hour, the duration of clinical effects may persist for greater than 6 hours. This persistence may be because of the higher affinity of zaleplon for specific α_2 and α_3 subunits of the GABA receptor, unlike zolpidem or zopiclone [74]. Clinical effects may include somnolence, dizziness, psychomotor, confusion, nervousness, rebound amnesia, and hallucinations. Higher doses ($>40–60$ mg) may cause increased CNS effects and impaired motor skills [44].

Eszopiclone

The precise mechanism of action of eszopiclone is unknown, but its effect is believed to result from its interaction with GABA-receptor complexes at binding domains located close to or allosterically coupled to benzodiazepine receptors. An average dose of 2 to 3 mg has a rapid onset of clinical symptoms occurring in approximately 30 minutes. Both immediate and extended-release forms are available. Clinical effects may include dizziness, psychomotor dysfunction, confusion, nervousness, amnesia, and hallucinations. Nausea, vomiting, and anticholinergic effects have been reported in less than 10% of patients [75]. By itself, eszopiclone has not been reported to cause respiratory depression, but it may produce additive CNS-depressant effects when coadministered with other sedatives. The clinical effects of eszopiclone are longer in duration compared with zopiclone or zolpidem, with a $t_{1/2}$ of 6 hours [67].

Zopiclone

Zopiclone is not currently available in the United States. It is the racemic mixture of two stereoisomers; the active stereoisomer is eszopiclone. Clinical effects therefore are similar to eszopiclone.

Laboratory analysis

Because of the amnesic properties of these drugs, victims often may not report the sexual assault for several days. Sensitive analytic techniques are necessary to detect these drugs and their metabolites in urine or hair samples after a single dose. Unfortunately, the drug screens found in most hospital laboratories do not detect the new generation short-acting class of sleep aids called nonbenzodiazepine hypnotics. Although numerous private facilities are now capable of detecting nonbenzodiazepine drugs, most state forensic laboratories integrate these HPLC-MS/MS amine-detection tests into their repertoire of available toxicologic screens. Because testing of nonbenzodiazepine drugs is a third tier of testing in many state forensic laboratories, only cases containing documentation suspecting drugs other than alcohol or common drugs of abuse may be analyzed in this manner.

γ-hydroxybutyrate, 1,4-butanediol, and γ-butyrolactone

Since March 2000, GHB and the synthetic precursor compounds, 1,4-butanediol (1,4-BD) or γ-butyrolactone (GBL), have been schedule I agents in the United States. The availability of GHB has been restricted in numerous countries, such as Australia, Brunei, Canada, Finland, France, Italy, Japan, New Zealand, Norway, the United States, South Africa, Sweden, Switzerland, and the United Kingdom. GHB can be illegally purchased as an odorless and colorless liquid form or an off-white powder that easily dissolves in liquids. GHB is sold on the street under various names, including Liquid ecstasy, Liquid X, Liquid E, Gib, Natural sleep-500, Somatomax, Georgia home boy, Grievous bodily harm, Soap, Scoop, Easy lay, Salty water, G-riffick, Cherry menth, and Organic Quaalude.

Sexual assault perpetrators have used GHB as a fast and effective means of intoxication for their victims. Although national statistics are not available to estimate the prevalence of GHB used to facilitate sexual assault, recent publications estimate approximately 4% of alleged sexual assault cases in the United States are positive for GHB [7,9,21,76]. Numerous GHB-related DFSA cases have also been published in the United Kingdom and France [21,70,77,78]. Sexual assault cases report victims have either voluntarily or unwillingly ingested GHB on a date, at social parties, or in "rave" dance party settings.

GHB is a naturally occurring substance produced in the brain. GHB is reversibly metabolized to GABA through multiple endogenous enzymes (Fig. 3) [79–81]. Illicit consumption of GHB, or the synthetic GHB

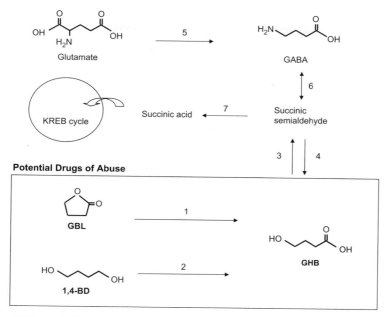

Fig. 3. GHB metabolism. In the brain, γ-hydroxybutyrate (GHB) is reversibly metabolized into γ-aminobutyric acid (GABA) using the endogenous enzyme GABA transaminase. Illicit consumption of 1,4-butanediol (1,4-BD) or γ-butyrolactone (GBL) may also be metabolized into GABA by way of multiple endogenous enzyme systems. The endogenous metabolic enzymes involved are (*1*) lactonase, or nonenzymatic ester hydrolysis; (*2*) alcohol dehydrogenase or aldehyde dehydrogenase; (*3*) GHB dehydrogenase; (*4*) succinic semialdehyde reductase or NADPH-dependent aldehyde reductase; (*5*) glutamic acid decarboxylase; (*6*) GABA transaminase; (*7*) succinic semialdehyde dehydrogenase. Potential drugs of abuse are boxed and in bold.

precursor compounds 1,4-BD or GBL, promotes GABA activity [81]. In addition to increased metabolism to GABA, GHB has direct effects on the CNS by binding GHB-specific receptors. Animal studies support the existence of distinct GHB receptors in the CNS, because GHB can still act as a neuromodulator even in the presence of the GABA$_B$-specific inhibitor baclofen and in GABA$_B$ receptor knockout mice [82–84]. GHB is suggested to increase dopamine levels in the substantia nigra, potentiate the endogenous opioid system, and mediate GABA transmission [81].

GHB, 1,4-BD, and GBL are frequently sold on the street and at rave dance parties in liquid form and are colorless and tasteless. These drugs can be easily masked in drinks and consumed by willing or unwilling victims of sexual assault.

Clinical effects

Onset of GHB effects occurs in approximately 15 to 30 minutes, depending on the dose (average 1–5 g) and chemical purity. Clinical effects are augmented in the presence of coadministered drugs, such as alcohol and other sedative drugs [85]. The clinical effects are dose dependent and typically last 3 to 6 hours. Initial symptoms include drowsiness, disorientation, and dizziness. Low dose (<1 g) produces mild symptoms, such as CNS depression, amnesia, hypotonia, and reduced inhibitions (similar to alcohol). Larger doses, 1 to 2 g, cause increased somnolence, drowsiness, dizziness, bradycardia, and bradypnea. High doses (>2 g) often interfere with motor coordination and balance, induce significant respiratory depression and bradypnea, Cheyne-Stokes respiration, nausea, vomiting, diminished cardiac output, coma, and death [73,86,87].

Laboratory monitoring

GHB is metabolized quickly ($t_{1/2} \sim 30$ minutes) and is not detected on most routine urine and serum toxicology screens. Several state and private laboratories have the ability to perform analyses on blood, urine, and hair samples using GC-FID or GC-MS [30,76,88]. Testing sensitivity is not the primary issue with GHB; timely collection of sample collection is. Because of its rapid metabolism, plasma samples should be collected less than 6 to 8 hours after ingestion and urine samples collected in less than 10 to 12 hours. Urine and plasma may exhibit endogenous levels of GHB within 8 to 12 hours after ingestion (<1 mg/dL in urine, <4 mg/L in blood/plasma) [89]. Samples reaching endogenous levels make it difficult to legally prove GHB doping in sexual assault cases. Exogenous levels of GHB have been detected in hair samples at 7 days postintoxication [70]. The timely presentation of the patient for medical attention and physician recognition of GHB symptoms presented by sexually assaulted victims are essential for prosecution of sexual offenders.

Ketamine

Ketamine (ketamine hydrochloride) is an analgesic and general anesthetic that produces a rapid-acting dissociative effect. It was first synthesized in1962 as a medical anesthetic for humans and animals. Today ketamine is approved for use in emergency medicine, critical care, and veterinary medicine. The prosecution of a ketamine-facilitated sexual assault perpetrator in 1993 and the increase in its illicit use prompted the DEA to restrict ketamine as a schedule III drug in August 1999. Ketamine is outlawed in the United Kingdom and classified as a schedule I narcotic in Canada. Ketamine is available by prescription as a tablet or a parenteral solution. On the street, ketamine is sold under various names, including K, Ket, Special K, Super acid, Super C, Spesh, Vitamin K, Smack K, Kit-kat, Keller, Barry Keddle, HOSS, The Hoos, Hossalar, Kurdamin, Kiddie, Wonk, Regreta, and Tranq. Ketamine generally is sold illegally as either a colorless, odorless liquid or as a white or off-white powder. Liquid ketamine can be rapidly injected intramuscularly. Either liquid or powder form can be easily disguised in a victim's beverage. Ketamine powder can even be sprinkled onto marijuana or tobacco and smoked.

Clinical effects

The onset of action after oral ingestion can be as little as 20 minutes [90]. Hallucinatory effects may be short-acting (<1 hour) but so intense that the victim may have trouble discerning reality [77]. Ketamine produces effects similar to phencyclidine and dextromethorphan. The onset of clinical effects is rapid and depends on route of administration. Anesthesia effects by way of intramuscular injection take as little 20 to 30 seconds, oral ingestion about 30 minutes, and nasal insufflation approximately 10 minutes [44,91,92]. The $t_{1/2}$ for ketamine is 2 to 3 hours [93]. Duration of anesthetic effects is dose dependent (usually <1 hour) and effects on the senses, judgment, and coordination can have a longer duration (~6–24 hours). Ketamine can cause delirium, amnesia, dissociative anesthesia hallucinations, hypersalivation, nystagmus, impaired motor function, hypertension, and potentially fatal respiratory problems. Effects on blood pressure and respiratory depression can be significantly enhanced when coingested with alcohol.

Laboratory monitoring

No immunoassays are available to detect ketamine at this time. Ketamine and its active metabolites norketamine and dehydronorketamine can be detected in urine samples using GC-MS or LC-MS analyses. The limit of detection is 1 ng/mL [94,95].

Barbiturates

Barbiturates can produce a wide range of CNS depression, ranging from mild sedation to general anesthesia. They are categorized based on their ultrashort-acting, short-acting, medium-acting, or long-acting duration of clinical effects (Table 1). Barbiturates are classified as schedule II to IV drugs based on their rapid time of onset and duration and their abuse potential. They can inhibit excitatory or enhance inhibitory synaptic transmission. Barbiturates inhibit excitatory synaptic transmission by reducing glutamate-induced depolarizations [96]. Barbiturates enhance the effectiveness of GABA transmission by directly activating chloride channels and depressing synaptic transmission at virtually all synapses. Barbiturates effect the duration, not frequency, of GABA channel opening, thereby hyperpolarizing and decreasing the firing rate of neurons [97].

The estimated prevalence of barbiturates used to facilitate sexual assault is only about 1%, because of limited availability in recent years [7]. The

Table 1
Characterization of barbiturates

Chemical name	Duration	DEA scheduled classification
Thiamylal	Ultrashort	Schedule III
Thiopental ("truth serum")	Ultrashort	Schedule III
Methohexital	Ultrashort	Schedule IV
Amobarbital	Short	Schedule II
Aprobarbital	Short	Schedule II
Butabarbital	Short	Schedule II
Pentobarbital	Short	Schedule II
Secobarbital	Short	Schedule II
Butalbital	Medium	Schedule II
Cyclobarbital	Medium	Schedule III
Talbutal	Medium	Schedule II
Methylphenobarbital	Long	Schedule IV
Mephobarbital	Long	Schedule IV
Phenobarbital	Long	Schedule IV

ultrashort-acting barbiturate thiopental was recently reportedly used to facilitate a sexual assault in Italy [98]. The slang terms for these drugs are barbs, barbies, sleepers, blue bullets, nembies, pink ladies, and red devils.

Clinical effects

Onset of clinical symptoms varies (15–40 minutes) and the degree of symptoms is dose and drug dependent. Clinical effects may consist of CNS and respiratory depression, hypothermia, bullous skin lesions, aspiration pneumonia, nystagmus, dysarthria, ataxia, drowsiness hypothermia, renal failure, muscle necrosis, hypotension, hypoglycemia, coma, and death [44]. Coingestion with alcohol or other CNS depressants enhances toxic effects. Duration of effects depends on the dose and the specific drug itself.

Laboratory monitoring

Detection periods for barbiturates vary greatly depending on the specific barbiturate being used. Each barbiturate has a different half-life in the body. Ultrashort- and short-acting barbiturates (thiopental, secobarbital) may only be detected in the urine for 1 to 4 days, whereas longer-duration barbiturates (phenobarbital) can be detected for 2 to 3 weeks. Many larger hospital facilities can detect most barbiturates from urine samples with an extensive toxicology screen using competitive fluorescence polarization immunoassays [99]. Detection depends on the dose and half-life of the specific drug being tested. State forensic laboratories have extremely sensitive assays, such as HPLC-MS/MS and GC/MS-MS, capable of detecting very low concentrations of barbiturates from urine and hair samples that can greatly expand the window of detection [98].

Opioids

Several opioid drugs are included in the analysis for date-rape drugs. Although these drugs are highly regulated or only available by prescription, illicit use of these drugs is still common nationwide. Opiates are the naturally derived narcotics, such as heroin, morphine, and codeine. These are isolated from the poppy plant *Papaver somniferum*. Heroin is the only opiate currently listed as a schedule I drug, primarily owing to the rapid onset of action, clinical effects (euphoria and sedation), and its high abuse potential. Metabolism of codeine to morphine is required for its analgesic effects (Fig. 4). Opioids include the semisynthetic compounds, such as hydrocodone, hydromorphone, oxycodone, and fentanyl. These drugs all have potent analgesic and sedative properties but different pharmacokinetic properties. These drugs are available in powder or tablet forms having a slightly bitter taste. Either form can be hidden in a beverage, smoked, or inhaled. These drugs can easily be used to incapacitate a sexual assault victim.

Clinical effects

The major clinical effects of opioids are analgesia, sedation, pinpoint pupils (miosis), euphoria, and respiratory depression [44]. Pinpoint pupils may not always be seen in all and should not be solely relied on for the diagnosis. The onset of clinical symptoms varies with the drug and the method of administration. Onset of effects for oral ingestion of opioids varies, but most are within 30 to 60 minutes; inhalation or injection is more rapid (within 5 minutes). Duration of clinical effects depends on the specific opioid drug. Naloxone reversal of sedation may clue the health care team to the presence of opioids.

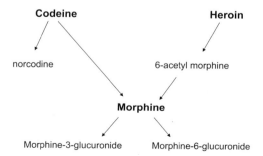

Fig. 4. The opiate metabolites detected by immunoassay and GC-MS. A small percentage of codeine is converted to active metabolites by CYP2D6 to norcodeine (~10%), morphine (~10%), and hydrocodone (<2%). Heroin is rapidly metabolized to 6-acetyl morphine and then hydrolyzed to morphine; both are active metabolites. Morphine is conjugated to inactive metabolite morphine-3-glucuronide and the potent metabolite morphine-6-glucuronide.

Laboratory monitoring

In the hospital setting commercial immunoassays are designed to detect naturally occurring opiates (morphine and codeine). Specific GC-MS analysis protocols are available for confirming natural, synthetic, and semisynthetic opioid compounds from urine specimens. In addition, specific immunoassays and GC-MS protocols are available for detection of methadone and propoxyphene. Documentation of suspected opioid-related clinical symptoms assists state laboratories in detecting and confirming a diverse array of opioid compounds potentially used to incapacitate a victim of sexual assault.

Over-the-counter medications

Several medications that may be used to facilitate sexual assault are legally available without a prescription. Although these medications are diverse in class, their clinical effects may be used to incapacitate a sexual assault victim. Sexual predators may use these drugs because their effects are exacerbated with alcohol and can easily be used to adulterate a victim's drink.

Dextromethorphan

Dextromethorphan is sold over the counter as an antitussive agent alone or in combination with other cough aids (pseudoephedrine, acetaminophen, chlorpheniramine). It is the *d*-isomer of the potent opiate analgesic 3-methoxy-N-methylmorphine (levorphanol). Although dextromethorphan is structurally related to opioids, it is devoid of analgesic or sedative effects at therapeutic doses. Dextromethorphan is metabolized by CYP2D6 to a more potent metabolite, dextrorphan [100,101]. Dextrorphan is a stronger noncompetitive antagonist than dextromethorphan for the N-methyl-D-aspartate glutamate receptor [102]. These properties promote its use in treatment of neuropathic and postoperative pain management [102–106].

Even though dextromethorphan has a strong safety profile at therapeutic concentrations, it is highly abused for its sedative, hallucinogenic, short-term memory loss, dissociative, and euphoric properties at high doses. Although no cases have been published using dextromethorphan in DFSA, large doses can impair a victim's sensory and motor skills making it a potential drug for use in DFSA. Dextromethorphan is widely available over the counter in liquid, tablet, and gel capsule formulations, or over the internet in a white power form [107]. Although liquid dextromethorphan has a bad taste, crystallized and powder forms can easily be disguised in drinks and consumed by an unknowing victim. Street names for dextromethorphan are Dex, DXM, Tuss, Robo, Skittles, Triple-C, and Syrup.

Despite the safety of dextromethorphan when used at the recommended dosage (<120 mg/day), higher doses can result in nausea, vomiting, seizure, loss of consciousness, irregular heartbeat, and death [108,109]. Serotonin syndrome may develop in patients on other serotoninergic drugs because of additive inhibition of serotonin reuptake by dextromethorphan [110]. Patients who have genetic variations in CYP2D6 causing rapid metabolism of dextromethorphan may present with greater clinical effects [111–113].

Anticholinergics

Scopolamine and atropine are anticholinergic agents of the belladonna alkaloid family. Scopolamine is used for motion sickness and as an adjunct to anesthesia to produce sedation and amnesia. Scopolamine produces a higher degree of sedation than atropine because of the higher degree of penetration into the CNS. The high potency, rapid onset, and amnestic effects of scopolamine have lead to its being included on testing for DFSA cases [114].

The major clinical effects of scopolamine are classic anticholinergic symptoms, such as dilated pupils (mydriasis), dry mouth, hallucinations, and slurred speech. Other clinical effects are tachycardia, vomiting, confusion, and amnesia. Large doses can result in coma, seizures, and death. The onset of clinical symptoms is fast (within 15–30 minutes) and duration of effects may last up to 2 to 3 days.

Antihistamines

Antihistamines are typically used in the treatment of allergies or insomnia. First-generation antihistamines (diphenhydramine, chlorpheniramine) readily cross the blood-brain barrier, producing greater CNS effects than second-generation antihistamines (fexofenadine). First-generation antihistamines hit central and peripheral histamine (H_1 and H_2) receptors, but are still widely used because they are effective and inexpensive [115]. Few cases have documented the use of diphenhydramine in DFSA [32], yet the anticholinergic proprieties of antihistamines make this a class of drugs feasible for DFSA.

First-generation antihistamines can cause CNS depression and anticholinergic symptoms, such as sedation, hallucinations, confusion, agitation, and psychosis. Onset of action is 15 to 60 minutes and clinical symptoms typically last 4 to 6 hours [116]. Large doses can exacerbate these effects and can even result in cardiotoxicity, coma, and seizures [117]. Coingestion with alcohol or other sedative-hypnotic drugs may increase some or all of these clinical symptoms. Victims may have difficulty distinguishing events of a sexual assault because of the anticholinergic effects of the drugs. A victim may not present for hours or days after a sexual assault, therefore, because of the clinical effects of the drugs themselves.

Laboratory monitoring

Analysis of blood or urine antihistamine levels is not typically performed in the health care setting. Because these nonprescription drugs are commonly used by the general public, interpretation of a positive test result is problematic. Dextromethorphan cross-reacts with most immunoassays for opioid compounds. Confirmation protocols for dextromethorphan are available using GC-MS. Most anticholinergics are detected using GC-MS. Urine specimens are sufficient for the highly specific GC-MS and HPLC-MS/MS analyses [47,118]. When a victim of sexual assault reports or presents with specific signs and symptoms, it is imperative that the medical staff document these findings and relay this information to the laboratory on collecting the necessary biologic samples. Without such documentation, state forensic laboratories may overlook the need to specifically analyze biologic specimens for these agents.

Summary

DFSA is a complex and ever-prevalent problem presenting to North American emergency departments. Emergency personnel should consider DFSA in patients who are amnestic to the specific details of the event following a reported sexual assault. The presence of ethanol or a positive routine drug screen in a sexual assault victim does not exclude the potential for another drug being present. In addition, a negative routine drug screen does not exclude all potential agents that are used in DFSA. It is imperative for emergency personnel to clearly document the history and the presenting signs and symptoms to assist laboratory personnel to hone in and detect the agent used in a DFSA.

References

[1] Anonymous. ACOG issues report on sexual assault - American College of Obstetricians and Gynecologists - special medical reports. American Family Physician March 1, 1998.

[2] Rose VL. National Criminal Victimization Survey, 2003. In: Bureau of Justice Statistics: U.S. Department of Justice; 2004.

[3] Kilpatrick DG, Edmonds CN, Seymour A. Rape in America: a report to the Nation. Arlington (VA): National Center for Victims of Crime and Crime Victims Research and Treatment Center; 1992.

[4] Fisher BS, Cullen FT, Turner MG. The sexual victimization of college women. Washington, DC: Department of Justice (US), National Institute of Justice; 2000. NCJ 182369.

[5] Grunbaum JA, Kann L, Kinchen S, et al. Youth risk behavior surveillance—United States, 2003. MMWR Surveill Summ 2004;53(2):1–96.

[6] Tjaden P, Thoennes N. Full report of the prevalence, incidence, and consequences of violence against women: findings from the National Violence Against Women Survey. Washington, DC: National Institute of Justice; 2000. NCJ 183781.

[7] ElSohly MA, Salamone SJ. Prevalence of drugs used in cases of alleged sexual assault. J Anal Toxicol 1999;23(3):141–6.

[8] Hindmarch I, ElSohly M, Gambles J, et al. Forensic urinalysis of drug use in cases of alleged sexual assault. J Clin Forensic Med 2001;8(4):197–205.

[9] Slaughter L. Involvement of drugs in sexual assault. J Reprod Med 2000;45(5):425–30.

[10] Negrusz A, Juhascik M, Gaensslen RE. Estimate of the incidence of drug-facilitated sexual assault in the U.S. U.S. Department of Justice; 2005.

[11] Fitzgerald N, Riley KJ. Drug-facilitated rape: looking for the missing pieces. National Institute of Justice Journal 2000;243:8–15.

[12] Anonymous. Personal crimes of violence. In: US Justice Department of Justice- Bureau of Justice Statistics Criminal Victimization in the United States; 2004.

[13] Marc B, Baudry F, Vaquero P, et al. Sexual assault under benzodiazepine submission in a Paris suburb. Arch Gynecol Obstet 2000;263(4):193–7.

[14] McGregor MJ, Lipowska M, Shah S, et al. An exploratory analysis of suspected drug-facilitated sexual assault seen in a hospital emergency department. Women Health 2003; 37(3):71–80.

[15] McGregor MJ, Du Mont J, Myhr TL. Sexual assault forensic medical examination: is evidence related to successful prosecution? Ann Emerg Med 2002;39(6):639–47.

[16] Campbell R. Rape survivors' experiences with the legal and medical systems: do rape victim advocates make a difference? Violence Against Women 2006;12(1):30–45.

[17] Burgess AW, Fehder WP, Hartman CR. Delayed reporting of the rape victim. J Psychosoc Nurs Ment Health Serv 1995;33(9):21–9.

[18] Plumbo MA. Delayed reporting of sexual assault. Implications for counseling. J Nurse Midwifery 1995;40(5):424–7.

[19] Adamowicz P, Kala M. Date-rape drugs scene in Poland. Przegl Lek 2005;62(6):572–5 [in Polish].

[20] Goulle JP, Anger JP. Drug-facilitated robbery or sexual assault: problems associated with amnesia. Ther Drug Monit 2004;26(2):206–10.

[21] Scott-Ham M, Burton FC. Toxicological findings in cases of alleged drug-facilitated sexual assault in the United Kingdom over a 3-year period. J Clin Forensic Med 2005;12(4): 175–86.

[22] Rennison C. Rape and sexual assault: reporting to police and medical attention, 1992–2000. In: Rand MaG L, editor. Washington, DC: U.S. Department of Justice; 2002. p. 1–4.

[23] Cybulska B, Forster G. Sexual assault: examination of the victim. Medicine 2005;33(9): 23–8.

[24] Feldhaus KM, Houry D, Kaminsky R. Lifetime sexual assault prevalence rates and reporting practices in an emergency department population. Ann Emerg Med 2000;36(1):23–7.

[25] Anonymous. A National protocol for sexual assault medical forensic examinations: adults/adolescents. Office for violence against women. In: US Department of Justice; 2004. NCJ 206554.

[26] Kintz P, Villain M, Cirimele V. Hair analysis for drug detection. Ther Drug Monit 2006; 28(3):442–6.

[27] Cone EJ. Legal, workplace, and treatment drug testing with alternate biological matrices on a global scale. Forensic Sci Int 2001;121:7–15.

[28] Negrusz A, Gaensslen RE. Analytical developments in toxicological investigation of drug-facilitated sexual assault. Anal Bioanal Chem 2003;376(8):1192–7.

[29] Negrusz A, Moore CM, Kern JL, et al. Quantitation of clonazepam and its major metabolite 7-aminoclonazepam in hair. J Anal Toxicol 2000;24(7):614–20.

[30] Kintz P, Villain M, Ludes B. Testing for the undetectable in drug-facilitated sexual assault using hair analyzed by tandem mass spectrometry as evidence. Ther Drug Monit 2004; 26(2):211–4.

[31] Anonymous. Percent distribution of victimizations by perceived drug or alcohol use by offender. Table 32. Personal crimes of violence; 2004.

[32] Dyer J, Kim SY. Drug facilitated sexual assault: a review of 24 incidents [abstract]. J Toxicol Clin Toxicol 2004;42(4):519.

[33] Abbey A, Zawacki T, Buck PO, et al. How does alcohol contribute to sexual assault? Explanations from laboratory and survey data. Alcohol Clin Exp Res 2002;26(4): 575–81.

[34] Murdoch D, Pihl RO, Ross D. Alcohol and crimes of violence: present issues. Int J Addict 1990;25(9):1065–81.

[35] Ledray LE. The clinical care and documentation for victims of drug-facilitated sexual assault. J Emerg Nurs 2001;27(3):301–5.

[36] LeBeau M, Andollo W, Hearn WL, et al. Recommendations for toxicological investigations of drug-facilitated sexual assaults. J Forensic Sci 1999;44(1):227–30.

[37] Mohler-Kuo M, Dowdall GW, Koss MP, et al. Correlates of rape while intoxicated in a national sample of college women. J Stud Alcohol 2004;65(1):37–45.

[38] Cole TB. Rape at US colleges often fueled by alcohol. JAMA 2006;296(5):504–5.

[39] Holford NH. Clinical pharmacokinetics of ethanol. Clin Pharmacokinet 1987;13(5): 273–92.

[40] Smith GD, Shaw LJ, Maini PK, et al. Mathematical modeling of ethanol metabolism in normal subjects and chronic alcohol misusers. Alcohol Alcohol 1993;28(1):25–32.

[41] Taylor P. The time course of drug action. In: Pratt WB, editor. Principles of drug action. 3rd edition. Philadelphia: Churchill Livingstone; 1990. p. 297–364.

[42] Wasfi IA, Al-Awadhi AH, Al-Hatali ZN, et al. Rapid and sensitive static headspace gas chromatography-mass spectrometry method for the analysis of ethanol and abused inhalants in blood. J Chromatogr B Analyt Technol Biomed Life Sci 2004;799(2):331–6.

[43] Macchia T, Mancinelli R, Gentili S, et al. Ethanol in biological fluids: headspace GC measurement. J Anal Toxicol 1995;19(4):241–6.

[44] Rumack B, Toll L, Gelman C. Chloral hydrate. Micromedex healthcare series. vol. 129. Englewood (CO): Thomson Healthcare I, Micromedex Inc.; 2006.

[45] Breimer DD. Clinical pharmacokinetics of hypnotics. Clin Pharmacokinet 1977;2(2): 93–109.

[46] Ni YC, Wong TY, Lloyd RV, et al. Mouse liver microsomal metabolism of chloral hydrate, trichloroacetic acid, and trichloroethanol leading to induction of lipid peroxidation via a free radical mechanism. Drug Metab Dispos 1996;24(1):81–90.

[47] Miyaguchi H, Kuwayama K, Tsujikawa K, et al. A method for screening for various sedative-hypnotics in serum by liquid chromatography/single quadrupole mass spectrometry. Forensic Sci Int 2006;157(1):57–70.

[48] Schmitt TC. Determination of chloral hydrate and its metabolites in blood plasma by capillary gas chromatography with electron capture detection. J Chromatogr B Analyt Technol Biomed Life Sci 2002;780(2):217–24.

[49] Humbert L, Jacquemont MC, Leroy E, et al. Determination of chloral hydrate and its metabolites (trichloroethanol and trichloroacetic acid) in human plasma and urine using electron capture gas chromatography. Biomed Chromatogr 1994;8(6):273–7.

[50] Roset PN, Farre M, de la Torre R, et al. Modulation of rate of onset and intensity of drug effects reduces abuse potential in healthy males. Drug Alcohol Depend 2001;64(3): 285–98.

[51] Saum CA, Inciardi JA. Rohypnol misuse in the United States. Subst Use Misuse 1997;32(6): 723–31.

[52] Ohshima T. A case of drug-facilitated sexual assault by the use of flunitrazepam. J Clin Forensic Med 2006;13(1):44–5.

[53] Joynt BP. Triazolam blood concentrations in forensic cases in Canada. J Anal Toxicol 1993;17(3):171–7.

[54] Cheze M, Duffort G, Deveaux M, et al. Hair analysis by liquid chromatography-tandem mass spectrometry in toxicological investigation of drug-facilitated crimes: report of 128 cases over the period June 2003–May 2004 in metropolitan Paris. Forensic Sci Int 2005; 153(1):3–10.

[55] Waltzman ML. Flunitrazepam: a review of "roofies". Pediatr Emerg Care 1999;15(1): 59–60.

[56] Mattila MA, Larni HM. Flunitrazepam: a review of its pharmacological properties and therapeutic use. Drugs 1980;20(5):353–74.

[57] Chiu TH, Rosenberg HC. Comparison of the kinetics of [3H]diazepam and [3H]flunitraze-pam binding to cortical synaptosomal membranes. J Neurochem 1982;39(6):1716–25.

[58] Mattila MA, Saila K, Kokko T, et al. Comparison of diazepam and flunitrazepam as adjuncts to general anaesthesia in preventing arousal following surgical stimuli. Br J Anaesth 1979;51(4):329–37.

[59] Seppala T, Nuotto E, Dreyfus JF. Drug-alcohol interactions on psychomotor skills: zopiclone and flunitrazepam. Pharmacology 1983;27(Suppl 2):127–35.

[60] Drummer OH, Syrjanen ML, Cordner SM. Deaths involving the benzodiazepine flunitrazepam. Am J Forensic Med Pathol 1993;14(3):238–43.

[61] Kintz P, Villain M, Dumestre-Toulet V, et al. Drug-facilitated sexual assault and analytical toxicology: the role of LC-MS/MS A case involving zolpidem. J Clin Forensic Med 2005; 12(1):36–41.

[62] Mastrovitch TA, Bithoney WG, DeBari VA, et al. Point-of-care testing for drugs of abuse in an urban emergency department. Ann Clin Lab Sci 2002;32(4):383–6.

[63] Wu YH, Tan JY, Xia Y. [Determination of 7-aminoflunitrazepam, the major metabolite of flunitrazepam in urine by high performance thin-layer chromatography]. Se Pu 2002;20(2): 182–4 [in Chinese].

[64] elSohly MA, Feng S, Salamone SJ, et al. A sensitive GC-MS procedure for the analysis of flunitrazepam and its metabolites in urine. J Anal Toxicol 1997;21(5):335–40.

[65] Wang PH, Liu C, Tsay WI, et al. Improved screen and confirmation test of 7-aminoflunitrazepam in urine specimens for monitoring flunitrazepam (Rohypnol) exposure. J Anal Toxicol 2002;26(7):411–8.

[66] Wagner J, Wagner ML, Hening WA. Beyond benzodiazepines: alternative pharmacologic agents for the treatment of insomnia. Ann Pharmacother 1998;32(6):680–91.

[67] Sanna E, Busonero F, Talani G, et al. Comparison of the effects of zaleplon, zolpidem, and triazolam at various GABA(A) receptor subtypes. Eur J Pharmacol 2002;451(2):103–10.

[68] Anonymous. Product Information: Lunesta(TM), eszopiclone. Marlborough (MA): Sepracor; 2005.

[69] Anderson IB, Kim SY, Dyer JE, et al. Trends in gamma-hydroxybutyrate (GHB) and related drug intoxication: 1999 to 2003. Ann Emerg Med 2006;47(2):177–83.

[70] Goulle JP, Cheze M, Pepin G. Determination of endogenous levels of GHB in human hair. Are there possibilities for the identification of GHB administration through hair analysis in cases of drug-facilitated sexual assault? J Anal Toxicol 2003;27(8):574–80.

[71] Juhascik M, Le NL, Tomlinson K, et al. Development of an analytical approach to the specimens collected from victims of sexual assault. J Anal Toxicol 2004;28(6):400–6.

[72] Anonymous. Product Information: Ambien CR(TM), zolpidem tartrate extended-release tablets. New York: Sanofi-Synthelabo Inc.; 2005.

[73] Gock SB, Wong SH, Nuwayhid N, et al. Acute zolpidem overdose—report of two cases. J Anal Toxicol 1999;23(6):559–62.

[74] George CF. Pyrazolopyrimidines. Lancet 2001;358(9293):1623–6.

[75] Anonymous. Product Information: Lunesta(TM), eszopiclone tablets. Marlborough (MA): Sepracor Inc.; 2004.

[76] Elliott SP, Burgess V. Clinical urinalysis of drugs and alcohol in instances of suspected surreptitious administration ("spiked drinks"). Sci Justice 2005;45(3):129–34.

[77] Smith KM. Drugs used in acquaintance rape. J Am Pharm Assoc (Wash) 1999;39(4):519–25 [quiz: 581–3].

[78] Dorandeu AH, Pages CA, Sordino MC, et al. A case in south-eastern France: a review of drug facilitated sexual assault in European and English-speaking countries. J Clin Forensic Med 2006;13(5):253–61.

[79] Vayer P, Mandel P, Maitre M. Conversion of gamma-hydroxybutyrate to gamma-aminobutyrate in vitro. J Neurochem 1985;45(3):810–4.

[80] Maitre M. The gamma-hydroxybutyrate signalling system in brain: organization and functional implications. Prog Neurobiol 1997;51(3):337–61.

[81] Drasbek KR, Christensen J, Jensen K. Gamma-hydroxybutyrate—a drug of abuse. Acta Neurol Scand 2006;114(3):145–56.

[82] Koek W, Carter LP, Lamb RJ, et al. Discriminative stimulus effects of gamma-hydroxybutyrate (GHB) in rats discriminating GHB from baclofen and diazepam. J Pharmacol Exp Ther 2005;314(1):170–9.

[83] Kaupmann K, Cryan JF, Wellendorph P, et al. Specific gamma-hydroxybutyrate-binding sites but loss of pharmacological effects of gamma-hydroxybutyrate in GABA(B)(1)-deficient mice. Eur J Neurosci 2003;18(10):2722–30.

[84] Wu Y, Ali S, Ahmadian G, et al. Gamma-hydroxybutyric acid (GHB) and gamma-aminobutyric acidB receptor (GABABR) binding sites are distinctive from one another: molecular evidence. Neuropharmacology 2004;47(8):1146–56.

[85] Cook CD, Biddlestone L, Coop A, et al. Effects of combining ethanol (EtOH) with gamma-hydroxybutyrate (GHB) on the discriminative stimulus, locomotor, and motor-impairing functions of GHB in mice. Psychopharmacology (Berl) 2006;185(1):112–22.

[86] Marwick C. Coma-inducing drug GHB may be reclassified. JAMA 1997;277(19): 1505–6.

[87] Viera AJ, Yates SW. Toxic ingestion of gamma-hydroxybutyric acid. South Med J 1999; 92(4):404–5.

[88] McCusker RR, Paget-Wilkes H, Chronister CW, et al. Analysis of gamma-hydroxybutyrate (GHB) in urine by gas chromatography-mass spectrometry. J Anal Toxicol 1999; 23(5):301–5.

[89] Yeatman DT, Reid K. A study of urinary endogenous gamma-hydroxybutyrate (GHB) levels. J Anal Toxicol 2003;27(1):40–2.

[90] Green SM, Johnson NE. Ketamine sedation for pediatric procedures: Part 2, Review and implications. Ann Emerg Med 1990;19(9):1033–46.

[91] Hersack RA. Ketamine's psychological effects do not contraindicate its use based on a patient's occupation. Aviat Space Environ Med 1994;65(11):1041–6.

[92] Louon A, Lithander J, Reddy VG, et al. Sedation with nasal ketamine and midazolam for cryotherapy in retinopathy of prematurity. Br J Ophthalmol 1993;77(8):529–30.

[93] Clements JA, Nimmo WS, et al. Bioavailability, pharmacokinetics, and analgesic activity of ketamine in humans. J Pharm Sci 1982;71(5):539–42.

[94] Moore KA, Sklerov J, Levine B, et al. Urine concentrations of ketamine and norketamine following illegal consumption. J Anal Toxicol 2001;25(7):583–8.

[95] Anonymous. An overview of club drugs: drug intelligence brief. In: DEA; 2000. Available at: http://www.drugwatch.org/research/gbighb.htm.

[96] Macdonald RL, McLean MJ. Cellular bases of barbiturate and phenytoin anticonvulsant drug action. Epilepsia 1982;23(Suppl 1):S7–18.

[97] Hobbs WR, Rall TW, Verdoorn TA. Hypnotics and sedatives: ethanol. In: Harman JG, Limbird LE, editors. Goodman & Gilman's the pharmacological basis of therapeutics. 9th edition. New York: McGraw-Hill; 2002. p. 361–96.

[98] Frison G, Favretto D, Tedeschi L, et al. Detection of thiopental and pentobarbital in head and pubic hair in a case of drug-facilitated sexual assault. Forensic Sci Int 2003;133(1–2): 171–4.

[99] Schwenzer KS, Pearlman R, Tsilimidos M, et al. New fluorescence polarization immunoassays for analysis of barbiturates and benzodiazepines in serum and urine: performance characteristics. J Anal Toxicol 2000;24(8):726–32.

[100] Kupfer A, Schmid B, Pfaff G. Pharmacogenetics of dextromethorphan O-demethylation in man. Xenobiotica 1986;16(5):421–33.

[101] Motassim N, Decolin D, Le Dinh T, et al. Direct determination of dextromethorphan and its three metabolites in urine by high-performance liquid chromatography using a precolumn switching system for sample clean-up. J Chromatogr 1987;422:340–5.

[102] Palmer GC. Neuroprotection by NMDA receptor antagonists in a variety of neuropathologies. Curr Drug Targets 2001;2(3):241–71.

[103] Price DD, Mao J, Frenk H, et al. The N-methyl-D-aspartate receptor antagonist dextrome-thorphan selectively reduces temporal summation of second pain in man. Pain 1994;59(2): 165–74.

[104] Hughes AM, Rhodes J, Fisher G, et al. Assessment of the effect of dextromethorphan and ketamine on the acute nociceptive threshold and wind-up of the second pain response in healthy male volunteers. Br J Clin Pharmacol 2002;53(6):604–12.

[105] Ilkjaer S, Bach LF, Nielsen PA, et al. Effect of preoperative oral dextromethorphan on im-mediate and late postoperative pain and hyperalgesia after total abdominal hysterectomy. Pain 2000;86(1–2):19–24.

[106] Sindrup SH, Jensen TS. Pharmacologic treatment of pain in polyneuropathy. Neurology 2000;55(7):915–20.

[107] Schwartz RH. Adolescent abuse of dextromethorphan. Clin Pediatr (Phila) 2005;44(7): 565–8.

[108] Hanzlick R. National Association of Medical Examiners Pediatric Toxicology (PedTox) Registry Report 3. Case submission summary and data for acetaminophen, benzene, car-boxyhemoglobin, dextromethorphan, ethanol, phenobarbital, and pseudoephedrine. Am J Forensic Med Pathol 1995;16(4):270–7.

[109] Carlsson KC, Hoem NO, Moberg ER, et al. Analgesic effect of dextromethorphan in neu-ropathic pain. Acta Anaesthesiol Scand 2004;48(3):328–36.

[110] Navarro A, Perry C, Bobo WV. A case of serotonin syndrome precipitated by abuse of the anticough remedy dextromethorphan in a bipolar patient treated with fluoxetine and lith-ium. Gen Hosp Psychiatry 2006;28(1):78–80.

[111] Li L, Pan RM, Porter TD, et al. New cytochrome P450 2D6*56 allele identified by geno-type/phenotype analysis of cryopreserved human hepatocytes. Drug Metab Dispos 2006; 34(8):1411–6.

[112] Chen SQ, Cai WM, Wedlund PJ. [Distinguishing CYP2D6 homozygous and heterozygous extensive metabolizers by dextromethorphan phenotyping]. Yao Xue Xue Bao 1997;32(12): 924–7.

[113] Manaboriboon B, Chomchai C. Dextromethorphan abuse in Thai adolescents: a report of two cases and review of literature. J Med Assoc Thai 2005;88(Suppl 8):S242–5.

[114] Anonymous. Recommended maximum detection limits for common DFSA drugs and me-tabolites in urine samples. Mesa (AZ): Drug Facilitated Sexual Assault Committee - Society of Forensic Toxicologists; 2005. p. 1–4.

[115] Tomassoni AJ, Weisman RS. Antihistamines and decongestants. In: Flomenbaum NE, Goldfrank LR, Hoffman RS, et al, editors. Goldfrank's toxicologic emergencies. 8th edi-tion. New York: McGraw-Hill; 2005. p. 785–93.

[116] Albert KS, Hallmark MR, Sakmar E, et al. Pharmacokinetics of diphenhydramine in man. J Pharmacokinet Biopharm 1975;3(3):159–70.

[117] Sharma AN, Hexdall AH, Chang EK, et al. Diphenhydramine-induced wide complex dys-rhythmia responds to treatment with sodium bicarbonate. Am J Emerg Med 2003;21(3): 212–5.

[118] Hasegawa C, Kumazawa T, Lee XP, et al. Simultaneous determination of ten antihistamine drugs in human plasma using pipette tip solid-phase extraction and gas chromatography/ mass spectrometry. Rapid Commun Mass Spectrom 2006;20(4):537–43.

ELSEVIER
SAUNDERS

Emerg Med Clin N Am 25 (2007) 527–548

EMERGENCY
MEDICINE
CLINICS OF
NORTH AMERICA

Bringing Order Out of Chaos: Effective Strategies for Medical Response to Mass Chemical Exposure

Mark A. Kirk, MD[a],*, Michael L. Deaton, PhD[b]

[a]Blue Ridge Poison Center, Division of Medical Toxicology, Department of Emergency
Medicine, University of Virginia, P.O. Box 800744, Charlottesville, VA 22908-0774, USA
[b]Integrated Science and Technology, MSC 4102, James Madison University,
Harrisonburg, VA 22807, USA

An accident releasing hazardous chemicals or a deliberate chemical terrorism attack will create chaos and confusion that complicates the emergency response. Time is of the essence when administering treatment to the victims of hazardous chemical emergencies. Clinicians are challenged to urgently treat patients needing care, even before a chemical is confirmed.

Every day in the emergency department (ED), physicians routinely diagnose and simultaneously treat life-threatening conditions based on the best information available at the moment. Most often, basic clinical information such as physical findings and a few rapid point-of-care diagnostic tests provide sufficient information to empirically treat a critically ill patient. As time passes, the patient's condition is more clearly defined because additional information becomes available. Hazardous chemical emergencies, especially those caused by highly toxic chemical threat agents[1], such as nerve agents and cyanide, must be handled in the same way if health care providers are to save lives from the potent toxic effects. Hence, in the face of a chemical attack or accident, the medical response must be quick to recognize specific conditions that need urgent medical interventions.

---

* Corresponding author.
E-mail address: mak4z@virginia.edu (M.A. Kirk).

[1] Chemical threat agents are toxic chemicals that could be used in a terrorist attack against civilians, or chemicals that could be released at toxic levels by accident or natural disaster. This is a term used by federal and Department of Defense agencies such as United States Army Medical Institute of Chemical Defense (USAMICD), Center for Disease Control (CDC), National Institute of Health (NIH), and Department of Homeland Security (DHS).

0733-8627/07/$ - see front matter © 2007 Published by Elsevier Inc.
doi:10.1016/j.emc.2007.02.005

emed.theclinics.com

Coupling basic toxicology concepts to a thorough understanding of the nature of hazardous chemical accidents can provide a framework for an effective emergency response strategy.

The chaos and confusion: anticipating the "most likely" challenges

The consequences of hazardous chemical accidents and chemical terrorism attacks are chaos, confusion, and seeming unpredictability [1–6]. How can those responding to the scene or awaiting the arrival of victims at the hospital gain a sense of control? Everyone involved can hope it will not happen in their locale, and hope, if it does, that the "all-hazards" plan will suffice.

Being proactive by anticipating the "most likely" challenges, and preparing for them may provide some sense of control. However, each incident is unique and it is impossible to be prepared for every challenge that may arise during the response. Nonetheless, common themes become evident when incidents are evaluated using evidence-based disaster planning [7]. By analyzing past events, challenges can be identified that are likely to occur in any emergency response. Therefore, one of the first steps toward preparedness requires learning from the past to attempt to answer two questions: (1) what are the most common challenges likely to occur? and (2) how are people likely to behave during these events?

Despite the observations from evidence-based disaster research and reports of recurring challenges during incidents, the literature shows that many lessons are "learned" over and over [7–9]. In addition, an often-overlooked factor in planning is anticipating and managing the behaviors of large groups of victims, first responders, care providers, and the community as a whole [10]. Managing large groups of people after an incident requires anticipating their likely behaviors during a crisis and designing response plans that are robust in the face of such behavior. Auf der Heide [8] suggests, "Plan for what people are *likely* to do, not what they *should* do."

All large-scale disasters have predictable and recurring patterns [7–9]. In addition to common patterns, hazardous chemical events have unique predictable and recurring patterns that are independent of their cause (accident or deliberate attack) or scale (# casualties, size of region affected).

The inability of the medical system to adequately prepare for these recurring patterns is at least partially due to several commonly accepted misconceptions or myths about what will happen in the presence of a toxic chemical release. These myths are listed in Box 1.

These myths represent what emergency planners *hope* would happen in such events. These myths also represent underlying assumptions that shape how communities prepare for toxic chemical releases. Unfortunately, the reality is much different. As a consequence, emergency planning that is based on these assumptions can be woefully inadequate. To illustrate, four case studies are presented.

Box 1. Common myths about chemical disasters

Myth 1. Hospitals will be notified in advance of arrival of chemically exposed patients.

Myth 2. The offending toxin will be rapidly identified so that on-scene and emergency department care providers will give specific and appropriate treatment.

Myth 3. Dispatchers will send emergency response units to the scene so that trained personnel will triage, treat, and decontaminate victims.

Myth 4. Casualties will be transported by ambulance and they will first transport the most serious patients already decontaminated.

Four case studies

South Carolina train derailment

At 2:40 AM on January 6, 2005, a Norfolk Southern freight train wrecked in Graniteville, South Carolina. The train contained 42 cars including tankers filled with chlorine. The chlorine escaped and created a large toxic cloud that covered a large populated area including a textile mill with 500 night shift workers inside. The consequences of the event: 9 deaths, 529 sought medical care, 18 were treated at area physicians' offices, and 5400 were forced to evacuate in a 1-mile radius of the crash [11]. The Regional Poison Center was initially contacted by a person living near the crash site. She smelled a chemical odor and complained of burning eyes. The poison center promptly called the local ED and found on duty a single emergency physician, who was already overwhelmed with 1 critically ill patient, 6 patients who had pulmonary edema, and 100 patients in the waiting room [2]. The public safety officer at the accident scene notified the ED and suggested that the accident involved a release of sodium nitrate. The poison center researched sodium nitrate's expected health effects from poisoning and found that patients did not exhibit those symptoms. Fifteen minutes later, the chemical was thought to be methanol. Finally, over 1 hour later, the chemical was confirmed to be chlorine. By then the poison center already gave the ED physician human health effects information and treatment recommendations based on the victims' reported clinical presentations.

Tokyo sarin gas attack

On March 20, 1995, at 7:55 AM, terrorists released the nerve agent sarin into the Tokyo subway system [5,12–16]. People became immediately ill and many people rushed from the train cars and subway platforms to the streets. Published accounts of this incident demonstrate a gap between clinicians rendering care and accurate information needed to guide their decisions [5,12,13]. On-scene emergency responders reported to hospitals that an explosion occurred in the subway and they should prepare for victims who have smoke inhalation and carbon monoxide poisoning. The closest hospital, St. Luke's International Hospital, received 500 patients during the first hour of the event. Only 23% of the patients arrived by ambulances while most arrived by walking, taxi, or private vehicle. The first patient arrived by foot and was the hospital's best information source at that time. A delay in identifying the substance and lack of effective communication left hospital staff "blind" until 3 hours after the incident began. Health care providers treated patients without the benefit of knowing the causative agent. They relied on their clinical observations and the scanty and inaccurate information from the scene. Because sarin was not suspected, patients were brought into waiting rooms and other parts of the hospital for treatment without any attention to decontamination. At 11:30 AM, hospitals received word that the victims were exposed to the nerve agent, sarin, a military chemical weapon. They received the information by way of television news broadcast [13]. In the final analysis, approximately 1200 people had signs and symptoms suggestive of at least mild nerve agent poisoning, and 12 died. However, approximately 5500 people sought medical care [4,6]. Also, reports suggest 135 (10%) prehospital providers and 110 (23%) hospital staff developed symptoms of nerve agent poisoning [12,13].

Indianapolis, Indiana industrial accident

In Indianapolis in 1995, the fire department evacuated nearby neighborhoods after realizing that a burning building contained cyanide. Even though air monitoring found no evidence of cyanide, 80 employees at a distant warehouse began to complain of chest tightness, nausea, and dizziness. Patients were transported to the hospital and two patients were treated using the cyanide antidote kit. One patient required ICU admission, not from cyanide toxicity, but from the administered antidote's (sodium nitrite) resulting hypotension and ischemic electrocardiogram changes [4].

Desert storm SCUD attacks

In 1991, during the United States–led Desert Storm operation, 39 Iraqi SCUD missiles landed in Israel [17,18]. These attacks caused over 1000 casualties. One half of the casualties were diagnosed with acute psychologic reactions or acute anxiety. Because it was unknown if chemical weapons were part of the missiles' payload, it appeared that people anticipated toxic chemicals and without verification began to treat themselves. One fourth of the casualties were due to inappropriate autoinjection of atropine because of fear that a chemical nerve agent attack had occurred. Another 40 patients were injured while rushing to a sealed room to avoid chemical exposure. At least 11 deaths were attributed to the missile attacks, although only 2 were from missile trauma. Seven patients (including 1 child) reportedly suffocated from improper use of gas masks, and 4 died of myocardial infarctions.

What really happens in a chemical event?

When a large-scale chemical event happens, the reality is different than the ideal described in Box 1. The authors describe five "*myth-buster*" realities that give a more realistic picture of how a community (people + emergency resources) is likely to respond to a chemical event. These five realities are summarized in Box 2 and further described in this section.

The inevitable consequence of these realities is that the medical response surge capacity can be quickly overwhelmed when faced with a large-scale chemical event [1–6]. This can lead to numerous problems that can significantly erode the effectiveness of the medical response, including (1) failure to treat the most seriously injured patients, (2) mistaken diagnoses, (3) medication errors, and (4) misdirected or squandered medical response resources.

Reality 1: medical personnel are often left in the dark

During the early stages of many chemical events, medical personnel may find themselves operating "in the blind" with little or no understanding about the nature of the crisis they are facing. We refer to this initial period of uncertainty as the *silent gap* because clinicians are left to make critical decisions with little useful input about the nature of the event from

---

Box 2. What really happens in a chemical event?

Reality 1. Medical personnel must often "operate in the blind" during the early stages of an event.

Reality 2. The offending chemical may not be identified for hours, or even days.

Reality 3. Emergency response personnel seldom have adequate tools or resources to effectively triage, decontaminate, and treat the large numbers of victims of a large-scale chemical exposure.

Reality 4. The first victims arriving at the hospital often arrive under their own power without direct involvement from emergency response personnel on the scene.

Reality 5. The general public can behave in ways that significantly erode the effectiveness of the emergency medical response.

knowledgeable informed sources that are "on the scene" or receive guidance about clinical findings and treatment from clinical experts.

During the silent gap, confirmatory diagnostic test results are unavailable. At this point, clinicians seldom even know what tests to run. Rumors fly as fearful or panic-stricken bystanders and real exposure victims arrive at the hospital with their own (often confused) reports about what has happened or how they feel [10]. During this stage, missing or misleading information about the alleged chemical is common, possibly leading to unnecessary or even inappropriate and harmful therapies. Hospital staff can themselves suffer injury if they fail to use adequate personal protection (as was the case in the Tokyo sarin incident whereby several hospital staff experienced symptoms of nerve agent poisoning through inappropriate handling of victims) [13]. Medical personnel on the scene and at the hospital need clinical guidance from experts. Without such guidance, they are left to improvise, and critical health care resources are misdirected, wasted, or even incapacitated.

Reality 2: the offending chemical may not be identified for hours, or even days

Based on literature published on the case of the Tokyo sarin gas attack, it was over 3 hours before the hospital personnel knew what chemical agent was involved, and this knowledge came from watching the national television news! [13]. After the Graniteville, South Carolina train derailment, the correct identification of the chemical agent came over 1 hour after the event and after several hundred patients had already arrived at the nearest hospital [2].

In the absence of such information, hospital personnel are left to rely upon whatever information they can get from patients (many of whom are merely stunned and bewildered or suffering from acute anxiety), rumor, news reports, and so forth. Such information can be extensive and contradictive.

Reality 3: emergency response personnel seldom have adequate tools or resources to effectively triage, decontaminate, and treat the large numbers of victims of chemical exposure

Many chemical agents commonly produced, transported, or used in the United States are toxic enough to rapidly produce life-threatening conditions. Because the offending agent is often unknown at the beginning, the first responders would need to have ready access to expert guidance to adequately triage, decontaminate, and treat victims at the scene of the event. Unfortunately, responders are often unaware of valuable and readily available information resources, or those resources may not be immediately available because of inadequate development of emergency communication networks [13,19].

It is well understood that the training of medical personnel for response to chemical events should be based on community-specific risk analysis that takes into account the chemicals posing the greatest risk in the community, as well as the potential high-impact scenarios involving those chemicals [20,21]. Unfortunately, most current training and preparation is poorly targeted to community-specific risks [22]. Because this training and preparedness is too generic, specific knowledge, information resources, equipment, and therapeutics may not be available in supplies sufficient to deal with the most likely scenarios.

Reality 4: the first victims arriving at the hospital often arrive under their own power without direct involvement from emergency response personnel on the scene

Following the release of methyl isocyanate in Bhopal, India, an estimated 200,000 people sought medical care [1]. After the sarin attack in the Tokyo subway, 5500 people arrived at nearby health care facilities for medical care [13]. The train derailment releasing chlorine gas in Graniteville, South Carolina caused the evacuation of 5400 people and 529 to seek medical care [2]. In all these cases, many of the first victims to arrive at the hospital come under their own power. Many of these individuals are upset and their fears fuel their sense that they have been somehow affected by an unknown and highly toxic agent. The information they provide to hospital staff can be confusing, contradictory, and misleading.

Reality 5: the general public can behave in ways that significantly erode the effectiveness of the emergency medical response

Abundant examples are found in the literature that demonstrate how a mass chemical exposure will prompt large numbers of people to seek medical care [1–6,23–26]. The greatest numbers of patients seeking care are often those who have or do not have symptoms that perceive they have been poisoned, but do not exhibit obvious signs or symptoms of poisoning. Although many patients experience symptoms based solely on fear or anxiety, some may have an illness that will result in adverse outcomes if not quickly diagnosed and treated. When this occurs during the silent gap (and it almost always does), the ability of the medical system to effectively triage and identify the most critically ill patients is jeopardized. All four of the incidents described earlier illustrate this phenomenon.

Events that subject people to a chemical exposure can be frightening. Many people fear that toxic chemical exposure will inevitably lead to long-lasting ill effects, like an internal chemical time bomb waiting to cause harm years later [12,16,27–30]. In the presence of a reported chemical release, this fear can cause many people to rapidly develop symptoms that do not have an organic etiology. This phenomenon has been called "mass hysteria," "mass sociogenic illness," and "mass psychogenic illness."

Hysteria and other terms deliver a negative connotation to patients. Some prefer "outbreaks of multiple unexplained symptoms" because of these negative connotations [31]. Anxiety is almost always present, but actual hysteria is not a common feature of these events [32]. The physical symptoms reported in these outbreaks are likely manifestations of distress. Affected persons mistake their distress as chemical exposure, which likely contributes to their anxiety and exacerbates symptoms [33].

The trigger is generally a presumption of an exposure to a chemical, and often an unusual odor believed to be associated with a highly toxic chemical induces symptoms [3,26,31,34–36]. Sometimes the inciting event involves exposure to an actual chemical or poisonous substance. At other times, the mere rumor of an exposure can induce symptoms. During an actual release, there will be victims of direct toxicity as well as those that suffer from symptoms that cannot be explained by the exposure [26,37,38]. In fact, some suggest that, after a terrorist incident, the number of individuals who have *not* experienced physical harm but still perceive that they have been exposed may be many times greater than those who are suffering the toxic effects of real exposure [12,13,26,39,40].

Which chemicals should we prepare for?

Common sources of chemical events

To be better prepared, emergency planners must focus on getting the right information into the right hands at the right time. One of the most critical pieces of information is the identity or nature of the offending chemical agent. Access to this information by medical personnel and on-site first responders would dramatically reduce the chaos and its consequences during the early stages of an event. This would give clinicians increased confidence in their therapeutic and disposition decisions.

Given the large numbers of toxic chemicals, this can seem like a daunting task. Before September 11, 2001, training and planning for anticipated deliberate toxic chemical attacks mainly concentrated on chemicals designed specifically as military weapons such as nerve agents, sulfur mustard, and phosgene. Until recently, not much attention was paid to the over 80,000 potentially toxic substances produced, stored, and moved for manufacturing, agriculture, and service industries throughout the United States. Any of these could be released accidentally or deliberately, putting many people in danger.

Because of their availability and toxicity, these chemicals in our communities are increasingly referred to as "weapons of opportunity"[41]. Upon release, many of these highly toxic chemicals are readily airborne, leading to inhalation exposure and toxic effects [20].

These chemicals are likely candidates for accidents and for hostile action by terrorists. CBS's *60 Minutes* aired a segment demonstrating the ease of entering an industrial facility to gain access to large quantities of toxic industrial chemicals [42]. Additionally, a report published by the Government Accounting Office stated that: "...industrial chemicals can cause mass casualties and require little if any expertise or sophisticated methods...can be bought on the commercial market or stolen, thus avoiding the need to manufacture them" [43].

It is unrealistic for first responders or emergency personnel to know these substances in enough detail to make confident decisions during the early phases of a crisis. This approach is not realistic and leads to training that is too generic to be of practical use during an event [22].

On the other hand, it is realistic to train medical personnel for response to chemical events based on community-specific risk analysis that takes into account the chemicals posing the greatest risks in the community, as well as the potential high-impact scenarios involving those chemicals [21,22]. In addition, first responders and medical personnel can learn to rapidly identify potential chemical classes based on toxic syndromes.

Applying basic principles of toxicology for clinical decision-making during mass chemical exposure

The four incidents described earlier make it clear that clinical decision making during an emergency response to a hazardous chemical accident or chemical terrorist attack can be complex and highly uncertain. To do the best for the most, clinicians need a system that rapidly identifies toxicity and guides early medical decisions and antidote therapy. Applying basic principles of toxicology can simplify decision making during mass exposures to toxic chemical events. Identifying toxic syndromes at the bedside and using the dose–response concept to assess toxic chemical exposure can be helpful.

Toxicology principle 1: using toxic syndrome recognition for rapid diagnosis and empiric therapy

Tens of thousands of chemicals are harmful to humans, and knowing the specific toxic effects of even a large portion of the possible chemical agents would be an impossible task. Toxic chemicals can often be grouped into classes, whereby all the chemicals in a given class cause similar human health effects. These constellations of toxic effects or *toxic syndromes* comprise a set of clinical "fingerprints" for groups of toxins [44–47]. Moreover, all the toxins associated with a given toxic syndrome are treated similarly. Hence, during the early phases of a toxic chemical emergency, when the exact chemical is often unknown, identification of the toxic syndromes that are present can be a useful decision-making tool that can overcome many of the problems associated with the silent gap. For example, narcotic overdoses that arise from substance abuse, accidental overmedication, or accidental ingestion of prescription medications cause a predictable constellation of clinical findings (pinpoint pupils, coma, and respiratory depression) that are well known and readily identified by all health care providers in the emergency medical system (first responders, paramedics, medical and nursing students, nurses, and physicians) [48]. The identification of this constellation of signs and symptoms is all that is needed to diagnose narcotic overdose. This immediately alerts the health care provider to a treatable life-threatening condition (eg, respiratory arrest). Once identified, any health care provider at the scene or in the hospital will take action by administering naloxone, the specific antidote for all narcotic overdoses. At this stage of treatment, it does not matter if the offending agent is morphine, heroin, oxycodone, or any other narcotic. The clinical condition is the same, the initial treatment is the same, and the anticipated complications are similar. Once the life-threatening crisis has been averted and time passes, more specific information from the history or diagnostic test results will guide additional therapeutic decisions and patient disposition.

Toxic syndromes are easily identified with only a few observations, such as:

- Vital signs
- Mental status
- Pupil size
- Mucous membrane irritation
- Lung exam for wheezes or rales
- Skin for burns, moisture, and color

Toxic syndrome recognition is important because it provides a tool for rapid detection of the suspected cause and can focus the differential diagnosis to consideration of only a few chemicals with similar toxic effects. Table 1 [49,50] lists readily recognized toxic syndromes that are likely to be observed in mass chemical exposures. By focusing on certain chemicals, specific diagnostic testing and empiric therapies can be rendered based on objective clinical evidence. Specifically during a mass exposure, recognition can provide a triage tool for identifying exhibiting toxic effects and also provide a common "language" so that emergency responders from the scene through to the hospital ED can clearly communicate a clinical message.

With the extraordinary number of chemicals in use, this tool does not apply to every chemical but to most of the commonly encountered chemicals reported in HazMat incidents. Other toxic effects caused by chemicals include hematologic injury such as methemoglobinemia or hemolysis, liver and kidney injury, and peripheral neuropathies. These less-common toxic effects may require the assistance of a medical toxicologist to guide work-up and medical management.

The use of toxic syndromes as a diagnostic tool is fundamental to an effective medical response. However, the degree to which the toxic symptoms present themselves depends on both the route of exposure and the dose.

Table 1
Common toxic syndromes observed in mass chemical exposures

Toxic syndrome	Common signs and symptoms	Examples
Irritant gas syndrome	Eye, nose, and throat irritation, cough, wheezes, shortness of breath, chest pain Caution: may have a delayed presentation	Ammonia, chlorine delayed presentation seen with phosgene and nitrogen dioxide
Chemical burns	Painful burning skin, mucous membrane irritation, systemic effects	Hydrochloric acid, hydrofluoric acid, hydrocarbon solvents such as degreasors and defatters
Organophosphate Insecticide poisoning (Cholinergic storm)	Pinpoint pupils, eye pain, shortness of breath, wheezes, rales, sweating skin, drooling, tearing, vomiting, diarrhea, fasciculations, coma, seizures	Organophosphate and carbamate insecticides, nerve agents
Acute solvent exposure	Headache, lightheadedness, nausea, mucous membrane irritation, confusion, syncope	Paint thinners, degreasors and lubricants, toluene, methylene chloride, trichloroethylene,
"Knock-down" or metabolic poisoning	Rapid loss of consciousness, seizures, hypotension, cardiac arrest	Cyanide, hydrogen sulfide, phosphine
Behavioral response to the fear of chemical exposure "The fear factor"	Lightheadedness, shortness of breath, chest pain, faint, nausea, sweating skin, palpitations, tremor	Often "fight or flight" stress response from fear. CAUTION: low level exposure to toxins can resemble this response

The toxic syndromes listed in this table are derived from expected clinical effects after exposure to those chemicals most often reported to be involved in accidental spills, those with likelihood of causing significant health impact upon release, and those with emergent treatments available (eg, cyanide and nerve agent poisoning) [20,49,50,58].

Toxicology principle 2: route of exposure is a determinant of toxicity

A chemical's physical state and the route of exposure influence toxicity [51]. The chemical's state often determines the route of exposure. Gases, vapors, airborne powders, and aerosolized liquids are inhalation risks. For many chemicals, the toxic effects occur at the site of absorption. For example, irritant gases attack the water in the respiratory mucosa and eye, causing burning pain, irritation, and copious secretions at the site of contact. Inhalation exposure also allows some rapid entry into the systemic circulation, causing toxic effects distant from the entry route. Hydrogen cyanide is a gas that rapidly enters the circulation through the lung and causes loss of consciousness, seizures, cardiac dysrhythmias, hypotension, and possible death in a matter of minutes after the exposure.

Chemicals in contact with the skin can cause local effect but may also enter the systemic circulation and cause effects at distant sites from the entry route. Organophosphate insecticides are fat-soluble chemicals that rapidly penetrate the skin and enter the blood stream to circulate to distant sites. Skin exposure can delay onset of systemic effects as compared with the rapid entry through the lung.

Toxicology principle 3: the dose makes the poison

Paracelsus, a 15th century scientist, made this claim: "What is it that is not poison? All things are poison and nothing is without poison. The right dose differentiates a poison from a remedy" [51]. Evaluating clinical effects based on the amount of exposure is a basic toxicology principle called dose–response [51]. The dose is the total amount of chemical absorbed during an exposure. It depends on the concentration of the chemical *and* duration (contact time) of the exposure. Chemicals cause predictable toxic effects based on the dose. Ethanol is a good example. Incremental increases in blood ethanol levels result in predictable increases in alteration of consciousness (signs of inebriation), poor coordination, and eventually coma/respiratory depression, and finally death [52].

One important factor affecting the dose is the duration of the exposure. High concentrations over a long duration are more likely to produce adverse health effects than the same or lower concentration over a shorter exposure period. An acid placed on the skin will cause more tissue destruction the longer it stays in contact with the tissues. If the acid is immediately washed off the skin, injury is limited [53]. The same is true for inhaled chemicals. The longer a victim is allowed to breathe toxic chemicals, the greater the dose of exposure.

Applying these dose–response principles can guide patient assessment to toxic chemical exposures. Patients who have higher concentrations and longer durations of exposure result in greater doses to the victim and will more likely have harmful effects. Those receiving larger doses need more urgent attention and possibly life-saving interventions than those receiving smaller doses (especially if asymptomatic).

The dose determines the poison during triage. Determining if a patient had direct contact (eg, splash or skin contact) and the relative distance from areas with the highest concentrations (eg, near the source of a leak or spill) can guide triage decisions, just like principles of radiation dose delivery (ie, time, shielding, distance) apply to many mass chemical events [54]. Obtaining history about the time a patient was in a toxic environment and the distance from the areas of greatest concentration can help to stratify patients into high-risk and low-risk groups. This approach is similar to using an account of the mechanism of injury to anticipate injuries even before the clinician touches the trauma patient. Understanding the different mechanisms of trauma (eg, speed of the vehicle, presence of fatalities in the same accident, or height of a fall) and the predictable pattern of injuries that may result will influence the patient's evaluation and affect care. This approach is not an absolute solution for poisonings but is potentially valuable for mass chemical exposures whereby triaging patients is critical to quickly find those most at risk for serious illness.

In addition to triage, the same principles can guide treatment strategies for hazardous chemical exposures. The most basic treatment objective is to limit exposure time and decrease concentration as rapidly as possible. Moving rapidly away from a vapor cloud in an accidental release is common sense and illustrates the point of decreasing concentration and duration of exposure. Similarly, deluging with water after splashing a concentrated sulfuric acid on the skin will decrease the chemical's concentration and the duration of exposure [53].

Doing the best for the most: a strategy for putting it all together

A community could devise an effective response strategy if it focused on: (1) planning for expected challenges to the emergency response and health care systems, (2) identifying the greatest chemical risks that could cause harm if accidentally or deliberately released, and (3) using critical decision pathways during the emergency response that apply basic toxicologic principles. Such a strategy should place a high priority on:

- Rapidly recognizing situations and clinical presentations suggesting a hazardous chemical accident or chemical terrorism attack is in play
- Taking actions to close the silent gap
  - Creating a community-specific risk assessment to determine the most likely chemicals to be involved in an accident
  - Use a tiered response strategy
  - Creating a communications network to effectively manage information
- Providing medical care that will do the best for the most victims of the incident

Rapidly recognizing situations and clinical presentations suggesting a hazardous chemical accident or chemical terrorism attack is in play

Much emphasis is placed on proper personal protective equipment and specific steps in the decontamination procedure [21,55,56]. Although these principles are important, *the single most important step toward protection and excellent patient care is to recognize suspicious situations and clinical presentations that are likely to be related to chemical exposure. This recognition will lead to ACTION!* Plans cannot be activated nor any actions taken unless a high-risk situation is recognized. After the sarin attack in the Tokyo subway, the first patient to arrive walked into the ED soon followed by over 500 additional patients [5]. For the first few hours, the staff did not recognize that the situation could be from a toxic chemical exposure and did not recognize the specific toxic syndrome caused by nerve agents [13]. Because they were unaware, patients were escorted into the hospital fully clothed.

Chemical contamination and toxic effects may often go unrecognized because health care providers are distracted during early stages of an incident by multiple victims who have traumatic injuries, sudden unconsciousness, or unexplained cardiac arrest, and by the large number of patients seeking care. Therefore, prehospital and ED personnel must be alert for high-risk situations. Triage personnel, in particular, should be trained to recognize high-risk situations that could send chemically contaminated patients to the ED. Nearly all ED evacuations/closures have been related to lack of early recognition and high levels of concern about the potential for secondary contamination, and not the lack of a written protocol or dedicated decontamination equipment [57].

Examples of situations that should raise the suspicion of a chemical exposure:

- Victims exhibiting signs and symptoms of specific toxic syndromes
- Industrial accidents, fires, or explosions
- Transportation accidents
- Agricultural accidents
- Clandestine drug laboratory accidents
- Sudden onset of illness in large groups of people from crowed areas (especially government, political, or religious places)
- Victims noticing chemical odor or vapor cloud

Recognizing a toxic syndrome serves as a detection tool or early alert system for recognizing a potential hazardous chemical exposure. Recognizing these syndromes should lead staff to take protective actions. Physicians assisting victims in the Tokyo sarin subway attack stated: "We suspected the cause of the victims' illness was some form of organophosphate agent exposure. We were puzzled as to why it had happened in the subway" [13]. They recognized the syndrome and empiric treatment followed.

Taking actions to close the silent gap: create a community-specific risk assessment to determine the most likely chemicals to be involved in an accident

Lessons from the past demonstrate the silent gap exists in most incidents involving hazardous chemicals. Specific preparedness activities and a structured response strategy can decrease this period of uncertainty about causative agents and give the clinician objective data to assist in critical clinical decisions, thus closing the silent gap.

Because a virtually limitless list of potentially devastating "weapons of opportunity" are available for use in a terrorist attack or are at risk of being accidentally released, an overwhelming body of knowledge is required for health care providers to master and use in this chaotic decision-making environment. Moreover, because events involving such agents are not an everyday occurrence in any given community, the benefits of training can rapidly decay through lack of use. Instead, a realistic strategy should focus on chemicals used, manufactured, or stored in the local community. Specific industrial activities are more prone to errors and chemical accidents. Burgess found that agricultural manufacturing; petroleum refining; industrial chemical manufacturing; electric, light, and power production; and paper mills had the highest number of hazardous chemical events [58]. Data like these should alert community planners to the industries (and their commonly used or manufactured chemicals) as the most sources of chemical accidents. Transportation accidents add a level of complexity to planning because of the vast array of chemicals that flow through a community by highway, rail, or waterway. Compared with other transportation accidents, railroad accidents are specifically prone to impact public health, and certain chemicals are readily identifiable that are carried in mass quantities by railand have a significant risk to public health if released in an accident [59].

Throughout history, inhalation of toxic gases has subjected the greatest number of people to harm [1,60,61]. Chemicals with specific characteristics are more likely to affect large numbers of people if released in an accident or used as chemical weapons of opportunity [20]. First, the chemical must have inherent toxicity. Next, it must readily become airborne allowing movement away from the point of origin. Finally, it must be available in quantities large enough to deliver dangerous concentrations to nearby large populations. Therefore, the highest priority planning must focus on those chemicals in each community with these characteristics. Knowing the high-risk chemicals in a community can direct emergency response planning and training efforts by providing advance knowledge of their unique characteristics, clinical effects, and therapies. Knowledge and preparation can shorten the silent gap.

Taking actions to close the silent gap: use a tiered response strategy

A crucial therapeutic goal of an emergency response to mass chemical exposure is the timely administration of appropriate life-saving treatments to patients most needing them. This goal is realistic if a response strategy is built around rapid detection of toxic syndromes. During mass exposures, it is not easy to distinguish patients most urgently needing care from the large number of patients that are likely to actually seek care. Delaying treatment of patients needing immediate care will result in increased morbidity and mortality.

Identifying toxic syndromes is an approach that will help bridge the silent gap by helping providers focus on the most critical empiric observations. This strategy eliminates the need for mastery of detailed information about a multitude of chemicals while still guiding rapid and appropriate actions that may make a difference in patients' outcomes.

Using toxic syndrome recognition as the foundation, a tiered community response strategy can be built. The elements in the strategy are:

1) Initial patient assessment: using toxic syndromes as a diagnostic frame-work, medical personnel identify the toxic syndrome(s) present in the victims.
2) Staff protection: based on the toxic syndrome(s) identified, medical personnel (prehospital care providers and hospital staff) refer to "just in time" training to guide efforts at personal protection and decontamination of staff and victims.
3) Empiric treatment and antidote administration: the knowledge of the toxic syndrome immediately identifies the most appropriate treatment options including time urgent and life-saving antidotes (eg, Mark 1 kits and cyanide antidotes).
4) Confirmation of causative chemicals: the toxic syndrome narrows down the list of potential causative chemical agents to a manageable level. This in turn provides guidance to clinicians about which tests to run to identify and confirm the specific agents involved, thereby assuring that laboratory resources are applied in the most effective way possible. In addition, over time, several lines of investigation, such as scene anal-yses or factual details of the incident, will help to clarify/confirm the identity of the causative chemical.
5) Chemical-specific therapies: once the specific causative agents are iden-tified, medical personnel are able to administer any chemical-specific therapies that might be needed and make more informed decisions about patient disposition.

This tiered strategy presupposes that hospital staff has on hand the ap-propriate antidotes, protective equipment, and so forth to adequately re-spond to any given chemical event. Unfortunately, this is often not the case [22,62]. Gursky [63], Rubin [64], and Treat and colleagues [65] indicate that most hospitals are woefully unprepared for and unaware of chemicals that pose the greatest threats and potential for casualties in their communi-ties (either by attack or accident). Moreover, during the early stages of a chemical event (ie, during the silent gap), the effectiveness of the medical response depends on the diagnostic capabilities of personnel "on the scene" who often have limited medical training. The community-specific risk assess-ment can direct advance planning for the medical response community so they possess specific knowledge, equipment, and antidotes for the most likely events. Moreover, applying toxic syndrome recognition to a tiered re-sponse will give clinicians a higher degree of certainty about causative agents and objective data to assist in critical clinical decisions. Applying the tiered response to this level of preparedness and certainty will close the silent gap, thus optimizing the emergency response capabilities.

Taking actions to close the silent gap: create a communications network to effectively manage information

The case examples previously described demonstrate the susceptibility of communications to fail and is often reported in "lessons learned" analyses [7–9]. In hazardous chemical accidents, accurate and reliable information is a resource, and information management is a key component of an effective response. Responders and health care providers at all levels must be able to readily exchange information. This requires a common "language" with which to describe events as they unfold. The use of toxic syndrome identification provides that common language and set of diagnostic criteria for staff located at the hospital and for emergency personnel who are at the scene of the event.

Information gathered by on-scene personnel must be relayed to hospitals before the wave of patients converges on the ED. To provide the best care possible, clinicians must rapidly access reliable information regarding human health effects and treatment. In response to the Tokyo subway sarin attack in 1994, physicians suggested ways to correct the observed problems during their emergency response [13–15]. They observed that the most significant problems with communications were a lack of an efficient chemical disaster information network and that poison information centers should act as regional mediators of all toxicologic information. They suggested that police, fire departments, self-defense forces, poison information centers, and hospitals need to form an information network. The regional poison centers' abilities to acquire and disseminate information in a crisis makes it a critical information resource in the communications network [13,19].

Providing medical care that will do the best for the most victims of the incident

"Doing the best for the most" is challenging when confronted with a mass chemical exposure. For the most part, medical management requires the sequential recognition of four different classes of medical needs.

I: Patients needing decontamination

It is essential to recognize patients who have harmful chemicals still in contact with their skin and clothing. The purpose of decontamination is to prevent further harm to the patient and to swiftly deliver a "clean" patient to the treatment area. A toxic chemical's contact time and concentration are determinants of the extent of injury [51,53]. Therefore, decontamination is a FIRST AID procedure. Rapidly remove contaminated clothing, and copiously irrigate contaminated skin or eyes with water. The second reason to decontaminate a patient is to prevent the spread of contamination away from the scene and avoid secondary contamination to health care providers. Every patient at a hazardous chemical incident does *not* need a full decontamination [66]. Deciding to decontaminate every victim at the scene will overwhelm the response system and impede medical care. A detailed discussion about patient decontamination is beyond the scope of this article but is reviewed in detail elsewhere [21,55,56,66].

II: Patients needing immediate life-saving care (advanced life-support measures)

After decontamination, treatment of victims exposed to toxic chemicals primarily involves symptomatic and supportive care. Most critically ill poisoned patients have acute reversible conditions requiring supportive care measures. Many times, supportive care measures alone will improve the outcome of critically ill poisoned patients by focusing on maintaining a patent airway, preventing hypoxia, and treatment of shock. Valuable resources, such as antidotes, may be in limited supply during a mass chemical exposure. Decisions about aggressive resuscitation efforts and use of resources must take into account a patient's likelihood of survival.

III: Patients needing urgent antidote therapy or other specialized therapy

Few specific antidotes exist for hazardous chemical exposures; therefore, recognizing syndromes caused by chemicals treated with specific antidotes avoids blindly administering antidotes to patients who do not have clear indications. Clinicians must immediately recognize the toxic syndromes caused by nerve agents and cyanide and rapidly administer specific antidotes to give critically ill patients the best chance of survival.

IV: The psychologic needs of patients, families, care providers, media, and the community

The greatest diagnostic challenge for evaluating a patient who has potential poisoning is determining if the patient's problem is due to direct toxic effects of chemicals. Patients who have obvious contamination or signs of poisoning need immediate medical attention. Several patients will be asymptomatic but fearful of being poisoned and will seek medical care for reassurance. The greatest number of patients seeking care is often asymptomatic and symptomatic who are perceiving poisoning but not experiencing obvious signs or symptoms of poisoning [5,13]. Low-level exposure to highly toxic substances can cause nonspecific symptoms similar to those reported for perceived poisoning. For example, patients who have mild to moderate nerve agent poisoning after the 1995 Tokyo sarin attack reported nonspecific signs and symptoms such as chest tightness, dyspnea, tachycardia, nausea/vomiting, abdominal cramps, headache, and diaphoresis [5]. During a mass chemical exposure, the diagnosis of fear and anxiety is by exclusion only.

Nonspecific symptoms caused by the autonomic arousal from fear and anxiety seem to be contagious and has been called "crowd poison" [67]. Strategies to prevent spread include separating patients into small groups and removing patients from "line of sight" activities such as the presence of ambulances, fire trucks, television cameras, and workers in protective clothing. These sights and sounds signal that the situation is dangerous and enhance anxiety [34].

Delivering information and reassurance during a crisis requires risk communication skills [68–70]. The goal of risk communication is to provide people with accurate information and alleviate anxiety that stems from rumor and misinformation. Information is an antidote to fear, because those who have more knowledge regarding the risks of exposure improve their attitudes toward those exposures [31]. Important principles of risk communication include recognizing and responding to the emotional response (outrage) to risk mostly by listening to patients' concerns. People need a sense of control, and providing specific actions will give patients some sense of control [68].

Summary

An accident releasing hazardous chemicals or a deliberate chemical terrorism attack will create chaos, confusion, and seeming unpredictability that complicates the emergency response. Clinicians are challenged to urgently treat victims needing care, even before a chemical is confirmed. One of the first steps toward preparedness is to gain some sense of control by anticipating the "most likely" challenges learned from past events. Predictably, the medical response can be overwhelmed when faced with a large-scale chemical event leading to numerous problems that can significantly erode its effectiveness. An effective response strategy should: (1) plan for these predictable challenges to the emergency response and health care systems, (2) identify the greatest chemical risks that could cause harm if accidentally or deliberately released, and (3) use critical decision pathways during the emergency response that apply basic toxicologic principles. Emergency planning that focuses on these areas can bring a sense of order to the chaos and provide medical care that will do the best for the most victims of the incident.

References

[1] Dhara V, Dhara R. The Union Carbide disaster in Bhopal: a review of health effects. Arch Environ Health 2002;57(5):391–404.
[2] Eldridge D, Richardson W, Michels J, et al. The role of poison centers in a mass chlorine exposure. Clin Toxicol 2005;43:766–7.
[3] Jones T, Craig A, Hoy D, et al. Mass psychogenic illness attributed to toxic exposures at a high school. N Engl J Med 2000;342:96–100.
[4] Kirk M, Olinger M, et al. Medical mass hysteria. Clin Toxicol 1996;34:620.
[5] Okumura T, Takasu N, Ishimatsu S, et al. Report on 640 victims of the Tokyo subway sarin attack. Ann Emerg Med 1996;28(2):129–224.

[6] Wax P, Becker C, Curry S. Unexpected "gas" casualties in Moscow: a medical toxicology perspective. Ann Emerg Med 2003;41:700–5.

[7] Auf der Heide E. The importance of evidence-based disaster planning. Ann Emerg Med 2006;47:34–49.

[8] Auf der Heide E. Disaster response: principles of preparation and coordination. Available at: http://orgmail2.coe-dmha.org/dr/index.htm. Accessed January 10, 2007.

[9] Auf der Heide E. Disaster planning, part II: disaster problems, issues, and challenges identified in the research literature. Emerg Med Clin North Am 1996;14:453–80.

[10] Nanagas K, Kirk M. Perceived poisons. Med Clin North Am 2005;89:1359–78.

[11] Henry C, Belflower A, Drociuk D, et al. Public health consequences from hazardous substances acutely released during rail transit—South Carolina, 2005; selected states, 1999–2004. MMWR Morb Mortal Wkly Rep 2005;54(3):64–7.

[12] Ohbu S, Yamashina A, Takasu N, et al. Sarin poisoning on Tokyo subway. South Med J 1997;90(6):587–93.

[13] Okumura T, Suzuki K, Fukuda A, et al. The Tokyo subway sarin attack: disaster management, part 2: hospital response. Acad Emerg Med 1998;5(6):618–24.

[14] Okumura T, Suzuki K, Fukuda A, et al. The Tokyo subway sarin attack: disaster management, part 1: community emergency response. Acad Emerg Med 1998;5(6):613–7.

[15] Okumura T, Suzuki K, Fukuda A, et al. The Tokyo subway sarin attack: disaster management, part 3: national and international response. Acad Emerg Med 1998;5(6):625–7.

[16] Murakami H. Underground: the Tokyo gas attack and the Japanese psyche. New York: Random House; 2000.

[17] Bleich A, Dycian A, Koslowsky M, et al. Psychiatric implications of missile attacks on a civilian population: Israeli lessons from the Persian Gulf War. JAMA 1992;268(5):613–5.

[18] Karsenty E, Shemer J, Alshech I, et al. Medical aspects of the Iraqi missile attacks on Israel. Isr J Med Sci 1991;27:603–7.

[19] Baer A, Kirk M, Holstege C, et al. Obtaining medical information during a nuclear, biological, or chemical (NBC) incident: a survey study [abstract]. Clinical Toxicology 2004; 42:820.

[20] Hauschild V, Bratt G. Prioritizing industrial chemical hazards. J Toxicology and Env Health 2005;68(Part A):857–76.

[21] Occupational Safety and Health Administration. OSHA best practices for hospital-based first receivers of victims from mass casualty incidents involving the release of hazardous substances. Available at: http://www.osha.gov/dts/osta/bestpractices/firstreceivers_hospital.html. Accessed December 14, 2006.

[22] Fricker R, Jacobson J, et al. RAND Issue paper: measuring and evaluating local preparedness for a chemical or biological terrorist attack; 2002. Available at: http://www.rand.org/pubs/issue_papers/IP217. Accessed December 12, 2006.

[23] Ramalingaswami V. Psychosocial effects of the 1994 plague outbreak in Surat, India. Mil Med 2001;166(12 Suppl):29–30.

[24] Alexander DA, Klein S. Biochemical terrorism: too awful to contemplate, too serious to ignore: subjective literature review. Br J Psychiatry Suppl 2003;183:491–7.

[25] Clauw DJ, Engel CC Jr, Aronowitz R, et al. Unexplained symptoms after terrorism and war: an expert consensus statement. J Occup Environ Med 2003;45(10):1040–8.

[26] Hyams KC, Murphy FM, Wessely S. Responding to chemical, biological, or nuclear terrorism: the indirect and long-term health effects may present the greatest challenge [see comment]. J Health Polit Policy Law 2002;27:273–91.

[27] Collins DL. Human responses to the threat of or exposure to ionizing radiation at three mile island, Pennsylvania, and Goiania, Brazil. Mil Med 2002;167(2 Suppl):137–8.

[28] Kawana J, Ishimatsu S, Kanda K. Psycho-physiological effects of the terrorist sarin attack on the Tokyo subway system. Mil Med 2001;166:23–6.

[29] Pastel RH. Radiophobia: long-term psychological consequences of Chernobyl. Mil Med 2002;167(Suppl 1):134–6.

[30] Kovalchick D, Burgess J, Kyes K, et al. Psychological effects of hazardous materials exposures. Psychosom Med 2002;64:841–6.

[31] Pastel RH. Collective behaviors: mass panic and outbreaks of multiple unexplained symptoms. Mil Med 2001;166(12 Suppl):44–6.

[32] Bartholomew R, Goode E. Mass delusions and hysterias: highlights from the past millennium. Skeptical Inquirer 2000;24(3):20–8.

[33] Bartholomew RE, Wessely S. Protean nature of mass sociogenic illness: from possessed nuns to chemical and biological terrorism fears. Br J Psychiatry 2002;180:300–6.

[34] Boss LP. Epidemic hysteria: a review of the published literature. Epidemiol Rev 1997;19(2): 233–43.

[35] Bowler R, Mergler D, Huel G, et al. Aftermath of a chemical spill: psychological and physiological sequelae. Neurotoxicology 1994;15(3):723–9.

[36] Lees-Haley P, Brown R. Biases in perception and reporting following a perceived toxic exposure. Percept Mot Skills 1992;75:531–44.

[37] Holloway HC, Norwood AE, Fullerton CS, et al. The threat of biological weapons. Prophylaxis and mitigation of psychological and social consequences. JAMA 1997;278(5):425–7.

[38] Norwood AE, Holloway HC, Ursano RJ. Psychological effects of biological warfare. Mil Med 2001;166(12 Suppl):27–8.

[39] Romano J, King J. Psychological casualties resulting from chemical and biological weapons. Mil Med 2001;166(Suppl 2):21–2.

[40] Knudson G. Nuclear, biological, and chemical training in the US Army Reserves: mitigating psychological consequences of weapons of mass destruction. Mil Med 2001;166:63–5.

[41] Bennett M. TICs, TIMs, and terrorists. Today's Chemist at Work 2003; Available at: www.tcawonline.org. Accessed November 12, 2003.

[42] Kroft SUS. Plants: open to terrorists. 60 minutes finds lax security at many U.S. Chem facilities. Available at: http://www.cbsnews.com/stories/2003/11/13/60minutes/main583528.shtml. Accessed December 30, 2006.

[43] Combating terrorism: need for comprehensive threat and risk assessments of chemical and biological attacks. Available at: http://www.gao.gov/archive/1999/ns99163.pdf.

[44] Goldfrank L, Flomenbaum N, Lewin N, et al. Vital signs and toxic syndromes. In: Goldfrank L, editor. Goldfrank's toxicologic emergencies. seventh edition. New York: McGraw-Hill; 2002. p. 255–60.

[45] Kirk MA, et al. Care of the chemically contaminated patient. In: Ford M, Delaney K, Ling L, editors. Clinical toxicology. Philadelphia: W.B. Saunders Co; 2001. p. 115–26.

[46] Patel M, Schier J, Belson M, et al. Recognition of illness associated with exposure to chemical agents—United States, 2003. MMWR Morb Mortal Wkly Rep 2003;52(39):938–40.

[47] Kales S, Christiani D. Acute chemical emergencies. N Engl J Med 2004;350(8):800–8.

[48] Hoffman J, Schriger D, Luo J. The empiric use of naloxone in patients with altered mental status: a reappraisal. Ann Emerg Med 1991;20(3):246–52.

[49] Horton D, Berkowitz Z, Kaye W. Surveillance of hazardous materials events in 17 states, 1993–2001: a report from the Hazardous Substances Emergency Events Surveillance (HSEES) system. Am J Ind Med 2004;45(6):539–48.

[50] Walter FG, Dedolph R, Kallsen GW, et al. Hazardous materials incidents: a one-year retrospective review in central California. Prehospital Disaster Med 1992;7:151–6.

[51] Eaton D, Klaassen C. Principles of toxicology. In: Klaassen D, editor. Casarett and Doull's toxicology: the basic science of poisons. 6th edition. New York: McGraw-Hill; 2001. p. 11–34.

[52] Garriott J. Pharmacology and toxicology of ethyl alcohol. In: Garriott J, editor. Medicallegal aspects of alcohol. Tucson (AZ): Lawyers and Judges Publishing; 2003. p. 23–38.

[53] Leonard LG, Scheulen JJ, Munster AM. Chemical burns: effect of prompt first aid. J Trauma 1993;22:420–3.

[54] Bushberg J, Kroger L, Hartman M, et al. Nuclear/radiological terrorism: emergency department management of radiation casualties. J Emerg Med 2007;32(1):71–85.

[55] Hick JL, Hanfling D, Burstein JL, et al. Protective equipment for health care facility decontamination personnel: regulations, risks, and recommendations. Ann Emerg Med 2003; 42(3):370–80.

[56] Hick JL, Penn P, Hanfling D, et al. Establishing and training health care facility decontamination teams. Ann Emerg Med 2003;42(3):381–90.

[57] Burgess JL, Kirk MA, Borron SW, et al. Emergency department hazardous materials protocol for contaminated patients. Ann Emerg Med 1999;34:205–12.

[58] Burgess JL, Kovalchick DF, Harter L, et al. Hazardous materials events: an industrial comparison. J Occup Environ Med 2000;42(5):546–53.

[59] Orr M, Kaye W, Zeitz P, et al. Public health risks of railroad hazardous substance emergency events. J Occup Environ Med 2001;43:94–100.

[60] Baxter PJ, Kapila M, Mfonfu D. Lake Nyos disaster, Cameroon, 1986: the medical effects of large scale emission of carbon dioxide. BMJ 1989;298:1437–41.

[61] Wing JS, Brender JD, Sanderson LM, et al. Acute health effects in a community after a release of hydrofluoric acid. Arch Environ Health 1991;46:155–60.

[62] Dart RC, Stark Y, Fulton B, et al. Insufficient stocking of poisoning antidotes in hospital pharmacies. JAMA 1996;276(18):1508–10.

[63] Gursky E. *Hometown hospitals: the weakest link? Bioterrorism Readiness in America's Rural Hospitals*: the center for Technology and National Security Policy The National Defense University; 2004.

[64] Rubin J. Recurring pitfalls in hospital preparedness and response. Available at: http://www.homelandsecurity.org/journal/Articles/rubin.html. Accessed December 14, 2007.

[65] Treat K, Williams J, Furbee P, et al. Hospital preparedness for weapons of mass destruction incidents: an initial assessment. Ann Emerg Med 2001;38(5):562–5.

[66] Levitin H, Siegelson H, Dickinson S, et al. Decontamination of mass casualties re-evaluating existing dogma. Prehospital Disaster Med 2003;18(3):200–7.

[67] Wessely S. Mass hysteria: two syndromes? Psychol Med 1987;17(1):109–20.

[68] Sandman P. Crisis communication: guidelines for action. Available at: http://www.psandman.com/handouts/AIHA-DVD.htm. Accessed January 16, 2005.

[69] Sandman P. Responding to community outrage: strategies for effective risk communication. Fairfax American Industrial Hygiene Association; 1993.

[70] US Department of Health and Human Services. Communicating in a crisis: risk communication guidelines for public health officials; 2002.

ELSEVIER
SAUNDERS

EMERGENCY
MEDICINE
CLINICS OF
NORTH AMERICA

Emerg Med Clin N Am 25 (2007) 549–566

Unusual But Potential Agents of Terrorists

Christopher P. Holstege, MD[a,b,*],
Laura K. Bechtel, PhD[a,b], Tracey H. Reilly, MD[a],
Bram P. Wispelwey[c],
Stephen G. Dobmeier, BSN[b]

[a]Division of Medical Toxicology, Department of Emergency Medicine,
University of Virginia, P.O. Box 800744, 1222 Jefferson Park Avenue,
4th Floor, Charlottesville, VA 22908-0774, USA
[b]Blue Ridge Poison Center, University of Virginia Health System, P.O. Box 800744,
Charlottesville, VA 22908-0774, USA
[c]Critical Incident Analysis Group, Department of Psychiatry, University of Virginia,
1510 Oxford Road, Charlottesville, VA 22903, USA

Emergency personnel are tasked with the daunting job of being the first to evaluate and manage victims of a terrorist attack. Numerous potential chemical agents could be used by terrorists. For example, the Centers for Disease Control and Prevention (CDC) lists over 80 chemical agents (Box 1) that pose risk and can be found at http://www.bt.cdc.gov/agent/agentlistchem.asp. The challenge for first responders and local hospital emergency personnel is to prepare for a terrorist event that might use one or more of these agents. As part of that preparation, emergency physicians should have a basic understanding of potential chemical terrorist agents. It is beyond the scope of this article to review all potential terrorist agents. Rather, four potential agents have been chosen for review: sodium monofluoroacetate, trichothecene mycotoxins, vomiting agents, and saxitoxin.

Sodium monofluoroacetate (compound 1080)

Sodium monofluoroacetate (SMFA) is both chemically and toxicologically identical to the fluoroacetate found in certain poisonous plants in

---

* Corresponding author. Division of Medical Toxicology, Department of Emergency Medicine, University of Virginia, P.O. Box 800744, 1222 Jefferson Park Avenue, 4th Floor, Charlottesville, VA 22908-0774.

E-mail address: ch2xf@virginia.edu (C.P. Holstege).

0733-8627/07/$ - see front matter © 2007 Elsevier Inc. All rights reserved.
doi:10.1016/j.emc.2007.02.006
emed.theclinics.com

Box 1. A partial listing of potential chemical agents that pose a terrorist-use risk

Abrin
Acids
Adamsite
Ammonia
Arsenic
Arsine
Barium
Benzene
Brevetoxin
Bromine
Bromobenzylcyanide
Bz
Carbon monoxide
Caustics
Chlorine
Chloroacetophenone
Chlorobenzylidenemalononitrile
Chloropicrin
Colchicine
Cyanide
Cyanogen chloride
Dibenzoxazepine
Digitalis
Diphosgene
Ethylene glycol
Hydrogen fluoride
Lewisite
Long-acting anticoagulants
Mercury
Methyl bromide
Methyl isocyanate
Mustard
Nerve agents
Nicotine
Opioids
Organic solvents
Osmium tetroxide
Paraquat
Phosgene
Phosphine

Phosphorous
Saxitoxin
Sodium azide
Sodium monofluoroacetate
Stibine
Strychnine
Sulfuryl fluoride
Tear gas
Tetrodotoxin
Thallium
Trichothecene

Australia, South Africa, and South America [1,2]. SMFA is also known as "1080," referring to SMFA's catalog number that became its brand name. SMFA was discovered by German military chemists during World War II [3]. President Nixon banned the poison in the United States in 1972, but the Reagan administration reauthorized its use in the mid-1980s for livestock protection collars [2]. 1080 is manufactured by one United States company: Tull Chemical Co. in Oxford, Alabama, which has been manufacturing the poison since 1956 [4]. Much of Tull's 1080 is exported to other countries such as New Zealand, Mexico, Israel, and Australia for pest control. Accidental cases of ingestion of SMFA are rare but have occurred in China [5]. Also rare are cases of intentional (suicidal) ingestion in the United States [6]. There are no official reports that document the use of 1080 in a criminal manner.

In November 2004, Representative Peter DeFazio (D-OR) asked the Department of Homeland Security to halt production and use of compound 1080 because of its potential as a terrorist agent [7]. In May 2005, a United States report was released that included a photograph (taken May 2003) of a Tull 1080 can recovered by coalition troops in Iraq [4]. The Federal Bureau of Investigation, US Air Force, Canadian Security Intelligence Service, and US Homeland Security publicly list 1080 as a poison that terrorists could potentially use to contaminate public water supplies. In December 2005, Representative DeFazio introduced a bill "to prohibit the manufacture, processing, possession, or distribution in commerce of the poison sodium fluoroacetate," as well as to destroy existing stores of the poison [8]. The last action taken on this bill was in February 2006, when it was referred to the subcommittee on Crime, Terrorism, and Homeland Security.

Properties

The synthetic form of the SMFA (CAS # 62-74-8) exists as a white powder (similar in appearance to flour or powdered sugar) that remains stable for long periods of time. It is odorless, tasteless, and readily dissolves into water [1]. When present in natural water sources, it degrades within 7 days because of its metabolism by microorganisms within those environments. In water devoid of microorganisms, SMFA appears to remain stable [9]. It is insoluble in organic solvents such as ethanol or vegetable oils [6]. The only reported distinguishing characteristic is that it has a weak vinegar taste when mixed with water [6]. It is heat stable; it does not decompose until temperatures approach 200°C. SMFA is highly toxic to vertebrates, although the sensitivity of different species varies dramatically. In humans, the estimated lethal poisoning dose (LD50) ranges from 2 to 5 mg/kg body weight [6].

Routes of exposure

Compound 1080 is well absorbed from the gastrointestinal tract, the respiratory tract, open wounds, mucus membranes, and ocular exposure [1]. Most human exposures reported in the medical literature have been through ingestion. Toxicity has been reported to be the same whether it is administered orally, subcutaneously, intramuscularly, or intravenously [1]. Dusts containing SMFA are effectively toxic by inhalation [1].

Pathophysiology

The toxicologic mechanism of SMFA involves disruption of cellular energy production resulting in multisystem organ failure (Fig. 1) [10]. The parent compound, fluoroacetate, has low cellular toxicity. However, once ingested and absorbed, enzymatic reactions within cells convert fluoroacetate to fluoroacetyl-CoA. Fluoroacetyl-CoA, in the presence of oxaloacetate, is converted by citrate synthase to fluorocitrate, a potent inhibitor of the enzyme aconitase [10]. Aconitase catalyzes the reversible Krebs cycle reaction converting citrate to isocitrate. The inhibition of aconitase results in the interruption of the energy producing Krebs cycle and the buildup of citrate. Fluorocitrate also inhibits transport of citrate in and out of mitochondria, contributing the buildup of citrate. Elevated citrate levels disrupt energy production by way of glycolysis by inhibiting the enzyme phosphofructokinase. Elevated citrate levels may also cause life-threatening hypocalcemia. Because it takes time for the metabolic conversion of fluoroacetate to fluorocitrate, there is a delay from the time that the poison is ingested to the initial onset of signs and symptoms [11].

Clinical manifestations

Clinical signs and symptoms associated with SMFA poisoning are nonspecific. SMFA poisoning is characterized by a latent period of 30 minutes to 3 hours following the administration of the compound by any route [2,11,12]. However, delayed onset of symptoms has been reported up to 20 hours [6]. Even massive doses do not elicit immediate responses, although

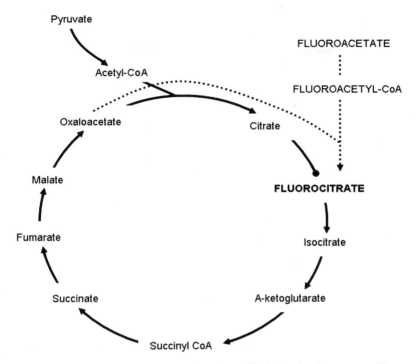

Fig. 1. Krebs cycle demonstrating the region of inhibition by fluoroacetate [1].

the latent period may be reduced. In animal studies, the early stages of poisoning are typically reported as displaying a range of signs including: lethargy, vomiting, trembling, excessive salivation, incontinence, muscular weakness, incoordination, hypersensitivity to nervous stimuli, and respiratory distress. Early neurologic signs include muscular twitches often affecting the face, such as nystagmus and blepharospasm. These then progress to generalized seizures, initially tonic and then becoming cyclically tonic–clonic with periods of lucidity in between [12]. Partial paralysis may be seen that lasts for prolonged time periods. Death typically results from depression of the respiratory center, cardiovascular failure, and/or ventricular fibrillation [2,12,13]. On autopsy, there are no characteristic lesions associated with SMFA poisoning [1].

Numerous human reports exist in the literature. Trabes and colleagues [12], for example, described a 15-year-old who attempted suicide by ingesting SMFA. She developed nausea, vomiting, and abdominal pain within 30 minutes of ingestion followed by a grand mal seizure 1 hour later with associated tachycardia (150 beats per minute) and profuse diaphoresis. She was described as disorientated, demonstrated signs of psychomotor agitation, and over the ensuing 4 hours, developed three additional grand mal seizures and then became comatose. Her cerebral spinal fluid was unremarkable with normal opening pressures. She recovered, but developed a chronic cerebellar ataxia and computerized topography findings of moderate diffuse brain atrophy.

Robinson and colleagues [6] reported the case of a 47-year-old male who ingested SMFA in a suicide attempt. He developed nausea and vomiting initially, and at 4 hours after ingestion, he experienced tonic–clonic seizures. At 34 hours postingestion, he responded to only noxious stimuli with an electroencephalaogram demonstrating mild diffuse slowing. At 48 hours he became febrile, tachypneic, and unresponsive to painful stimuli and placed on a ventilator. His chest radiograph revealed pulmonary edema. Over the following 3 days, he was minimally responsive to external stimuli, with decline in his renal function (serum creatinine peaked at 4.3 mg/dL). Two days later, he was discharged with no sequelae. Reigart and colleagues [13a] described an 8-month-old who developed two episodes of nausea and vomiting after ingesting SMFA, but was otherwise asymptomatic until seizures developed 20 hours postingestion.

Chi and colleagues [14] described two cases of SMFA intoxication. The first, a 26-year-old female, attempted suicide by swallowing 32 mL of 1% SMFA solution. She initially developed nausea and vomiting, and upon presentation was found to have a blood pressure of 80/40 mm Hg, respiratory rate of 32 breaths per minute, and a pulse of 120 beats per minute. Her initial labs were significant for a plasma creatinine of 1.8 mg/dL, potassium of 3.3 mmol/L, alanine aminotransferase 124 U/L and blood sugar of 248 mg/dL. Her initial arterial blood gas on 40% oxygen revealed: pH 7.342; pCO2 32.1; pO2 74.4, HCO3- 17.4; base excess -7.2. She developed progressive metabolic acidosis and subsequent hypotension and respiratory failure. She expired 48 hours after exposure. In the second case, a 62-year-old female presented 1 hour after ingestion of 16 mL of 1% SMFA solution. She immediately suffered nausea and vomiting. Her initial vitals signs were: blood pressure 167/78 mm HG, respiratory rate 19 breaths per minute, pulse 120 beats per minute. Her initial labs were significant for a plasma creatinine of 1.0 mg/dL, potassium of 2.8 mmol/L, alanine aminotransferase 65 U/L, and blood sugar of 478 mg/dL. Her initial arterial blood gas on 28% oxygen revealed: pH 7.296; PCO2 39.5; PO2 123, HCO3- 19.4; base excess -6.0. She developed progressive metabolic acidosis, hypotension, respiratory failure, and gastrointestinal bleeding, but survived and was discharged without sequelae 21 days after ingestion.

In a retrospective study of 38 human cases of SMFA poisoning, Chi and colleagues [5] noted the most frequent symptom to be nausea and/or vomiting (74%). Electrocardiograph changes were variable ranging from mild nonspecific ST and T wave abnormalities (72%) to ventricular tachycardias and asystole. The most common electrolyte abnormalities included hypocalcemia (42%) and hypokalemia (65%). Seven of the 38 patients died in this series. Discriminate analysis identified hypotension, increased serum creatinine, and decreased pH as the most important predictors of mortality, with sensitivity of 86% and specificity of 96%.

Laboratory testing

The CDC has created a multilevel laboratory response network to provide surge capacity testing for exposure to chemical or biological terrorist agents. The laboratory response network links 126 clinical laboratories to public health agencies in all states by providing state-of-the-art facilities that can analyze potential biological and chemical terrorist agents. At the onset of an event, state laboratories are capable of performing some initial testing. More specialized analyses from one of the seven CDC-funded level 1 facilities may be required. Furthermore, the CDC directly may employ a "rapid toxic screen" to analyze human blood and urine samples for a large number of potential terrorist agents. If medical personnel suspect patient exposure to a chemical or biological terrorist agent, the health care team should immediately contact their respective state or local health department (http://www.cdc.gov/doc.do/id/states). Most detection methods require collection and shipping of human specimens as specified by the CDC Laboratory Information for Chemical Emergencies' web page (http://www. bt.cdc.gov/chemical/lab.asp).

Chemical detection methods are currently used to detect SMFA in human blood specimens. Derivatized extracts are analyzed using gas chromatography mass spectroscopy (GCMS) or gas chromatography with electron-capture detection. Because the exact mechanism for SMFA metabolism has not been elucidated, rapid collection of blood specimens should be obtained and immediately stored at 4°C in suspected cases.

Treatment

There is no specific antidote for SMFA toxicity, and therapy is primarily focused at supportive care. Even though activated charcoal does appear to bind SMFA, it does not appear to affect either the area under the curve of serum fluoroacetate levels versus time or decrease mortality rates [15]. Several different treatments have been explored for SMFA toxicity. Because SMFA induces hypocalcemia, calcium supplementation through administration of either calcium gluconate or calcium chloride has been shown to be of benefit [16,17]. In animal models, sodium succinate has been shown to be of benefit as a potential antidote to revive the Krebs cycle [16]. Because of the reported potential for delayed clinical effects, patients who have known oral exposure to SMFA should be observed for a minimum of 24 hours following oral exposure.

Trichothecene mycotoxins

Select mycotoxins are potential weapons and include such potent agents as aflatoxin, fumonisin, ochratoxin, and the trichothecenes (ie, T-2 toxin and vomitoxin) [18,19]. The trichothecene mycotoxins constitute a family of more than 60 compounds produced by several fungi, including *Fusarium,*

Myrothecium, Phomopsis, Stachybotrys, Trichoderma, and Trichothecium [19]. All trichothecenes contain a common 12,13-epoxytrichothene skeleton and are subdivided into four chemical groups (type A, B, C, D). T-2 toxin is the most extensively studied of the trichothecenes.

The trichothecene mycotoxins have a long and sorted history. In the Ukraine in 1931, a unique disease to horses was recognized that was characterized by lip edema, stomatitis, oral necrosis, rhinitis, and conjunctivitis [20]. The clinical effects often progressed through well-defined stages including pancytopenia, coagulopathy, neurologic compromise, superinfections, and death. When autopsies were performed on the afflicted animals, the entire alimentary tract was found to have diffuse hemorrhage and necrosis, giving rise to the name *alimentary toxic aleukia* [19,21]. During World War II, a large population within Orenburg, Russia became ill following the ingestion of overwintered grain colonized by mold, giving a similar disease pattern as noted in previous animal outbreaks [22]. In 1940, Soviet scientists coined the term *stachybotryotoxicosis* to describe the acute syndrome (sore throat, bloody nasal discharge, dyspnea, cough, and fever) resulting from the inhalation of *Stachybotrys* mycotoxins [22]. These outbreaks subsequently lead to the discovery of the trichothecene mycotoxins, with T-2 toxin isolated in 1968.

The name "yellow rain" is derived from incidents beginning in 1975, when two communist governments in Laos and Cambodia (allied with the Soviet Union) retaliated against Hmong tribes that sided with the United States during the Vietnam War [19]. The supposed chemical attacks were delivered by low-flying aircraft that dropped a yellow oily liquid that lead to adverse effects by those exposed. In 1983, a United States report summarized the history of T-2 development in the Soviet Union, 2 years after United States chemical weapons experts matched samples from the attack to trichothecene signatures. These charges have since been disputed by Harvard biologist and biological weapons opponent Matthew Meselson and others, who believe that T-2 mycotoxins occur naturally in the Laos region and suggested that the yellow rain was the harmless fecal matter of honey bees [19]. In Meselson's view, the poisoning from T-2 mycotoxins was the result of eating moldy foods and was simply coincidental with the natural bee droppings. As of 2007, this matter has not been resolved, and much key information and data from the incidents remain classified [23].

Properties

The trichothecene mycotoxins are extremely stable proteins that are resistant to heat, autoclaving, hypochlorite, and ultraviolet light. However, when exposed to sodium hydroxide, the toxins are rendered inactive [24]. Of the naturally occurring trichothecenes, T-2 is one of the most potent toxins in animal studies and the most extensively studied. These toxins can be delivered as dusts, droplets, aerosols, or smoke from various dispersal systems and exploding munitions. They are highly soluble in several organic solvents, such as ethanol, and only slightly soluble in water. T-2 toxin is distributed rapidly to tissues, with the hepatobiliary system being the major route for the metabolism and elimination. The reported LD50 of T-2 toxin is approximately 1 mg/kg [25].

Routes of exposure

The trichothecene mycotoxins are well absorbed by topical, oral, or inhalational routes.

Pathophysiology

The trichothecene mycotoxins are markedly cytotoxic [26]. These agents have multiple cellular actions. For example, these toxins bind to the 60S ribosomal subunit and inactivate its peptidyl transferase activity at the transcription site, thereby inhibiting protein synthesis [19]. Actively proliferating cells are particularly sensitive. As a result, these toxins have both cytotoxic effects and immunosuppressive effects.

Clinical manifestations

The various trichothecenes cause a wide range of clinical effects on nearly every organ system when studied in animals [27]. The trichothecene mycotoxins can cause mucosal and skin irritation if exposed topically. Cutaneous signs include erythema, edema, pain, pruritis, and blisters [21]. Ultimately, necrosis and sloughing of large areas of skin may occur [22]. Severe ocular irritation and corneal ulceration may also be seen. Acute trichothecene intoxication may result in vomiting, hemorrhagic diathesis, and cardiovascular dysfunction resembling endotoxic shock [20]. Airway and intestinal necrosis may occur depending upon the route and dose of exposure. Soon after exposure, leukocytosis may be seen [20]. However, with increasing toxicity, pancytopenia may develop, predisposing to bleeding and sepsis [20]. Symptoms develop within a few hours of exposure. There are no human trichothecene exposure case reports published in the literature.

Laboratory testing

The parental compound T-2 is rapidly metabolized to HT-2, T2-triol, and T-2 tetraol within hours after consumption. Therefore, detection methods have been developed that measure T-2 metabolites that have intrinsically longer half-lives [28,29]. Current methods rely on inexpensive and rapid enzyme-linked immunoassays for T-2 metabolite detection in urine samples within 1 week after exposure [30,31]. Results from the enzyme-linked immunoassays assay can be available within hours.

T-2 metabolites can be detected in blood samples for as long as 1 month using a highly sensitive modified liquid chromatography tandem mass spectroscopy analysis (LCMS/MS) [30,32]. Results may take hours to days using the LCMS/MS method. Because of the high equipment cost, requirement of highly trained personnel, and lack of quality standard controls, LCMS/MS is not the preferred analytical method. Unfortunately, until other methods are available for analyzing T-2 and T-2 metabolites outside the 1-week collection window, LCMS/MS will continue to be used. With this in mind, development of bioassays for cytotoxic screening of T-2 metabolites is currently being investigated [33].

Treatment/disposition

Adsorbents such as activate charcoal may be useful in treatment if used early following oral exposure [24]. Washing the exposed skin with water and detergent promptly after the exposure may remove some of the agent and limit its absorption [21]. No specific antidote is currently available, and care is focused on symptomatic and supportive treatment. Steroids, such as methyl prednisolone and dexamethasone, may be of benefit following skin exposure.

Vomiting agents

The chemicals classified as vomiting agents include the chemical warfare agents diphenylchlorarsine (DA), diphenylcyanoarsine (DC), and diphenylaminearsine (DM, adamsite) [34,35]. DM was the first of these to be synthesized by German chemist Heinrich Wieland in 1915. American chemist Robert Adams independently developed the same compound in 1918 and named it adamsite. The first reported use of a vomiting agent in warfare came in 1917 when German troops used DA. It was not well filtered by standard issue masks and forced opposing troops to remove their masks during combat. Once the masks were removed because of nausea and vomiting, Germany's enemies were exposed to the toxic effects of other agents including chlorine gas and phosgene. Although the Germans also produced DC and DM at this time, documentation of their use in World War I is limited. Vomiting agents are reportedly produced for riot control purposes, but only questionable accounts exist of foreign nations using them in this manner.

In June 2003, letters containing DM (adamsite) were sent to the United States, British, and Saudi Embassies; Belgium's Prime Minister Guy Verhofstadt; the Court of Brussels; a Belgian ministry; the Oostende airport; and the Antwerp port authority [36]. At least two postal workers and five policemen were hospitalized with symptoms of skin irritation, eye irritation, and difficult breathing after exposure to the substance. Three people who were exposed in Oostende were also hospitalized. Belgium police suspected a 45-year-old Iraqi political refugee opposed to the United States–Iraq War. Upon searching his residence, antiterrorism investigators found a plastic bag containing powder. The investigators suffered similar symptoms to those who were exposed to the letters, and the Iraqi was charged with premeditated assault. No other instances of vomiting agent use have been reported, although buried adamsite has been found in one of many chemical weapons dumping sites in Shikhany, Russia [37].

Properties

DA appears as colorless crystals, DC as a white solid, and DM as light yellow-to-green crystals [34]. DA and DM are odorless; DC reportedly has an odor similar to garlic or bitter almonds. All 3 agents are insoluble in water [38].

DM is the most toxic agent of this group, with an estimated LCt50 of 11,000 mg/min/m^3 (ie, an estimated 50% lethality for a group of patients breathing air with a concentration of 11,000 mg/m^3 for 1 min) [34]. Other factors also are important, such as the exposed patient's preexisting health status and the time from exposure to medical care.

Routes of exposure

Vomiting agents typically are disseminated as aerosols. The primary route of absorption is through the respiratory system. Exposure also can occur by ingestion, dermal absorption, or eye contact [38].

Clinical manifestations

The effects of the vomiting agents by any route of exposure are slower in onset and longer in duration than typical riot control agents [34]. On initial exposure, vomiting agents are irritants. This irritation is delayed for several minutes after contact. As a result of this delay, vomiting agents do not have early warning properties. By the time symptoms of irritation occur and personnel consider donning their protective equipment, significant contamination already may have occurred. Systemic signs and symptoms subsequently follow the initial irritation and consist of headache, nausea, vomiting, diarrhea, abdominal cramps, and mental status changes. Symptoms typically persist for several hours after exposure. Damage to the skin may ensue if prolonged contact occurs [39]. Death has been reported with excessive exposure [34]. The autopsy of this individual found severe airway and lung damage.

Laboratory testing

These agents are enzyme inhibitors that have high affinity for sulfhydryl groups. Following absorption, DA and DC are rapidly hydrolyzed to diphenylarsinic (DPAA), then conjugated to glutathione (DPAA-GS), and excreted. Therefore, blood and urine samples should be collected within 24 hours. Current methods can quantitate DPAA and DPAA-GS levels within hours using gas chromatography and mass spectroscopy analysis (GCMS/MS) [40]. Inadequate data are available regarding DM metabolic products, thereby limiting GCMS/MS methods to the parental DM molecule and creating a shorter collection window predominantly from blood samples [41]. The collection window can be opened significantly when measuring organic arsenic levels as opposed to specific metabolites in blood or tissue samples using GCMS. Arsenic levels in combination with a patient's cytogenetic profile and clinical presentation may help pinpoint exposure to specific organoarsenic agents [42].

Treatment/disposition

The initial care of patients exposed to vomiting agents primarily is supportive. No specific antidotes are available. Care is focused on relieving irritant and systemic effects (ie, antiemetics).

Saxitoxin

Saxitoxin (STX) is associated with the syndrome known as *paralytic shellfish poisoning* and it poses a worldwide health problem [43]. STX is formed by dinoflagellates, which cause a phenomenon known as a *red tide*. Marine life (mollusks, crabs, and fish) may feed on these and bioaccumulate the dinoflagellate toxins. Humans may inadvertently consume intoxicated seafood [43,44]. Numerous outbreaks of paralytic shellfish poisoning have been reported worldwide. Paralytic shellfish poisoning is caused by not only saxitoxin, but also other chemical variations of saxitoxin, for example decarbamoyl STX (dc-STX) and N-sulfocarbamoyl (B1) toxin.

Governments reportedly began experimenting with saxitoxin in the 1950s. In 1969, President Richard Nixon banned biological weapons. Subsequently, nearly all the United States STX produced was destroyed. However, in 1975, approximately 10 g of STX was discovered in a storage facility, triggering a US Senate investigation and a redistribution of the remaining STX to universities for research purposes.

In recent years, terrorist events have resulted in increased regulations of STX [45]. STX has been listed in the "Select Agent Program" by the United States (Box 2). The US Department of Health and Human Services and the US Department of Agriculture published final rules, which implement the provisions of the USA Patriot Act and Public Health Security and Bioterrorism Preparedness and Response Act of 2002. These rules set forth the requirements for possession, use, and transfer of select agents and toxins. The select chemical toxins identified in the final rules have the potential to pose a severe threat to public health and safety, to animal and plant health, or to animal and plant products. The CDC regulates the possession, use, and transfer of these select agents and toxins that have the potential to pose a severe threat to public health and safety. The CDC Select Agent Program oversees these activities and registers all laboratories and other entities in the United States that possess, use, or transfer a select agent or toxin.

Box 2. Health and human services select agent toxins

Abrin
Conotoxins
Ricin
Shigatoxin
T-2 toxin
Botulism toxins
Diacetoxyscirpenol
Saxitoxin
Staphylococcal enterotoxins
Tetrodotoxin

Saxitoxin is also currently listed in schedule 1 of the Chemical Weapons Convention as one of the most potent toxins known. Saxitoxin and ricin are the only two naturally occurring toxins classified as schedule 1 of the Chemical Weapons Convention.

Properties

STX is a naturally occurring toxin. STX has also been synthesized using various different methods [46]. STX is water-soluble, heat stable, and unaffected by cooking [44]. The LCt_{50} of STX is 5 mg/min/m^3 and is reportedly 2000 times more toxic than sodium cyanide by weight [47].

Routes of exposure

STX toxicity can occur by either ingestion or inhalation. Contamination of food or water with STX are viewed as viable concerns for mass human exposure [48]. In animal experiments, inhalational routes of administration are more potent than oral routes, causing death within minutes compared with hours for oral [49].

Pathophysiology

STX is a specific high-affinity blocking ligand of voltage-dependent sodium channels [50]. STX binds competitively to a site on the external surface of the channel, named toxin site 1. This binding inhibits sodium flux through these ion channels rendering excitable tissues such as nerves and muscle nonfunctional.

Clinical manifestations

There are no published reports of saxitoxin being used by terrorists, though concern remains high pertaining to its potential use, its marked toxicity, and its natural availability. There are numerous reports in the literature of saxitoxin being ingested in contaminated food, which sheds light on the clinical manifestations of STX toxicity.

In two separate outbreaks reported in 1990, nine fisherman developed symptoms within 2 hours following consumption of STX-contaminated shellfish [44]. Reported symptoms included numbness of the mouth (six of nine), vomiting (four of nine), paresthesias of the extremities (seven of nine), numbness and tingling of the tongue (two of nine), numbness of the face (five of nine), low-back pain (six of nine), and periorbital edema (one of nine). Two hours following the onset of symptoms, one of the fishermen suffered a "cardiopulmonary arrest" and died. Of the remaining eight, only two required hospitalization. The duration of neurologic symptoms was less than 24 hours, and those who had low back pain approximately 3 days. Of those who survived, all recovered uneventfully.

In 1994, nine people, 38 to 80 years old, presented to the ED 6 to 18 hours after the first symptoms of STX toxicity occurred [51]. In all cases, symptoms began 60 to 90 minutes after ingestion of contaminated shellfish and consisted of dizziness, ataxia, paresthesias (oral–facial and extremity), but no gastrointestinal complaints. Six people had progressive impairment of gait, confining them to a wheelchair after 6 to 8 hours. All had normal vital signs on arrival with axial ataxia and bilateral dysmetria. Four had bilateral nystagmus, and three had dysarthria. All had distal stocking and glove superficial impairment and bilateral moderate position and vibratory sense impairment, with preservation of tendon jerks. Hematology and biochemistry routine testing were normal in all patients. Cerebral spinal fluid from two patients was normal. None developed respiratory involvement, and all were discharged from the hospital within 3 days. Within 2 weeks, all recovered but still complained of fatigue, paresthesias, and memory loss, which persisted up to 3 months. There were no long-term sequelae.

In 2000, a 65-year-old female reportedly ingested STX-contaminated blowfish and within minutes developed tingling of her lips and tongue, which intensified over the ensuing 2 hours [52]. She developed increasing chest pain and had mild tachycardia and hypertension (160/70 mm Hg) requiring treatment with topical nitroglycerin [53]. Six to 8 hours after ingestion, she developed ascending paralysis and declining pulmonary function requiring intubation. Over the following day she regained reflexes, and voluntary movement and was extubated 72 hours later.

In 2002, two fishermen died following STX-contaminated shellfish ingestion [54]. Symptoms before demise included lip paresthesias, nausea, extremity weakness, and "tongue immobilization." The forensic examination of both victims did not show pathologic abnormalities with the exception of the lungs, which revealed pulmonary edema. STX was detected in gastric contents, body fluids, and tissue samples.

In summary, following oral exposure, STX causes prominent paresthesias, often beginning circumorally and spreading to the limbs. This can then progress to paralysis with retention of reflexes [49]. Cranial nerve dysfunction, hypersalivation, diaphoresis, respiratory failure, hypertension, and hypotension have all been reported.

Laboratory testing

Measuring levels of saxitoxin in human samples requires early acquisition of samples. Saxitoxin undergoes minimal metabolism, but is rapidly excreted into the urine. Saxitoxin can also concentrate in liver, spleen, and central nervous system tissues [55]. Because of the extremely rapid excretion profile of saxitoxin compounds, urine samples are preferred rather than serum samples. All saxitoxin testing should be performed by a state health department laboratory where high performance LCMS/MS is used. These LCMS/MS methods can provide saxitoxin fingerprint analyses to determine if the saxitoxin agent was derived from an organic source (shellfish ingestion) or a purified saxitoxin source (biological warfare agent). Any cases suspected of saxitoxin exposure should collect urine specimens within 24 hours of exposure. Higher levels of saxitoxin exposure can extend detection times for several days [56]. Alternatively less sensitive methods are available for detecting saxitoxin in human samples, such as high-performance liquid chromatography and receptor binding assays [57,58].

State facilities may request submission of shellfish samples, if the physician suspects saxitoxin exposure due to ingestion of contaminated shellfish. Current United States Food and Drug Administration (USFDA) guidelines require all shellfish sold in the United States be tested for paralytic shellfish toxins. The mouse bioassay is the current gold standard method approved by the USFDA for detection and quantitation of paralytic shellfish toxins in shellfish marketed to human consumers [59]. This method identifies paralytic shellfish toxins by injecting mice with 1 ml of an acidic extract, then measuring time of death as a measurement of toxicity (5–15 min). The toxicity of the sample is then calculated with reference to dose–response curves established with saxitoxin standards and expressed in mouse units. Specificity for saxitoxin is based on the extremely rapid toxicity profile compared with other paralytic shellfish toxins. This method is not used to determine levels in humans.

Treatment/disposition

There is no known antidote for STX toxicity. Most patients will recover if they receive adequate and timely supportive care.

Summary

It will be a challenge for emergency personnel to diagnose and direct appropriate therapy for victims who develop an unexpected illness resulting from the intentional release of a chemical substance. There are numerous potential chemical agents that could be used by terrorists. Emergency health care providers should have a general understanding of these agents and should be able to recognize the signs and symptoms of a presenting sentinel case.

References

[1] Egekeze JO, Oehme FW. Sodium monofluoroacetate (SMFA, compound 1080): a literature review. Vet Hum Toxicol 1979;21(6):411–6.

[2] Eason C. Sodium monofluoroacetate (1080) risk assessment and risk communication. Toxicology 2002;181–182:523–30.

[3] Abraham K. Defazio bill bans poison. The Eugene Weekly. January 12, 2006. Available at: http://www.predatordefense.org/EugeneWeekly.pdf.

[4] Milstein M. Iraq's tests of coyote poison surface: Rep. Peter DeFazio says use of the poison he had tried to have banned underscores loose US controls of lethal agents. The Oregonian. May 28, 2005. Available at: http://www.globalsecurity.org/org/news/2005/050528-iraq-poison.htm.

[5] Chi CH, Chen KW, Chan SH, et al. Clinical presentation and prognostic factors in sodium monofluoroacetate intoxication. J Toxicol Clin Toxicol 1996;34(6):707–12.

[6] Robinson RF, Griffith JR, Wolowich WR, et al. Intoxication with sodium monofluoroacetate (compound 1080). Vet Hum Toxicol 2002;44(2):93–5.

[7] Milstein M. Wolf poison raises alarms about its terrorism potential. The Oregonian. November 3, 2004.

[8] De Fazio P. Sodium fluoroacetate elimination act. In: Congress US, editors. vol. 109. 2005:H.R. 4567.

[9] Booth LH, Ogilvie SC, Wright GR, et al. Degradation of sodium monofluoroacetate (1080) and fluorocitrate in water. Bull Environ Contam Toxicol 1999;62(1):34–9.

[10] Twigg LE, Mead RJ, King DR. Metabolism of fluoroacetate in the skink (Tiliqua rugosa) and the rat (Rattus norvegicus). Aust J Biol Sci 1986;39(1):1–15.

[11] Sherley M. The traditional categories of fluoroacetate poisoning signs and symptoms belie substantial underlying similarities. Toxicol Lett 2004;151(3):399–406.

[12] Trabes J, Rason N, Avrahami E. Computed tomography demonstration of brain damage due to acute sodium monofluoroacetate poisoning. J Toxicol Clin Toxicol 1983;20(1):85–92.

[13] Ando J, Shiozu K, Kawasaki H. A selective blockade of the cardiac inotropic effect of adrenaline by sodium monofluoroacetate. Bull Osaka Med Sch 1966;12(1):1–4.

[13a] Reigart JR, Brueggeman JL, Keil JE. Sodium Fluoroacetate poisioning. Am J Dis Child 1975;129(10):1224–6.

[14] Chi CH, Lin TK, Chen KW. Hemodynamic abnormalities in sodium monofluoroacetate intoxication. Hum Exp Toxicol 1999;18(6):351–3.

[15] Norris WR, Temple WA, Eason CT, et al. Sorption of fluoroacetate (compound 1080) by Colestipol, activated charcoal and anion-exchange in resins in vitro and gastrointestinal decontamination in rats. Vet Hum Toxicol 2000;42(5):269–75.

[16] Omara F, Sisodia CS. Evaluation of potential antidotes for sodium fluoroacetate in mice. Vet Hum Toxicol 1990;32(5):427–31.

[17] Taitelman U, Roy A, Raikhlin-Eisenkraft B, et al. The effect of monoacetin and calcium chloride on acid-base balance and survival in experimental sodium fluoroacetate poisoning. Arch Toxicol Suppl 1983;6:222–7.

[18] Stark AA. Threat assessment of mycotoxins as weapons: molecular mechanisms of acute toxicity. J Food Prot 2005;68(6):1285–93.

[19] Bennett JW, Klich M. Mycotoxins. Clin Microbiol Rev 2003;16(3):497–516.

[20] Parent-Massin D. Haematotoxicity of trichothecenes. Toxicol Lett 2004;153(1):75–81.

[21] Cieslak TJ, Talbot TB, Hartstein BH. Biological warfare and the skin I: bacteria and toxins. Clin Dermatol 2002;20(4):346–54.
[22] Etzel RA. Mycotoxins. JAMA 2002;287(4):425–7.
[23] Wannemacher R, Weiner S. Trichothecene mycotoxins. In: Sidell F, editor. Textbook of military medicine. Washington, DC: TMM Publications; 1997. p. 655–9.
[24] Paterson RR. Fungi and fungal toxins as weapons. Mycol Res 2006;110(Pt 9):1003–10.
[25] Chan PK, Gentry PA. LD50 values and serum biochemical changes induced by T-2 toxin in rats and rabbits. Toxicol Appl Pharmacol 1984;73(3):402–10.
[26] Coulombe RA Jr. Biological action of mycotoxins. J Dairy Sci 1993;76(3):880–91.
[27] Rosenbloom M, Leikin JB, Vogel SN, et al. Biological and chemical agents: a brief synopsis. Am J Ther 2002;9(1):5–14.
[28] Beasley VR, Swanson SP, Corley RA, et al. Pharmacokinetics of the trichothecene mycotoxin, T-2 toxin, in swine and cattle. Toxicon 1986;24(1):13–23.
[29] Babich H, Borenfreund E. Cytotoxicity of T-2 toxin and its metabolites determined with the neutral red cell viability assay. Appl Environ Microbiol 1991;57(7):2101–3.
[30] Zheng MZ, Richard JL, Binder J. A review of rapid methods for the analysis of mycotoxins. Mycopathologia 2006;161(5):261–73.
[31] McKean C, Tang L, Billam M, et al. Comparative acute and combinative toxicity of aflatoxin B1 and T-2 toxin in animals and immortalized human cell lines. J Appl Toxicol 2006;26(2):139–47.
[32] Biselli S, Hummert C. Development of a multicomponent method for Fusarium toxins using LC-MS/MS and its application during a survey for the content of T-2 toxin and deoxynivalenol in various feed and food samples. Food Addit Contam 2005;22(8): 752–60.
[33] Widestrand J, Lundh T, Pettersson H, et al. A rapid and sensitive cytotoxicity screening assay for trichothecenes in cereal samples. Food Chem Toxicol 2003;41(10): 1307–13.
[34] Zajtchuck R, editor. Textbook of military medicine. Washington, DC: TMM Publications; 2002. Other riot control compounds.
[35] Pitten FA, Muller G, Konig P, et al. Risk assessment of a former military base contaminated with organoarsenic-based warfare agents: uptake of arsenic by terrestrial plants. Sci Total Environ 1999;226(2–3):237–45.
[36] Appendix A-Chronology of significant terrorist incidents, 2003. Patterns of Global Terrorism. The Office of the Coordinator for Counterterrorism; 2004.
[37] Katsva M. Threat of chemical and biological terrorism in Russia. Nonproliferation, demilitarization, and arms control. Center for International Trade and Security at the University of Georgia [special issue]. The Monitor 1997;3(2):14–16.
[38] Ellison D. Handbook of chemical and biological warfare agents. Boca Raton (FL): CRC Press LLC; 2000.
[39] McGown EL, van Ravenswaay T, Dumlao CR. Histologic changes in nude mouse skin and human skin xenografts following exposure to sulfhydryl reagents: arsenicals. Toxicol Pathol 1987;15(2):149–56.
[40] Ishii K, Tamaoka A, Otsuka F, et al. Diphenylarsinic acid poisoning from chemical weapons in Kamisu, Japan. Ann Neurol 2004;56(5):741–5.
[41] Haas R, Tsivunchyk O, Steinbach K, et al. Conversion of adamsite (phenarsarzin chloride) by fungal manganese peroxidase. Appl Microbiol Biotechnol 2004;63(5): 564–6.
[42] Ochi T, Suzuki T, Isono H, et al. In vitro cytotoxic and genotoxic effects of diphenylarsinic acid, a degradation product of chemical warfare agents. Toxicol Appl Pharmacol 2004; 200(1):64–72.
[43] Landsberg JH, Hall S, Johannessen JN, et al. Saxitoxin puffer fish poisoning in the United States, with the first report of Pyrodinium bahamense as the putative toxin source. Environ Health Perspect 2006;114(10):1502–7.

[44] Paralytic shellfish poisoning—Massachusetts and Alaska, 1990. MMWR Morb Mortal Wkly Rep 1991;40(10):157–61.

[45] Llewellyn LE. Saxitoxin, a toxic marine natural product that targets a multitude of receptors. Nat Prod Rep 2006;23(2):200–22.

[46] Fleming JJ, Du Bois J. A synthesis of (+)-saxitoxin. J Am Chem Soc 2006;128(12):3926–7.

[47] Wang J, Salata JJ, Bennett PB. Saxitoxin is a gating modifier of HERG K+ channels. J Gen Physiol 2003;121(6):583–98.

[48] Gleick P. Water and terrorism. Water Policy 2006;8:481–503.

[49] Donaghy M. Neurologists and the threat of bioterrorism. J Neurol Sci 2006;249(1):55–62.

[50] Penzotti JL, Fozzard HA, Lipkind GM, et al. Differences in saxitoxin and tetrodotoxin binding revealed by mutagenesis of the Na+ channel outer vestibule. Biophys J 1998;75(6): 2647–57.

[51] de Carvalho M, Jacinto J, Ramos N, et al. Paralytic shellfish poisoning: clinical and electrophysiological observations. J Neurol 1998;245(8):551–4.

[52] Wong M, Ruck B, Shih R, et al. Two cases of suspected saxitoxin poisoning from puffer fish ingestion. J Toxicol Clin Toxicol 2002;40(5):613–4.

[53] Neurologic illness associated with eating Florida pufferfish–2002. Can Commun Dis Rep 2002;28(13):108–11.

[54] Garcia C, del Carmen Bravo M, Lagos M, et al. Paralytic shellfish poisoning: post-mortem analysis of tissue and body fluid samples from human victims in the Patagonia fjords. Toxicon 2004;43(2):149–58.

[55] Andrinolo D, Michea LF, Lagos N. Toxic effects, pharmacokinetics and clearance of saxitoxin, a component of paralytic shellfish poison (PSP), in cats. Toxicon 1999;37(3):447–64.

[56] Stafford RG, Hines HB. Urinary elimination of saxitoxin after intravenous injection. Toxicon 1995;33(11):1501–10.

[57] Bell P, Gessner B, Hall G, et al. Assay of saxitoxin in samples from human victims of paralytic shellfish poisoning by binding competition to saxiphilin and block of single sodium channels [abstract]. Toxicon 1996;34(3):337.

[58] Doucette M, Logan F, Dolah F, et al. Analysis of samples from a human PSP intoxication event using a saxitoxin receptor assay and HPLC [abstract]. Toxicon 1996;34(3):337.

[59] Van Egmond HP, Van Den Top HJ. Worldwide regulations for marine phycotoxins. Presented at the CNEVA, Proceedings of Symposium of Marine Biotoxins. Paris, January 30–31, 1991.

ELSEVIER
SAUNDERS

EMERGENCY
MEDICINE
CLINICS OF
NORTH AMERICA

Emerg Med Clin N Am 25 (2007) 567–595

Chemical Terrorism Attacks: Update on Antidotes

David T. Lawrence, DO*, Mark A. Kirk, MD

Blue Ridge Poison Center, Division of Medical Toxicology, Department of Emergency Medicine, University of Virginia, P.O. Box 800744, Charlottesville, VA 22908-0774, USA

Few true antidotal therapies are available for acute poisonings. Most toxicologic emergencies are managed with attention to good supportive care. There has been increasing concern that biological, chemical, or radioactive agents will be used by terrorists. In this article, the authors explain the rationale, indications, and practical application of several antidotes that will become necessary in the event of a criminal or terrorist attack using one of several potential agents. These antidotes will often need to be initiated before the completion of confirmatory tests. Therefore, the toxin must be suspected based on clinical presentation, and empiric therapy must be initiated swiftly to minimize morbidity and mortality.

Nerve agents

Background

Nerve agents were designed for use on the battlefield. Though rarely employed in warfare, recent documented use includes the Iraqi military's use against Iranian troops and the Kurds in the 1980s [1] and the Aum Shinrikyo cult's release in Japan in 1994 and 1995 [2]. Nerve agents are acetylcholinesterase enzyme inhibitors similar to organophosphate insecticides. The action of acetylcholine released into a synaptic cleft or neuromuscular junction is normally terminated when the enzyme acetylcholinesterase cleaves acetylcholine into choline and acetic acid [3]. Organophosphorous nerve agents are irreversible inhibitors of the cholinesterase enzymes. This inhibition causes an increase in the acetylcholine concentration and a marked

---

* Corresponding author.
E-mail address: dtl4n@virginia.edu (D.T. Lawrence).

0733-8627/07/$ - see front matter © 2007 Published by Elsevier Inc.
doi:10.1016/j.emc.2007.02.002

emed.theclinics.com

hyperstimulation of the cholinergic system, which is responsible for the predominant signs of toxicity [4].

There are two types of cholinergic receptors: muscarinic and nicotinic. Muscarinic receptors are found on organs innervated by the parasympathetic nervous system and in the central nervous system (CNS). Nicotinic receptors are found at the neuromuscular junction, the autonomic ganglia (sympathetic and parasympathetic), and in the CNS (Fig. 1) [3].

Peripheral muscarinic overstimulation causes systemic toxic effects. In the eye, contraction of the iris causes miosis, and contraction of the ciliary muscle causes eye pain and lack of accommodation [4]. Miosis was seen in 99% of the victims who had moderate to severe nerve agent exposure from the Tokyo sarin incident, and darkness of visual field was the most common subjective complaint. After exposure to sarin, many patients from the Matsumoto and Tokyo sarin attacks complained of eye pain, blurry vision, and headache [2].

Rhinorrhea, salivation, sweating, lacrimation, abdominal cramping, vomiting, and diarrhea are prominent symptoms [4]. Respiratory distress is caused by increased respiratory secretions and bronchospasm [5]. Overstimulation of the muscarinic system causes bradycardia. However, nicotinic effects, hypoxia, and/or anxiety may predominate and patients will instead be

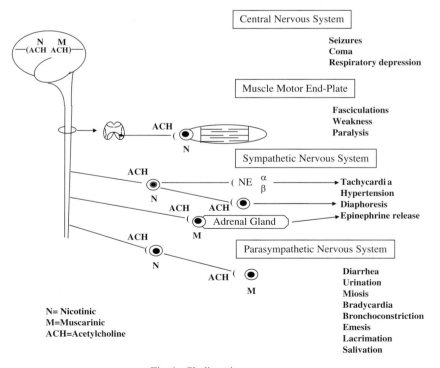

Fig. 1. Cholinergic receptors.

tachycardic [2]. Peripheral nicotinic effects include the sympathomimetic effects tachycardia and hypertension [6,7]. Effects at the neuromuscular junction cause muscle fasciculations, which can rapidly progress to fatigue and paralysis [3]. CNS effects are not specific and can present as anxiety; giddiness; headache; and cognitive changes, which can progress to coma, seizures, and central apnea [3,4]. Nerve agent intoxication therefore presents as a mixture of parasympathetic effects, sympathomimetic effects, neuromuscular failure, and CNS impairment.

The great majority of deaths due to nerve agents occur secondary to respiratory failure. This is due to bronchospasm and increased respiratory secretions, paralysis of the muscles of respiration, and central apnea [7]. A recent study using an animal model supports the importance of CNS effects in acute respiratory failure [8].

Seizures are a major cause of morbidity and mortality due to nerve agent poisoning. Nerve agent–induced seizures are believed to progress through three stages. In the first 5 minutes, seizures appear to be due to cholinergic overstimulation. During this period, an agent with central anticholinergic properties can abort or prevent seizures. After 5 minutes, other changes are noted including decrease in brain norepinephrine, increased glutaminergic response, and activation of N-methyl-D-aspartate (NMDA) glutamate receptors. At this point, a mixed cholinergic and noncholinergic stage is entered, and anticholinergic treatment alone will not terminate seizures. After 40 minutes, continuing seizure activity is mediated by noncholinergic mechanisms and results in structural neuronal injury [9–11].

Route of exposure

Patients will respond differently depending on the route of exposure [12]. Understanding the differences in presenting symptoms is vital for prompt, accurate diagnosis. Patients exposed to vapor will show symptoms within seconds to minutes. With a small vapor exposure, miosis, rhinorhea, and slight bronchospasm will be seen. This will progress to marked dyspnea with obvious secretions as the exposure continues. Those who have large exposures will progress to loss of consciousness, generalized fasciculations, convulsions, paralysis, and apnea [12].

Patients who have dermal exposure to liquid nerve agents may have delayed effects. The duration of the latent period depends on the amount to which the victim is exposed. Onset of symptoms may be delayed. There can be a delay of up to 18 hours before developing symptoms after dermal exposure to a nerve agent [12]. Contact with the skin will cause localized sweating and possibly fasciculations of the underlying muscles. Later patients will experience nausea, vomiting and diarrhea, generalized sweating, and fatigue. Symptoms can be seen earlier, within 2 to 30 minutes, with large exposures. The symptoms of larger exposures include those stated previously as well as loss of consciousness, convulsions, generalized fasciculations, increased secretions, paralysis, and apnea [12,13]. In contrast to vapor exposure, a dermal exposure will delay the development of miosis [12]. The delayed presentation and lack of miosis can make the diagnosis of a nerve agent exposure difficult. The extreme potency of these agents is illustrated by the fact that a droplet of the nerve agent VX less than one fifth of the size of the Lincoln Memorial on the back of a penny has the potential to kill the average human within 30 minutes if placed on unbroken skin [13].

Antidotal treatments

To minimize morbidity and mortality, several treatments must be initiated as soon as possible after recognition of nerve agent poisoning. Three antidotes with different mechanisms are available and act additively to combat the toxic effects of nerve agent poisoning.

Atropine

Mechanism. Atropine acts at muscarinic cholinergic receptors as a competitive antagonist. It is used to counter muscarinic effects, and administration will result in drying of secretions, alleviating bronchospasm, and reversing central apnea [4]. Given within the first 5 minutes, it can prevent organophosphate-induced seizures [14,15].

Indications. Atropine is indicated for any patient who has clinical signs and symptoms consistent with acetylcholinesterase inhibition and confirmed or suspected nerve agent exposure (Table 1). Miosis alone is not an indication for atropine administration [7].

Delivery. Atropine can be given either intravenous (IV) or intramuscular (IM) using the Mark 1 autoinjector kit (Survival Technology, Inc., Rockville, Maryland) (Fig. 2). Autoinjectors have been shown to be effective at administering certain medication, including atropine. Delivery by autoinjector is more effective than IM injections using a convential syringe [16]. The

Table 1
Indications for Atropine Treatment

Symptoms	Severity	Treatment	Disposition
None or isolated miosis	Minimal	None	Home after observation
Rhinorrhea, lacrimation, or mild dyspnea	Mild	Atropine	Home after recovery
Inability to ambulate, dyspnea, vomiting, fasiculations, weakness	Moderate	Atropine, 2-PAM, Benzodiazepines	Admit
Convulsions, coma, respiratory insufficiency	Severe	Atropine, 2-PAM, Benzodiazepines	Admit to ICU

(Adapted from [3,4,13,17,33]).

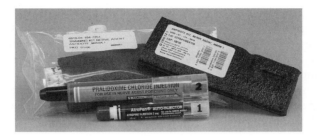

Fig. 2. Mark 1 kit.

autoinjectors also have the advantage of delivering a dose of medicine directly through clothing, including protective garments [16].

Additional atropine doses should be administered IV once access is obtained. The standard field treatment for severe poisoning is three autoinjectors or 6 mg initially with retreatment every 5 to 10 minutes. The initial intravenous dose should be 2 mg for adults or 0.02 mg/kg for children [17]. Additional dosing is based on clinical effects; therefore, there is no set dose for atropine in nerve agent poisoning. Atropine doses should be repeated every 5 minutes until the therapeutic endpoint is reached (ie, until pulmonary secretions are dried [reflected by improved oxygenation] and ease of breathing [or ease of ventilation]) [18]. From case reports, the typical total dose required after nerve agent poisoning has ranged from 5 to 20 mg [16,18]. However, similar to organophosphate insecticide poisoning, there are reports of larger doses (up to 200 mg) of atropine used to treat nerve agent casualties [2,19]. Tachycardia can occur in nerve agent poisoning due to stimulation of the sympathetic ganglia as well as respiratory distress and hypoxia. Tachycardia is not a contraindication to atropine administration [20].

Precautions. Excessive doses of atropine can result in deleterious effects including delirium, agitation, and tachycardia and hypertension. Atropine will likely not improve miosis or skeletal muscle paralysis; therefore, reversal of these effects is not a therapeutic endpoint. Attempting to reverse these findings with atropine can result in administration of excessive doses of atropine [17,21].

Benzodiazepines

Benzodiazepines are needed to prevent or treat nerve agent–induced seizures [22,23]. Aborting nerve agent–induced seizures is vital because it can prevent neuronal damage [24,25].

Mechanism. Benzodiazepines are potent gamma-aminobutyric acid (GABA) receptor agonists. They increase the effects of GABA at the GABA-A receptor, resulting in hyperpolarization of neurons from enhanced chloride entry [26]. The addition of benzodiazepine [27] therapy is necessary to terminate nerve agent–induced seizures because anticholinergic treatment is increasingly less effective from 5 minutes postexposure to 40 minutes [9]. Evidence suggests that pentobarbital may also terminate seizures and reduce neuronal damage because of its potent effects at the GABA-A receptor [9,10,28]. However, subsequent respiratory depression following this therapy would be impractical and unsafe in the field with a patient who is nonintubated. Fosphenytoin does not affect GABA-A and has been found to be ineffective in controlling nerve agent–induced seizures [29].

Indications. Benzodiazapines should be administered to any patient who has significant symptoms from nerve agent exposure. Benzodiazepines should be infused rapidly to unresponsive patients who have been exposed to nerve agents, because such patients may have nonconvulsive seizures due to the onset of paralysis [20]. Benzodiazapines are also useful for helping to alleviate the extreme anxiety many patients will be experiencing [30].

Delivery. The currently available autoinjectors deliver an IM dose of 10 mg of diazepam (Fig. 3). Once a patient arrives in the hospital, the benzodiazepine of choice should be midazolam [18]; although in resource-limited situations diazepam or lorazapam are acceptable alternatives. Several animal models demonstrate midazolam's superiority to other benzodiazepines [22,23]. Midazolam is also more readily absorbed after IM injection, a critically important route of administration until an IV is established.

Precautions. Benzodiazapines are sedatives and in large doses can cause respiratory depression. Therefore, caution must be used when administering to patients who do not have a protected airway. However, recent studies using animal models have indicated that benzodiazepines may help prevent apnea caused by nerve agents [31].

Pralidoxime
   Neither atropine nor benzodiazepines will alleviate symptoms affecting the nicotinic system. Over time, nerve agents will form an irreversible covalent bond with acetylcholinesterase in a process termed *aging*. Specific agents age at different rates. For example, soman rapidly and permanently

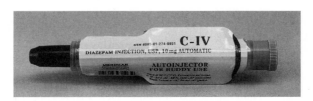

Fig. 3. Diazepam autoinjector.

disables the acetylcholinesterase enzyme in 2 to 6 minutes; sarin and VX age more slowly with 50% of affected acetylcholinesterase being permanently disabled in 5 hours and 48 hours, respectively. Once aging occurs, the patient will not regain vital functions, such as muscle strength or respiratory drive, until new enzyme is synthesized [30]. This may take weeks to months [3,20]. It is for this reason that oximes were developed. An oxime reactivates acetylcholinesterase if administered before aging. There are several oximes that have been tested as treatment for organophosphate toxicity [32]. Pralidoxime (2-PAM) is the only one currently approved for use in the United States.

Mechanism. Organophosphates form a covalent bond with the active site of acetylcholinesterase, preventing it from inactivating acetylcholine. 2-PAM is attracted to the active site of acetylcholinesterase, and its nucleophilic oxime moiety will attack the phosphate atom of the nerve agent. This will displace it from the active site, reactivating the enzyme (Fig. 4).

Indications. 2-PAM should be given to any patient exposed to an organophosphate nerve agent who is showing any systemic toxicity. This is particularly true if there are fasiculations or weakness.

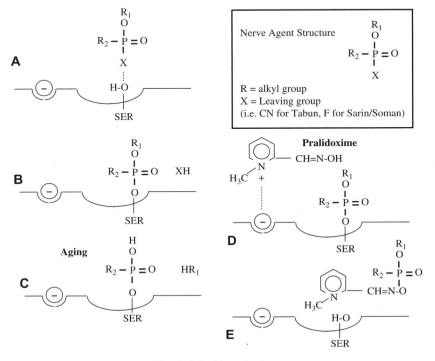

Fig. 4. 2-PAM mechanism.

Delivery. 2-PAM can be delivered IV (Fig. 5) or intramuscular IM. The preferred route is IV, although IM administration with a Mark 1 autoinjector is acceptable in the field before establishing an IV line. The initial dose should be given as quickly as possible to prevent aging [3].

The initial dose is 1 to 2 g diluted in 100 mL normal saline and given over 15 to 30 minutes. The initial pediatric dose is 20 to 50 mg/kg up to 2 g [33]. It has been generally recommended that a plasma concentration of 4 ug/ml be maintained [12,34]; although this absolute value has been disputed by some [30]. It is taken from older animal studies and the plasma concentrations will not be available for treatment decisions. However, it is important to note that 2-PAM is rapidly excreted by the kidney with a half-life of approximately 90 minutes and that 80% to 90% will be excreted within 3 hours [12]. Therefore, a continuous infusion is often recommended after the loading dose to maintain therapeutic levels [20,35,36]. The current World Health Organization recommendation is greater than a 30-mg/kg bolus followed by greater than an 8-mg/kg/hour infusion [37]. A study using healthy volunteers found that an infusion of 2-PAM was well tolerated and achieved consistent therapeutic levels [38]. Studies in patients who had moderate to severe toxicity from insecticide organophosphates have shown good results and no adverse effects with infusions of 500 mg/hour [36,39,40]. A series of pediatric patients showed no adverse effects to infusion rates of 9 to 19 mg/kg/hour [35]. A reasonable treatment regimen for severely poisoned patients would be 2 g IM or slow IV infusion over 15 to 30 minutes followed by a 500-mg/hour infusion.

Each Mark 1 autoinjector will deliver 600 mg of 2-PAM. It is recommended to administer three Mark 1 autoinjectors to severely poisoned patients delivering 1800 mg of 2-PAM, which is nearly the maximum recommended initial dose. Therefore, if a patient is still showing signs of cholinergic excess

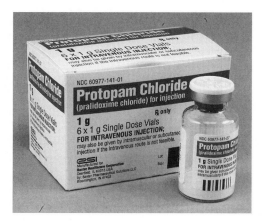

Fig. 5. Pralidoxime chloride single-dose vials.

after three Mark 1 kits, further treatment should include only the atropine portion of subsequent Mark 1 kits [41].

After initial 2-PAM administration, it is vital that additional atropine be given as necessary to reduce secretions and ease respirations [12].

Precautions. Delivering 2-PAM more rapidly than recommended can result in hypertension. This is usually self-limited, but in extreme cases, phentolamine 5 mg IV may be effective [3,12]. Laryngospasm and rigidity can also occur with rapid IV administration [33].

A recent series of studies shows a lack of benefit of 2-PAM and even potential harm when oximes are used in organophosphate poisoning [42–44]. However, these trials presented numerous variables, such as varying range of severity, varying time passed between exposure and treatment, and numerous other treatments rendered. Also, instead of studying nerve agent poisoning directly, these studied explored the use of oximes in organophosphate insecticide toxicity that are known to be less potent and have longer aging half times than nerve agents. At this point, given the body of evidence provided by in vitro and animal studies regarding the usefulness of 2-PAM and the significant clinical experience, the authors believe that there are not enough data to abandon using this antidote particularly when dealing with nerve agent poisoning.

Pediatrics

Children are a particular concern in regards to exposure to nerve agents. Their increased minute ventilation per body weight gives them a higher relative risk with exposure, and their smaller airways make respiratory difficulty more likely with bronchospasm and increased secretions. Children are also more prone to seizures [33]. Antidotes for nerve agent toxicity have not been well studied in children. Autoinjectors for 2-PAM and diazepam are marketed in adult doses only (600 mg and 10 mg, respectively). Atropine autoinjectors are manufactured in 2 mg (adult), 1 mg, and 0.5 mg sizes.

The dose for atropine can be up to 0.05 to 0.1 mg/kg either IV, IM, or intraosseous. Children over 40 kg can be administered an adult (2 mg) autoinjector. Children over 20 kg can receive a 1-mg autoinjector, and those over 10 kg can receive a 0.5-mg autoinjector.

The dose for 2-PAM is 25 to 50 mg/kg, up to a total of 2 g. A child over 12 kg will be able to tolerate the dose of one 600-mg 2-PAM autoinjector. Autoinjectors should be used with caution and the injection site should be carefully chosen in children because the needle is approximately 1 inch long [33]. Diazepam should be dosed at 0.05 to 0.3 mg/kg IV, and children over 30 kg can receive an adult autoinjector [33].

Undertreating a seriously poisoned patient is far more dangerous than causing mild toxicity from aggressive antidote administration [45,46]. Studies of accidental administration of adult atropine autoinjectors to children have shown that they can develop anticholoinergic symptoms, but no serious morbidity or mortality has been reported [46–48].

Strategy for mass exposures

CHEMPACK project

In the event of a chemical attack, immediate treatment of exposed individuals using appropriate antidotes is required. The large number of victims seeking medical care could easily overwhelm a hospital's resources. Many hospitals do not have sufficient stocks of antidotes to accommodate one or a few organophosphate insecticide–poisoned patients. Limited supplies of antidotes occur because the pharmaceuticals have variable shelf lives and replacing them is costly. For this reason, the US Centers for Disease Control implemented the CHEMPACK project. It is part of the US Centers for Disease Control Strategic National Stockpile, and its goal is to provide localities with antidotes to care for multiple victims exposed to nerve agents.

The containers holding the antidotes are kept at secure locations in selected localities. These containers keep a large number of Mark 1 autoinjectors; diazepam autoinjectors; and multidose vials of antidotes with syringes for injection, which can be deployed in a mass exposure. Local emergency planners and health departments are developing plans to integrate the CHEMPACK project into existing emergency response plans and preparedness efforts. More information can be obtained regarding the mechanism of mobilizing the CHEMPACK antidotes locally by contacting the community's emergency management organization.

Alternative sources of antidotes

If a facility begins to run low on atropine, there are several other agents that can be considered as substitutes. Glycopyrrolate is a peripherally acting antimuscarinic; it will dry secretions and help relieve bronchospasm but will have no central effects. Scopolamine has been used effectively [17,49,50]. Scopolamine may actually have an advantage because it has more potent central anticholinergic effects than atropine. Animal studies have demonstrated effectiveness of other anticholinergic agents including diphenhydramine [51] and jimsonweed extract [52].

Cyanide

Background

Cyanide is a potent poison with an extensive history as an agent of harm. It only takes a small amount to cause severe symptoms or death. Acute toxicity can occur through various routes, including inhalation, ingestion, dermal exposure, or parenteral administration [53]. Cyanide poisoning can result from many different sources including industrial accidents, ingestion of cyanide salts or substances that are biotransformed into cyanide, and from criminal poisoning [54]. Victims of smoke inhalation are also often exposed to significant amounts of cyanide in addition to carbon monoxide [55].

Because of its potency, cyanide has a potential as a weapon of terror. Methods of delivery could involve releasing cyanide in either a gaseous, liquid, or solid form. Weaponized cyanide has most often been delivered as the volatile liquids, hydrogen cyanide, or cyanogen chloride [56]. Alternatively, a solid cyanide salt, such as potassium cyanide, could be introduced to a mineral acid–releasing hydrogen cyanide gas [57,58]. At a concentration of 120 to 150 mg/m^3 (110–135 parts per million), cyanide can be fatal in approximately 30 minutes. A cyanide concentration of 300 mg/m^3 (270 parts per million) can cause immediate death [59]. Cyanide could also be introduced into food, drink, or medicines. An obvious example is the seven people killed by acetaminophen capsules adulterated with potassium cyanide [60]. An additional recent example: after being given 1.5 g of potassium cyanide, a 17-year-old male collapsed, seized, and developed profound hemodynamic instability after ingesting a tainted carbonated beverage containing 1.5 g of potassium cyanide. He died despite aggressive treatment [61]. An ingestion of as little as 50 mg could be fatal. Cyanide can cause systemic toxicity through dermal contact and can obviously cause toxicity when injected [62].

Cyanide exerts its toxic effects by inhibiting numerous enzymes. Cyanide's primary toxic action is inducing cellular hypoxia through inhibition of cytochrome oxidase. This enzyme is necessary for oxidative phosphorylation and therefore aerobic energy production [54]. This inhibition is accomplished when cyanide binds to the ferric ion of cytochrome aa3 and blocks oxygen's use in the last step of cellular respiration. The resulting shift from aerobic to anaerobic metabolism causes a depletion of cellular adenosine triphosphate and an accumulation of lactic acid [63].

The timing and extent of symptoms can vary depending on amount, duration, and route of exposure. Toxicity will usually manifest as CNS and cardiac toxicity because these are the most oxygen-sensitive systems. An exposure to a concentrated source of cyanide can cause death within seconds to minutes, making the provision of medical aid impossible. A lesser exposure can cause nonspecific symptoms including shortness of breath, hyperventilation, headache, weakness, and dizziness, which can be attributed to anxiety or other exposures [53].

The CNS signs and symptoms can progress to confusion, lethargy, seizures, and coma. It induces a neurally mediated tachypnea along with an initial rise in blood pressure. However, toxicity can progress to cardiac arrest heralded by bradycardia and hypotension. Classically, a cherry red skin color is described, secondary to increased venous O_2 saturation. However, this is not commonly seen and should not be relied on for diagnosis. Similar color between the arteries and veins has been visualized on fundiscopic examination [54].

Cyanide antidote kit

Mechanism

The only antidote currently available in the United States is the cyanide antidote kit. It consists of amyl nitrite, sodium nitrite, and sodium thiosulfate (Fig. 6). The nitrites (amyl and sodium) induce methemoglobinemia. Cyanide has a higher affinity for methemoglobin and will leave the mitochondria to bind to it and allow the mitochondria to resume oxidatitive phosphorylation. Sodium thiosulfate acts as a sulfhydryl donor for the enzyme rhodanese that converts cyanide to the less-toxic renally excreted thiocyanate [61,64].

Indications

Antidotal is indicated for any patient clinically suspected of having cyanide toxicity. Consider cyanide toxicity early in any patient who has sudden loss of consciousness and any combination of seizures, hemodynamic instability without a definitive cause. An elevated lactic acid is an important laboratory clue [63,65], although therapeutic actions may be needed before the results of diagnostic tests are available. An arterial or venous blood gas in a symptomatic patient will demonstrate metabolic acidosis. A narrowing of the oxygen saturation between an arterial and a mixed venous blood sample (narrow oxygen saturation gap) is highly suggestive of cyanide toxicity

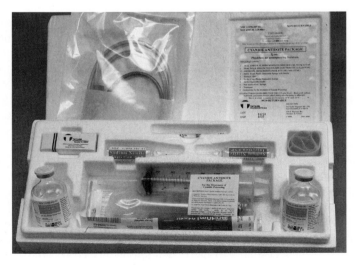

Fig. 6. Cyanide antidote kit.

[66]. Treatment should be initiated for patients who have these concerning presentations. Particularly, clusters of patients who present with rapid onset of a critical condition, victims of structural fires, or individuals involved in a high-risk activity (jeweler or lab worker) should be suspect. Cyanide levels can be obtained for later confirmation, but cyanide levels do not alter clinical management because of the time it takes for laboratory analysis. No rapid diagnostic tests are currently available to confirm cyanide poisoning. Therefore, clinicians must have a high index of suspicion based on clinical presentations and surrogate markers to initiate therapy.

Delivery

Amyl nitrite is supplied within glass pearls intended to be crushed and inhaled primarily through bag–valve mask–assisted ventilation. It is intended for use until an IV line is established. Administer pearls intermittently, 30 seconds per minute, and use a new pearl every 3 minutes ([53]). This initial step is meant to induce a methemoglobin level of approximately 3% to 5%, but amyl nitrite effects are unreliable [53]. Once an IV line is established, intravenous sodium nitrite is the preferred methemoglobin inducer. Sodium nitrite is more effective at inducing methemoglobinemia. Administer 10 mL of the 3% solution (300 mg) over 2 to 4 minutes [56]. In pediatric cases, it is imperative that the dose be carefully calculated. Children can develop excessive methemoglobinemia after nitrite administration [67]. Doses are calculated using the patient's weight and hemoglobin concentration. When hemoglobin is normal, a dose of 10 mg/kg is recommended. However, it is often not reasonable to wait for a hemoglobin level [54]. If the hemoglobin is unknown, it is reasonable to treat with 6 mg/kg because this will be safe even for a significantly anemic child [68].

Sodium thiosulfate should be delivered as an intravenous dose of 50 mL of a 25% solution. This provides 12.5 g of sodium thiosulfate. The pediatric dose is 1.65 mL/kg of the 25% solution given over 10 minutes [53]. Thiosulfate does not have any significant inherent toxicity; rare hypersensitivity reactions and rate-dependant hypotension may occur [64]. Although effective, sodium thiosulfate has a slow onset of antidotal action [59]. This can limit its usefulness as a monotherapy in severe poisonings. The combination of nitrite and thiosulfate is more effective (synergistic) compared with thiosulfate alone [56].

Early supportive treatment is essential. Assurance of airway protection, adequate ventilation, and optimizing oxygen are the first priority. Acidemia must be treated with adequate ventilation and bicarbonate. This will also enhance the efficacy of the antidote kit [54]. Delivery of high-level oxygen has synergistic anticyanide activity with sodium thiosulfate [69]. If the patient has an adequately protected airway, activated charcoal administration may be administered following oral exposures. Charcoal will bind cyanide, and any amount removed could have a significant impact on the clinical course or duration of treatment needed [54].

Precautions

Nitrite administration can result in several adverse reactions. Vasodilatation with hypotension and tachycardia can occur, particularly with rapid administration or supratherapeutic dosing [53]. This could limit its usefulness in already hemodynamically compromised patients [70]. Generating methemoglobinemia lowers the oxygen carrying capacity. This is especially concerning when treating cyanide-poisoned patients also suspected being poisoned by carbon monoxide, such as in victims of smoke inhalation [71]. Therefore, it is often recommended to forgo the nitrite portion of the antidote kit in smoke inhalation victims. There is evidence showing that giving the standard dose of sodium nitrite will raise the methemoglobin level to a maximum of 10.5%; this does not occur for 35 to 70 minutes, suggesting sodium nitrite may be safe to give to victims of smoke inhalation [72]. However, in those who have severe anemia or a confirmed high carbon monoxide level, the induction of significant methemoglobinemia may dangerously lower oxygen-carrying capacity. Consideration should be given to adjusting the dose or forgoing treatment with the nitrite portion of the kit.

Amyl nitrite is considered a pregnancy category X medication and should not be administered in the case of pregnancy [53]. Patients who have glucose-6-phosphate dehydrogenase deficiency have a risk of hemolysis if given thiosulfate [53]. In the presence of renal failure, thiocyanate can have toxic effects, including abdominal pain, vomiting, rash, and CNS dysfunction. If symptoms are severe enough, thiocyanate can be dialyzed [64,73].

Hydroxocobalamin

Because of the difficulty with availability and the complexity of administering the current cyanide antidote kit, an alternative antidote has been sought. Hydroxocobalamin has generated much interest as a potentially safer and simpler antidote for cyanide toxicity [57,71,74]. Hydroxocobalamin was recently approved in the United States by the US Federal Drug Administration (FDA) for treatment of cyanide poisoning. It has been investigated as a cyanide antidote for over 40 years [75–77], and it has been licensed as a cyanide antidote in France since 1996 [78].

Mechanism

Hydroxocobalamin combines with cyanide in an equimolar ratio to form cyanocobalamin [79]. Cyanocobalamin is also known as vitamin B-12; it is nontoxic and renally eliminated.

Indication

Hydroxocobalamin should be administered to any patient suspected of having cyanide toxicity. Its use should also be strongly considered in patients suffering the effects of smoke inhalation. Given its safety profile, there should be a low threshold to administer this treatment in patients who have possible cyanide exposures.

Delivery

Hydroxocobalamin is given as a 5-g IV dose. The pediatric dose is 70 mg/k up to 5 grams. This dose should be given over 15 minutes. Hydroxocobalamin is supplied in 250-mL vials, each containing 2.5 g of hydroxocobalamin, which are to be diluted in 100 mL of normal saline [80]. This amount will bind up to 250 mg of cyanide [57]. The dose can be repeated in a serious poisoning [59]. This antidote should be used in combination with sodium thiosulfate. They have synergistic effects, strengthening each other's antidotal efficacy [71]. Hydroxocobalamin can transiently raise blood pressure, a finding that has been seen in human [81,82] and animal [83,84] studies. This can potentially benefit those who are hemodynamically unstable due to cyanide toxicity and may help offset any hypotension induced by nitrite or sodium thiosulfate therapy. This effect is due to nitric oxide scavenging, which reduces the vasodilatation caused by cyanide toxicity [82]. It is recommended that hydroxocobalamin not be infused through the same site or at the same time as sodium thiosulfate. Thiosulfate binds hydroxocobalamin and renders it inactive [85]. It is recommended to give the faster acting hydroxocobalamin [86] first followed by sodium thiosulfate. This approach has been used successfully [87].

Precautions

Hydroxocobalamin is extremely safe when used as an antidote [71]. Allergic reactions are reported but only in patients receiving long-term treatment for pernicious anemia. Virtually every patient receiving a 5-g dose will develop red discoloration of the skin, mucous membranes, and urine. This discoloration typically resolves in 24 to 48 hours [57]. The same discoloration of the serum has been found to interfere with several laboratory tests [88]. These included serum iron, bilirubin, creatinine, and magnesium. Also a pustular rash developed in 11 of 66 subjects receiving a 5-g dose of hydroxocobalamin. The development was delayed until at least 1 week after infusion, and the rash resolved in 6 to 38 days [89].

Hydroxycobalamin's safety has been demonstrated in healthy volunteers [81,89] and has been used successfully to treat significantly poisoned patients [87,90,91]. Studies have shown it to be safe when administered empirically at fire scenes whether or not patients had cyanide poisoning [59,80]. If hydroxycobalamin were available, the combination of sodium thiosulfate and hydroxycobalamin could be given empirically as a safe and effective antidote in patients who have potential cyanide toxicity. This could eliminate the trepidation felt by many about giving the standard cyanide antidote kit to an unconfirmed exposure or to a victim of smoke inhalation.

Mass exposure

There is potential for a situation in which a large number of patients are exposed to cyanide and it will be likely that there are not adequate amounts of antidote kits [92,93]. The first step will be triage. Many patients who present will likely not in fact have significant cyanide toxicity. Those who present in cardiac arrest are unlikely to survive and treatment may have to be reserved for those who are more likely to survive.

It is reasonable to treat empirically with sodium thiosulfate alone. It is also important to realize that careful supportive care is extremely important even if there is inadequate antidote available. Although antidotal therapy is extremely important, supportive care alone has resulted in good outcome [94,95]. Careful attention to oxygenation, hemodynamic support, and correction of acidosis may be enough even without antidote availability.

Botulism

Background

Botulinum toxin is considered the most potent toxic substance. It has an LD50 of 1 ug/kg. Three distinct clinical entities exist for botulism: food bourne, infant, and wound [96]. There are seven distinct subtypes of clostridial neurotoxins (A, B, C1, D, E, F, and G) of which only A, B, E, and rarely F cause illness in humans [97–99].

Because of its extreme potency, botulism has gained attention as a possible bioterrorism agent. Potential modes of transmission are by introduction into food or water, aerosolization, or injection [99,100]. Recently a patient had a severe case of botulism after a cosmetic injection of unlicensed botulinum toxin [101].

After botulinum toxin is systemically absorbed, it attacks cholinergic presynaptic nerve ending. The toxin cannot cross the blood-brain barrier and therefore only affects the peripheral nervous system [96]. The toxin is taken up into the nerve by endocytosis and prevents the fusion of the synaptic vesicle with the nerve terminus [102]. Ultimately, the nerve cannot release acetylcholine, and neurotransmission is interrupted [103].

Clinical effects

The onset of symptoms is variable and delayed. Because of the delay, it can be challenging to identify the source. With food borne botulism, symptoms can appear as early as 2 hours postingestion but may not be noticed for up to 5 days. The time course for inhalational botulism is poorly understood, because of the small number of cases. However, the onset is believed to occur in approximately 3 days [104,105].

The presenting symptoms follow a typical pattern of descending weakness. This begins with cranial nerve dysfunction manifested as dysphagia, diplopia, and dysarthria. It progresses as a descending motor paralysis affecting the upper limbs, then the lower limbs. In severe cases, the intercostals and diaphragm are affected possibly necessitating mechanical ventilation [103,106]. Inhibition of muscarinic cholinergic function may be present such as: dry mouth, dilated pupils, and constipation [96]. Botulism transmitted by ingestion may also present with nausea and vomiting. These symptoms may precede neurologic symptoms [107]. Centrally, mentation is normal, and peripherally sensory involvement is lacking. This is helpful in distinguishing botulism from other neurologic conditions [107].

The paralysis caused by botulinum toxin will persist until the cleaved proteins are regenerated. Therefore, if a patient's condition progresses to the point of requiring mechanical ventilation, they can be ventilator-dependant for several months. For this reason, it is important to recognize botulism and initiate treatment with antitoxin as early as possible. Antitoxin treatment will not reverse any paralysis that has already occurred but will arrest the progression [105]. This can limit disability and prevent the need for intubation.

Antidote

The first step is careful supportive care, with attention to airway protection and ventilatory support. The definitive treatment for botulism is the administration of botulinum antitoxin. The standard antitoxin is a horse-derived serum with antibodies against subtypes A, B, and E. The antitoxin works by binding to and neutralizing any botulinum toxin that is free in the serum. It is important to initiate antitoxin therapy as soon as possible because the toxin must be neutralized before it is able to bind irreversibly to nerve terminus [106]. This therapy will be empiric, based on clinical suspicion, and no confirmatory tests will be readily available. There are several clues that should raise suspicion that an outbreak of botulism may have been caused by an intentional release of toxin: if there are a large number of patients; if there are multiple clusters without an identifiable source; when groups of patients share a common geographic connection; and outbreaks with the rare types C, D, F, G, or E [108].

A recent study found that patients who had food bourne botulism presenting with shortness of breath, impaired gag reflex, and no diarrhea had a high risk of death. In a situation with many victims and/or limited resources perhaps identifying this clinical syndrome could identify who needs more urgent antidotal therapy or transfer to a higher level of care [109].

Indication

Consider antitoxin administration in any patient who has a clinical presentation suspicious for botulism, particularly when a group of two or more presents with suggestive symptoms. Suspicious cases should be reported immediately to the local/state health department or contact the US Centers for

Disease Control directly to arrange antitoxin delivery [96,107]. The anti-toxin can only be obtained in this way, so notification should be initiated as soon as botulism is suspected. In addition, these public health agencies can initiate epidemiologic investigations to determine the source of poisoning.

Delivery

Administer 1 vial of immunoglobulin intravenously over 30 to 60 minutes after diluting 1:10 in normal saline [106].

Precautions

The antitoxin is a horse serum–derived product resulting in a significant chance of an allergic reaction. Historically, the incidence of allergic reactions has been reported to be 9%. Therefore, it is important to be well pre-pared in advance to treat any anaphylactic reaction [96]. Skin testing is recommended before administering the antitoxin [110]. However, further de-laying treatment to perform the skin test may not be feasible in some cases. Depending on the clinical scenario, the benefit of treating the illness as rapidly as possible may outweigh the risk of taking the additional time to skin test. Additionally, the rate of serious adverse reactions has declined to approximately 1% since the recommended dose was reduced to 1 vial [107]. Also, skin testing may not predict an adverse reaction. In one study, over half the patients who had an acute reaction had negative skin tests [111].

Other antidotes

The equine-derived antitoxin is not recommended to treat infant botu-lism. This is not only because of the high rate of adverse reactions, but also the fear of sensitizing infants against horses and horse-derived products for the rest of their lives. Recently, a human-derived immune globulin (baby-BIG) has been introduced [112,113] and should be used to treat infant botulism. It is effective for types A and B. In addition to infants, Baby-BIG can be considered for those who have had a serious reaction to the trivalent antibody and were not able to receive the full treatment or in those who have known severe allergy to equine-derived products [96]. Currently this baby-BIG antidote is only available from the California State Health De-partment (510-540-2646).

The United States army possesses an antitoxin against all seven (A–G) serotypes. It is an equine-derived immunoglobulin that has been cleaved by pepsin discarding the Fc (immunogenic portion) and leaving the F(ab')2 fragments specific for botulinum toxin. This therapy has a lower chance of adverse allergic reaction, but a skin test is still advised before ad-ministering this product [96,104].

Thallium

Background

Heavy metals are substances that have been considered as potential weapons of terror. Thallium is a less well-known toxic heavy metal but has many qualities making it ideal for mass poisonings. Thallium salts are odorless and tasteless, will dissolve completely in liquid, are easily absorbed, and can cause significant disability and even death [114]. There are numerous examples of thallium being used for deliberate poisoning [114–116]. A fatality was reported due to heroin tainted with thallium [117], and it has been introduced into a substance used as cocaine [118].

The minimum lethal dose is 12 mg/kg, meaning an absorbed ingestion of less than 1 gram can be fatal [119]. Thallium is absorbed rapidly from the gastrointestinal tract; it can be detected in the urine within 1 hour and may cause a green discoloration of the urine [120]. The exact mechanism of toxicity is unclear. Some suggest it is due to energy depletion from thallium's interference with the Krebs cycle, glycolysis, and oxidative phosphorylation. Others believe thallium forms stable complexes with the active sulfhydryl sites on enzymes [120–122].

Although neurologic symptoms are usually the most pronounced, thallium poisoning can cause many nonspecific clinical effects, making early diagnosis difficult [123]. The most reliable early clue for thallium toxicity is an ascending, rapidly progressive painful sensory peripheral neuropathy. Severe pain in the feet is often described [114,120,124]. This neuropathy can rarely affect the optic nerve, causing permanent blindness [125].

Alopecia is a key feature in diagnosing thallium poisoning. However, it may not be noticed for days to weeks after exposure, and it is not consistently present in all cases. Ideally, treatment should be initiated before the development of alopecia [115]. However, the clinical picture is often confusing, and thallium is often not considered until alopecia is noted.

Thallium causes many other nonspecific signs and symptoms. Gastrointestinal (GI) complaints have been reported [123] and typically precede neurologic symptoms. As opposed to arsenic poisoning, the GI symptoms are usually mild. Initially abdominal pain and diarrhea occur and are followed by constipation. Vomiting is usually not a prominent symptom [122]. The GI effects are helpful in distinguishing thallium toxicity from arsenic toxic [126]. Constipation is possibly due to thallium toxicity affecting the vagus nerve depressing intestinal motility and peristalsis [127].

Neurologic symptoms ranging from tremor, weakness, cranial nerve palsies to convulsions, coma, and death can be seen [123,124]. Cardiac manifestations include hypertension, tachycardia, and nonspecific ST and T wave changes can be present [119]. Renal toxicity evidenced by elevated serum urea nitrogen and creatinine along with proteinuria may occur [122].

Antidote

There is not a true antidote for thallium poisoning. However, Prussian blue can speed removal from the body and help lessen toxic effects. Prussian blue has a crystal lattice structure with a high affinity for thallium [128]. Thallium undergoes enteroenteric and enterohepatic circulation [129], meaning that it is absorbed, secreted back into the gut lumen, and reabsorbed. Prussian blue in the gastrointestinal tract can interrupt this enteroenteric circulation by attaching to the secreted thallium and enhancing its elimination from the body [120,128].

Numerous case reports have shown successful treatment with Prussian blue. Animal studies have supported the published clinical experience by showing increased elimination of thallium, as well as a decrease in brain thallium concentrations [121,130]. A recent study showed Prussian blue was safe and effective in reducing the radioactive thallium burden after thallium myocardial scintography [131].

Indications

Prussian blue is indicated for any patient who has thallium toxicity or known exposure to a toxic amount of thallium. The key is to suspect the diagnosis early in the course of poisoning. This will allow treatment to be initiated as soon as possible.

Delivery

The ideal dose of Prussian blue has never been fully determined. The manufacturer of Prussian blue recommends an adult dose of 9 g divided three times a day and a pediatric dose of 3 g divided three times a day [132]. However, doses of 150 to 250 mg/kg/day have been well tolerated since the first series describing its use in treating thallium toxicity [133] and have been used safely since [116,119,129]. Therefore, using this higher dose is reasonable and will likely have greater antidotal effect. Therapy is generally continued until urinary excretion falls below 0.5 mg/day [116,130].

Precautions

Prussian blue is an extremely safe antidote. No systemic adverse effects have been reported from its use [134]. It is believed that adverse effects are not observed because Prussian blue is not absorbed. However, it has been reported that patients receiving Prussian blue have developed a blue color in their tears, suggesting some systemic absorption [122]. Prussian blue causes constipation [131], which is also a possible manifestation of thallium toxicity [130]. It is recommended that Prussian blue be dissolved in 50 mL of 15% mannitol to act as a cathartic. Other cathartics may be effective. However, due to concerns over causing electrolyte disturbances with repeated doses agents containing magnesium or sorbitol, it is safest to use mannitol [132].

Alternate treatments

Activated charcoal will bind thallium. Due to the fact that thallium undergoes enterohepatic circulation, activated charcoal is capable of reducing the body's thallium burden. Activated charcoal is a reasonable alternative if Prussian blue is not available or if the number of victims is too great for the supply of Prussian blue [126,135].

Radiation emergencies

Perhaps the most feared terrorist attack is one involving a radioactive agent. Exposure to radioactive material can occur from discharge of a nuclear weapon, sabotage of a nuclear power plant, or detonation of a dirty bomb. The overall management of victims of a radioactive weapon attack is out of the scope of this article, but several excellent references are available [136–138]. Issues related to antidotes that may be beneficial in reducing long-term consequences in those exposed are addressed here.

Potassium iodide

Potassium iodide (Fig. 7) is indicated to help prevent the development of thyroid cancer in those exposed to radioactive iodine [139]. It functions by preventing thyroid uptake of radioactive iodine [140]. To provide a protective effect, it must be administered within a few hours of exposure [137]. Unfortunately potassium iodide does not provide total protection from radioactive iodine [140].

The FDA and the World Health Organization have similar guidelines on the administration of potassium iodide [141]. These guidelines take into

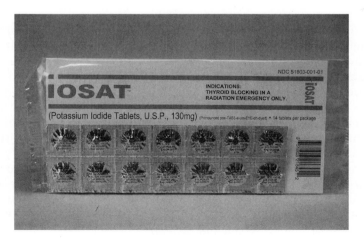

Fig. 7. Potassium iodide tablets.

account the fact that children have a far greater risk of developing cancer secondary to radioactive iodine exposure. Therefore, adults over 40 are generally not advised to take potassium iodide unless there is a projected thyroid dose of over 5 Gy [137]; children and pregnant or lactating women should receive prophylaxis for projected exposure of over .05 Gy [142].

The doses recommended by the FDA are: adults, 130 mg; children between 3 and 18 years, 65 mg; infants and children, 32 mg; and newborns up to 1 month, 16 mg [143] Daily dosing should continue until the risk of exposure is eliminated [142].

Potassium iodide is indicated for events such as a nuclear blast or a reactor meltdown. A dirty bomb would expose victims to gamma radiation and other radioactive agents for which potassium iodide provides no protection [143].

Prussian blue

Radiocesium (cesium-137) is readily available because of widespread use in radiotherapy and other medical and commercial devices. It is a principal constituent of radioactive fallout and is a likely source of contamination from a dirty bomb because of its ready availability [137,144]. Cesium contamination would cause a prolonged environmental hazard because it has a radioactive half-life of 30 years [144].

After being absorbed, cesium closely follows potassium, becoming uniformly distributed throughout the body. It is eliminated primarily through the kidney, with only approximately 10% normally excreted fecally [144]. The physiologic half-life varies, ranging from 50 to 150 days [128]. Victims generally present first with nausea, vomiting, and diarrhea. Dermal exposure can cause irritation, blistering, or necrotic lesions. Eventually exposure can lead to bone marrow suppression causing infection, hemorrhage, and death [128,144].

Prussian blue treats radiocesium exposure by a similar mechanism as for thallium poisoning. It binds to cesium secreted into the gut lumen, traps it, and allows it to be eliminated fecally. One study showed that patients urine/feces excretion ratio of 4:1 was reversed to 1:4 after administration of Prussian blue. Also, this study showed the half-life was reduced by approximately 43% [144].

The minimum effective dose for Prussian blue is 3 g/day. Larger doses, up to 10 g/day are well tolerated and may be more effective. The FDA recommends 3 g orally two times a day for adults and adolescents and 1 g three times a day for children 2 to 12 years old. The treatment should continue for at least 30 days [137]. The patient's serum potassium should be monitored. Also, Prussian blue can cause constipation, so it should be given with mannitol, and prophylactic administration of a laxative should be considered to prevent constipation and minimize the amount of time the radioactive matter in the feces is in contact with the intestines [144].

Prussian blue is considered nontoxic and has minimal if any absorption through an intact GI tract. Acute radiation illness can cause a marked esophagitis and enteritis. The use of Prussian blue in this situation has not been researched.

Summary

Many potential agents exist that can be used for the purpose of chemical terrorism. Recognizing the toxicity is the first step in assisting victims of such an attack. Careful decontamination and supportive care will be the most important steps along with recognizing the particular syndrome to guide antidotal treatment. Also, using antidotes appropriately and assuring access to safe antidotes is extremely important.

It is also important to realize that that the four toxins listed are more likely to be encountered in a nonterror-related incident (eg, pesticide exposure [organophosphates], exposure to improperly preserved foods [botulism], or smoke inhalation victims [cyanide]). Therefore, familiarity with these toxins' manifestations and antidotes is useful for general emergency medicine.

Acknowledgments

The authors thank Andre Berkin, RN for his photographic contributions to the article.

References

[1] Balali-Mood M, Shariat M. Treatment of organophosphate poisoning. Experience of nerve agents and acute pesticide poisoning on the effects of oximes. J Physiol Paris 1998;92(5-6): 375–8.

[2] Yanagisawa N, Morita H, Nakajima T. Sarin experiences in Japan: acute toxicity and long-term effects. J Neurol Sci 2006;249(1):76–85.

[3] Cannard K. The acute treatment of nerve agent exposure. J Neurol Sci 2006;249(1):86–94.

[4] Bajgar J. Complex view on poisoning with nerve agents and organophosphates. Acta Medica (Hradec Kralove) 2005;48(1):3–21.

[5] Lee EC. Clinical manifestations of sarin nerve gas exposure. JAMA 2003;290(5):659–62.

[6] Leikin JB, Thomas RG, Walter FG, et al. A review of nerve agent exposure for the critical care physician [see comment]. Crit Care Med 2002;30(10):2346–54.

[7] Newmark J. Therapy for nerve agent poisoning. Arch Neurol 2004;61(5):649–52.

[8] Bird SB, Gaspari RJ, Dickson EW. Early death due to severe organophosphate poisoning is a centrally mediated process. Acad Emerg Med 2003;10(4):295–8.

[9] McDonough JH Jr, Shih TM. Neuropharmacological mechanisms of nerve agent-induced seizure and neuropathology. Neurosci Biobehav Rev 1997;21(5):559–79.

[10] Myhrer T, Skymoen LR, Aas P. Pharmacological agents, hippocampal eeg, and anticonvulsant effects on soman-induced seizures in rats. Neurotoxicology 2003;24(3):357–67.

[11] Sanada M, Zheng F, Huth T, et al. Cholinergic modulation of periaqueductal grey neurons: does it contribute to epileptogenesis after organophosphorus nerve agent intoxication? Toxicology, in press.

[12] Sidell F. Nerve agents. In: Sidell F, Takafuji ET, Franz DR, editor. Medical aspects of chemical and biological warfare. Washington: Office of the Surgeon General at TMM publications; 1997. p. 129–80.

[13] Newmark J. Nerve agents. Neurol Clin 2005;23(2):623–41.

[14] McDonough JH Jr, Zoefel LD, McMonagle J, et al. Anticonvulsant treatment of nerve agent seizures: anticholinergics versus diazepam in soman-intoxicated guinea pigs. Epilepsy Res 1999;38(1):1–14.

[15] Shih TM, McDonough JH Jr. Organophosphorus nerve agents-induced seizures and efficacy of atropine sulfate as anticonvulsant treatment. Pharmacol Biochem Behav 1999; 64(1):147–53.

[16] Keyes D. Chemical nerve agents. Medical response to terrorism: preparedness and clinical practice. In: Keyes D, editor. 1st edition. Philadelphia: Lippincott Williams and Wilkins; 2005. p. 2–15.

[17] Weinbroum AA. Pathophysiological and clinical aspects of combat anticholinesterase poisoning. Br Med Bull 2005;72(1):119–33.

[18] Newmark J. Nerve agents: pathophysiology and treatment of poisoning. Semin Neurol 2004;24(2):185–96.

[19] Newmark J. The birth of nerve agent warfare: lessons from Syed Abbas Foroutan. Neurology 2004;62(9):1590–6.

[20] Holstege CP, Kirk M, Sidell FR. Chemical warfare. Nerve agent poisoning. Crit Care Clin 1997;13(4):923–42.

[21] Cosar A, Kenar L. An anesthesiological approach to nerve agent victims. Mil Med 2006; 171(1):7–11.

[22] Gilat E, Kadar T, Levy A, et al. Anticonvulsant treatment of sarin-induced seizures with nasal midazolam: an electrographic, behavioral, and histological study in freely moving rats. Toxicol Appl Pharmacol 2005;209(1):74–85.

[23] McDonough JH Jr, McMonagle J, Copeland T, et al. Comparative evaluation of benzodiazepines for control of soman-induced seizures. Arch Toxicol 1999;73(8-9):473–8.

[24] Hayward IJ, Wall HG, Jaax NK, et al. Decreased brain pathology in organophosphate-exposed rhesus monkeys following benzodiazepine therapy. J Neurol Sci 1990;98(1):99–106.

[25] Shih TM, Duniho SM, McDonough JH. Control of nerve agent-induced seizures is critical for neuroprotection and survival. Toxicol Appl Pharmacol 2003;188(2):69–80.

[26] Marrs TC. The role of diazepam in the treatment of nerve agent poisoning in a civilian population. Toxicol Rev 2004;23(3):145–57.

[27] Lallement G, Dorandeu F, Filliat P, et al. Medical management of organophosphate-induced seizures. J Physiol Paris 1998;92(5-6):369–73.

[28] Myhrer T, Anderson JM, Nguyen NH, et al. Soman-induced convulsions in rats terminated with pharmacological agents after 45 min: neuropathology and cognitive performance. Neurotoxicology 2005;26(1):39–48.

[29] McDonough J, Benjamin A, McMonagle J, et al. Effects of fosphenytoin on nerve agent-induced status epilepticus. Drug Chem Toxicol 2004;27(1):27–39.

[30] Eyer P. The role of oximes in the management of organophosphorus pesticide poisoning. Toxicol Rev 2003;22(3):165–90.

[31] Dickson EW, Bird SB, Gaspari RJ, et al. Diazepam inhibits organophosphate-induced central respiratory depression. Acad Emerg Med 2003;10(12):1303–6.

[32] Kassa J. Review of oximes in the antidotal treatment of poisoning by organophosphorus nerve agents. J Toxicol Clin Toxicol 2002;40(6):803–16.

[33] Rotenberg JS, Newmark J. Nerve agent attacks on children: diagnosis and management. Pediatrics 2003;112(3):648–58.

[34] Johnson MK, Vale JA, Marrs TC, et al. Pralidoxime for organophosphorus poisoning [comment]. Lancet 1992;340(8810):64.

[35] Farrar HC, Wells TG, Kearns GL. Use of continuous infusion of pralidoxime for treatment of organophosphate poisoning in children. J Pediatr 1990;116(4):658–61.

[36] Tush GM, Anstead MI. Pralidoxime continuous infusion in the treatment of organophosphate poisoning. Ann Pharmacother 1997;31(4):441–4.

[37] Bawaskar HS, Joshi SR. Organophosphorus poisoning in agricultural India–status in 2005 [comment]. J Assoc Physicians India 2005;53:422–4.

[38] Medicis JJ, Stork CM, Howland MA, et al. Pharmacokinetics following a loading plus a continuous infusion of pralidoxime compared with the traditional short infusion regimen in human volunteers. J Toxicol Clin Toxicol 1996;34(3):289–95.

[39] Kamha AA, Al Omary IY, Zalabany HA, et al. Organophosphate poisoning in pregnancy: a case report. Basic Clin Pharmacol Toxicol 2005;96(5):397–8.

[40] Shivakumar S, Raghaven K, Ishaq RM, et al. Organophosphorus poisoning: a study on the effectiveness of therapy with oximes. J Assoc Physicians India 2006;54:250–1.

[41] Tokuda Y, Kikuchi M, Takahashi O, et al. Prehospital management of sarin nerve gas terrorism in urban settings: 10 years of progress after the Tokyo subway sarin attack. Resuscitation 2006;68(2):193–202.

[42] Rahimi R, Nikfar S, Abdollahi M. Increased morbidity and mortality in acute human organophosphate-poisoned patients treated by oximes: a meta-analysis of clinical trials. Hum Exp Toxicol 2006;25(3):157–62.

[43] Peter JV, Moran JL, Graham P. Oxime therapy and outcomes in human organophosphate poisoning: an evaluation using meta-analytic techniques. Crit Care Med 2006; 34(2):502–10.

[44] Eddleston M, Szinicz L, Eyer P, et al. Oximes in acute organophosphorus pesticide poisoning: a systematic review of clinical trials. QJM 2002;95(5):275–83.

[45] Aaron C. Safety of adult nerve agent autoinjectors in children. J Pediatr 2005;146(1):8–10.

[46] Foltin G, Tunik M, Curran J, et al. Pediatric nerve agent poisoning: medical and operational considerations for emergency medical services in a large American city. Pediatr Emerg Care 2006;22(4):239–44.

[47] Amitai Y, Almog S, Singer R, et al. Atropine poisoning in children during the Persian Gulf crisis. A national survey in Israel. JAMA 1992;268(5):630–2.

[48] Kozer E, Mordel A, Haim SB, et al. Pediatric poisoning from trimedoxime (TMB4) and atropine automatic injectors. J Pediatr 2005;146(1):41–4.

[49] Krejcova G, Kassa J. Anticholinergic drugs–functional antidotes for the treatment of tabun intoxication. Acta Medica (Hradec Kralove) 2004;47(1):13–8.

[50] Kventsel I, Berkovitch M, Reiss A, et al. Scopolamine treatment for severe extra-pyramidal signs following organophosphate (Chlorpyrifos) ingestion. Clinical Toxicology 2005;43(7): 877–9.

[51] Bird SB, Gaspari RJ, Lee WJ, et al. Diphenhydramine as a protective agent in a rat model of acute, lethal organophosphate poisoning. Acad Emerg Med 2002;9(12):1369–72.

[52] Bania TC, Chu J, Bailes D, et al. Jimson weed extract as a protective agent in severe organophosphate toxicity. Acad Emerg Med 2004;11(4):335–8.

[53] Gracia R. Cyanide. In: Keyes D, editor. Medical response to terrorism: preparedness and clinical practice. 1st edition. Philadelphia: Lippincott Williams and Wilkins; 2005. p. 26–37.

[54] Holstege C, Isom GE, Kirk MA. Cyanide and hydrogen sulfide. In: Flomenbaum N, Goldfrank LR, Hoffman RS, et al, editors. Goldfrank toxicological emergencies. 8th edition. New York: The McGraw-Hill Companies, Inc; 2006. p. 1712–24.

[55] Eckstein M, Maniscalco PM. Focus on smoke inhalation–the most common cause of acute cyanide poisoning. Prehospital Disaster Med 2006;21(2 Suppl. 2):s49–55.

[56] Morocco AP. Cyanides. Crit Care Clin 2005;21(4):691–705.

[57] DesLauriers CA, Burda AM, Wahl M. Hydroxocobalamin as a cyanide antidote. Am J Ther 2006;13(2):161–5.

[58] Rotenberg JS. Cyanide as a weapon of terror. Pediatr Ann 2003;32(4):236–40.

[59] Megarbane B, Delahaye A, Goldgran-Toladano D, et al. Antidotal treatment of cyanide poisoning. J Chin Med Assoc 2003;66(4):193–203.

[60] Dunea G. Death over the counter. Br Med J (Clin Res Ed) 1983;286(6360):211–2.

[61] Peddy SB, Rigby MR, Shaffner DH. Acute cyanide poisoning. Pediatr Crit Care Med 2006; 7(1):79–82.

[62] Prieto I, Pujol I, Santiuste C, et al. Acute cyanide poisoning by subcutaneous injection. Emerg Med J 2005;22(5):389–90.

[63] Baud FJ, Borron SW, Megarbane B, et al. Value of lactic acidosis in the assessment of the severity of acute cyanide poisoning. Crit Care Med 2002;30(9):2044–50.

[64] Rebeca G, Greene S. Cyanide poisoning and its treatment. Pharmacotherapy 2004;24(10): 1358–65.

[65] LaPostolle F, Borron S, Baud F. Increased plasma lactate concentrations are associated with cyanide but not other types of acute poisoning. Clinical Toxicology 2006;44(5):777.

[66] Martin-Bermudez R, Maestre-Romero A, Goni-Belzunegui MV, et al. Venous blood arteriolization and multiple organ failure after cyanide poisoning. Intensive Care Med 1997; 23(12):1286.

[67] Geller RJ, Barthold C, Saiers J, et al. Pediatric cyanide poisoning: causes, manifestations, management, and unmet needs. Pediatrics 2006;118(5):2146–58.

[68] Howland A. Sodium and amyl nitrites. In: Flomenbaum N, Goldfrank LR, Hoffman RS, et al, editors. Goldfrank's toxicological emergencies. 8th edition. New York: The McGraw-Hill Company; 2006. p. 1725–30.

[69] Breen PH, Isserles SA, Westley J, et al. Effect of oxygen and sodium thiosulfate during combined carbon monoxide and cyanide poisoning. Toxicol Appl Pharmacol 1995;134(2): 229–34.

[70] Guidotti T. Acute cyanide poisoning in prehospital care: new challenges, new tools for intervention. Prehospital Disaster Med 2006;21(2 Suppl. 2):s40–8.

[71] Sauer SW, Keim ME. Hydroxocobalamin: improved public health readiness for cyanide disasters. Ann Emerg Med 2001;37(6):635–41.

[72] Kirk MA, Gerace R, Kulig KW. Cyanide and methemoglobin kinetics in smoke inhalation victims treated with the cyanide antidote kit. Ann Emerg Med 1993;22(9):1413–8.

[73] Baskin SI, Horowitz AM, Nealley EW. The antidotal action of sodium nitrite and sodium thiosulfate against cyanide poisoning. J Clin Pharmacol 1992;32(4):368–75.

[74] Dart R. Hydroxocobalamin for acute cyanide poisoning: new data from preclinical and clinical studies; new results from the prehospital emergency setting. Clinical Toxicology 2006;44(Suppl 1):1–3.

[75] Posner MA, Tobey RE, McElroy H. Hydroxocobalamin therapy of cyanide intoxication in guinea pigs. Anesthesiology 1976;44(2):157–60.

[76] Posner MA, Rodkey FL, Tobey RE. Nitroprusside-induced cyanide poisoning: antidotal effect of hydroxocobalamin. Anesthesiology 1976;44(4):330–5.

[77] Rose CL, Worth RM, Chen KK. Hydroxo-cobalamine and acute cyanide poisoning in dogs. Life Sci 1965;4(18):1785–9.

[78] Borron SW. Recognition and treatment of acute cyanide poisoning. J Emerg Nurs 2006; 32(4 Suppl. 1):S12–8.

[79] Mannaioni G, Vannacci A, Marzocca C, et al. Acute cyanide intoxication treated with a combination of hydroxycobalamin, sodium nitrite, and sodium thiosulfate. J Toxicol Clin Toxicol 2002;40(2):181–3.

[80] Fortin JL, Giocanti JP, Ruttiman M, et al. Prehospital administration of hydroxocobalamin for smoke inhalation-associated cyanide poisoning: 8 years of experience in the paris fire brigade. Clinical Toxicology 2006;44(Suppl 1):37–44.

[81] Forsyth JC, Mueller PD, Becker CE, et al. Hydroxocobalamin as a cyanide antidote: safety, efficacy and pharmacokinetics in heavily smoking normal volunteers. J Toxicol Clin Toxicol 1993;31(2):277–94.

[82] Gerth K, Ehring T, Braendle M, et al. Nitric oxide scavenging by hydroxocobalamin may account for its hemodynamic profile. Clinical Toxicology 2006;44(Suppl 1):29–36.

[83] Borron S, Stonerook M, Reid F. Efficacy of hydroxocobalamin for the treatment of acute cyanide poisoning in adult beagle dogs. Clinical Toxicology 2006;44(Suppl 1):5–15.

[84] Riou B, Bereaux A, Pussard E, et al. Comparison of the hemodynamic effects of hydroxo-cobalamin and cobalt edetate at equipotent cyanide antidotal doses in conscious dogs. Intensive Care Med 1993;19(1):26–32.

[85] Howland A. Hydroxocobalamin. In: Flomenbaum N, Goldfrank LR, Hoffman RS, et al, editors. Goldfrank's toxicological emergencies. 8th edition. New York: The McGraw-Hill company; 2006. p. 1731–3.

[86] Hall AHBH Rumack. Hydroxycobalamin/sodium thiosulfate as a cyanide antidote. J Emerg Med 1987;5(2):115–21.

[87] Froyshov S, Hoiseth G, Jacobsen D. Cyanide intoxication: course before and after treatment with antidote. Clinical Toxicology 2006;44(5):763.

[88] Curry SC, Connor DA, Raschke RA. Effect of the cyanide antidote hydroxocobalamin on commonly ordered serum chemistry studies. Ann Emerg Med 1994;24(1):65–7.

[89] Uhl W, Nolting A, Golor G, et al. Safety of hydroxocobalamin in healthy volunteers in a randomized, placebo-controlled study. Clinical Toxicology 2006;44(Suppl 1): 17–28.

[90] Bromley J, Hughes BGM, Leong DCS, et al. Life-threatening interaction between complementary medicines: cyanide toxicity following ingestion of amygdalin and vitamin C. Ann Pharmacother 2005;39(9):1566–9.

[91] Weng TI, Fang CC, Lin SM, et al. Elevated plasma cyanide level after hydroxocobalamin infusion for cyanide poisoning. Am J Emerg Med 2004;22(6):492–3.

[92] Dart RC, Stark Y, Fulton B, et al. Insufficient stocking of poisoning antidotes in hospital pharmacies. JAMA 1996;276(18):1508–10.

[93] Dart RC, Goldfrank LR, Chyka PA, et al. Combined evidence-based literature analysis and consensus guidelines for stocking of emergency antidotes in the United States. Ann Emerg Med 2000;36(2):126–32.

[94] Brivet F, Delfraissy JF, Duche M, et al. Acute cyanide poisoning: recovery with non-specific supportive therapy. Intensive Care Med 1983;9(1):33–5.

[95] Graham DL, Laman D, Theodore J, et al. Acute cyanide poisoning complicated by lactic acidosis and pulmonary edema. Arch Intern Med 1977;137(8):1051–5.

[96] Horowitz BZ. Botulinum toxin. Crit Care Clin 2005;21(4):825–39.

[97] Gupta A, Sumner CJ, Castor M, et al. Adult botulism type F in the United States, 1981–2002. Neurology 2005;65(11):1694–700.

[98] Keet CA, Fox CK, Margeta M, et al. Infant botulism, type F, presenting at 54 hours of life. Pediatr Neurol 2005;32(3):193–6.

[99] Timmons R, Carbone A. Botulism: the most toxic substance known. In: Keyes DC, editor. Medical response to terrorism: preparedness and clinical practice. 1st edition. New York: Lippincott Williams and Wilkins; 2005. p. 117–26.

[100] Patocka J, Splino M, Merka V. Botulism and bioterrorism: how serious is this problem? Acta Medica (Hradec Kralove) 2005;48(1):23–8.

[101] Souayah N, Karim H, Kamin SS, et al. Severe botulism after focal injection of botulinum toxin. Neurology 2006;67:1855–6.

[102] Grumelli C, Verderio C, Pozzi D, et al. Internalization and mechanism of action of clostridial toxins in neurons. Neurotoxicology 2005;26(5):761–7.

[103] Cherington M. Botulism: update and review. Semin Neurol 2004;24(2):155–63.

[104] Arnon SS, Schechter R, Inglesby TV, et al. Botulinum toxin as a biological weapon: medical and public health management [erratum appears in JAMA 2001 Apr 25;285(16):2081]. JAMA 2001;285(8):1059–70.

[105] Robinson RF, Nahata MC. Management of botulism. Ann Pharmacother 2003;37(1): 127–31.

[106] Villar RG, Elliott SP, Davenport KM. Botulism: the many faces of botulinum toxin and its potential for bioterrorism. Infect Dis Clin North Am 2006;20(2):313–27.

[107] Sobel J. Botulism. Clin Infect Dis 2005;41(8):1167–73.

[108] Penas SC, Faria OM, Serrao R, et al. Ophthalmic manifestations in 18 patients with botulism diagnosed in Porto, Portugal between 1998 and 2003. J Neuroophthalmol 2005;25(4): 262–7.
[109] Varma JK, Katsitadze G, Moiscrafishvili T, et al. Signs and symptoms predictive of death in patients with foodborne botulism–Republic of Georgia, 1980-2002 [see comment]. Clin Infect Dis 2004;39(3):357–62.
[110] Anonymous. Botulism: treatment overview for clinicians. 6/14/2006. Available at: www. bt.cdc.gov/agent/Botulism/clinicians/treatment.asp. Accessed October 9, 2006.
[111] Black RE, Gunn RA. Hypersensitivity reactions associated with botulinal antitoxin. Am J Med 1980;69(4):567–70.
[112] Arnon SS, Schechter R, Maslanka SE, et al. Human botulism immune globulin for the treatment of infant botulism [see comment]. N Engl J Med 2006;354(5):462–71.
[113] Fox CK, Keet CA, Strober JB. Recent advances in infant botulism. Pediatr Neurol 2005; 32(3):149–54.
[114] Rusyniak DE, Furbee RB, Kirk MA. Thallium and arsenic poisoning in a small midwestern town. Ann Emerg Med 2002;39(3):307–11.
[115] Pau PW. Management of thallium poisoning. Hong Kong Med J 2000;6(3):316–8.
[116] Vergauwe PL, Knockaert DC, Van Tittelboom TJ. Near fatal subacute thallium poisoning necessitating prolonged mechanical ventilation. Am J Emerg Med 1990;8(6):548–50.
[117] Questel F, Dugarin J, Dally S. Thallium-contaminated heroin. Ann Intern Med 1996; 124(6):616.
[118] Insley BM, Grufferman S, Ayliffe HE. Thallium poisoning in cocaine abusers. Am J Emerg Med 1986;4(6):545–8.
[119] Wainwright AP, Kox WJ, House IM, et al. Clinical features and therapy of acute thallium poisoning. Q J Med 1988;69(259):939–44.
[120] Malbrain MLNG, Lambrecht GLY, Zandijk E, et al. Treatment of severe thallium intoxication. Journal of Toxicology: Clinical Toxicolgy 1997;35(1):97–100.
[121] Rusyniak DE, Kao LW, Nanagas KA, et al. Dimercaptosuccinic acid and prussian blue in the treatment of acute thallium poisoning in rats. Journal of Toxicology: Clinical Toxicology 2003;41(2):137–42.
[122] Hoffman RS. Thallium toxicity and the role of prussian blue in therapy. Toxicol Rev 2003; 22(1):29–40.
[123] Jha S, Kumar R, Kumar R. Thallium poisoning presenting as paresthesias, paresis, psychosis and pain in abdomen. J Assoc Physicians India 2006;54:53–5.
[124] Tsai YT, Huang CC, Kuo HC, et al. Central nervous system effects in acute thallium poisoning. Neurotoxicology 2006;27(2):291–5.
[125] Tabandeh H, Crowston JG, Thompson GM. Ophthalmologic features of thallium poisoning. Am J Optho 1994;117(n2):243–5.
[126] Ibrahim D, Froberg B, Wolf A, et al. Heavy metal poisoning: clinical presentations and pathophysiology. Clin Lab Med 2006;26(1):67–97.
[127] Galvan-Arzate S, Santamaria A. Thallium toxicity. Toxicol Lett 1998;99(1):1–13.
[128] Thompson, DF, Callen ED. Soluble or insoluble prussian blue for radiocesium and thallium poisoning Ann Pharmacother, 2004;38(9):1509–14.
[129] Atsmon J, Taliansky E, Landau M, et al. Thallium poisoning in Israel. Am J Med Sci 2000; 320(5):327–30.
[130] Kamerbeek HH, Rauws AG, ten Ham M, et al. Prussian blue in therapy of thallotoxicosis. An experimental and clinical investigation. Acta Med Scand 1971;189(4):321–4.
[131] Bhardwaj N, Bhatnager A, Pathak DP, et al. Dynamic, equilibrium and human studies of adsorption of 201Tl by prussian blue. Health Phys 2006;90(3):250–7.
[132] Hoffman RS. Prussian blue. In: Flomenbaum N, Goldfrank LR, Hoffman RS, et al, editors. Goldfrank's toxicological emergencies. 8th edition. New York: The McGraw-Hill Companies, Inc; 2006. p. 1373–7.

[133] Stevens W, van Peteghem C, Heyndrickx A, et al. Eleven cases of thallium intoxication treated with prussian blue. Int J Clin Pharmacol Ther Toxicol 1974;10(1):1–22.

[134] Pearce J. Studies of any toxicological effects of prussian blue compounds in mammals– a review. Food Chem Toxicol 1994;32(6):577–82.

[135] Hoffman R, Hoffman R, Stringer J, et al. Comparative efficacy of thallium adsorption by activated charcoal, prussian blue, and sodium polystyrene sulfonate. J Toxicol Clin Toxicol 1999;37(7):833–7.

[136] Goans RE, Waselenko JK. Medical management of radiological casualties. Health Phys 2005;89(5):505–12.

[137] Koenig KL, Goans RE, Hatchett RJ, et al. Medical treatment of radiological casualties: current concepts. Ann Emerg Med 2005;45(6):643–52.

[138] Waselenko JK, MacVittie TJ, Blakely WF, et al. Medical management of the acute radiation syndrome: recommendations of the Strategic National Stockpile Radiation Working Group. Ann Intern Med 2004;140(12):1037–51.

[139] Cardis E, Kesminiene A, Ivanov V, et al. Risk of thyroid cancer after exposure to 131I in childhood. J Natl Cancer Inst 2005;97(10):724–32.

[140] Verger P, Aurengo A, Geoffroy B, et al. Iodine kinetics and effectiveness of stable iodine prophylaxis after intake of radioactive iodine: a review. Thyroid 2001;11(4):353–60.

[141] Schneider AB, Becker DV, Robbins J. Protecting the thyroid from accidental or terrorist-instigated 131I releases. Thyroid 2002;12(4):271–2.

[142] Anonymous. Guidance: potassium iodide as a thyroid blocking agent in radiation emergencies. December 10, 2001. Available at: www.fda.gov/cder/guidance/index.index. Accessed September 21, 2006.

[143] Vastag B. Experts advise on potassium iodide use: no protection against "dirty bombs. JAMA 2003;289(16):2058.

[144] Dennis FT, Chelsea OC. Prussian blue for treatment of radiocesium poisoning. Pharmacotherapy 2001;21(11):1364–7.

ELSEVIER
SAUNDERS

Emerg Med Clin N Am 25 (2007) 597–602

EMERGENCY
MEDICINE
CLINICS OF
NORTH AMERICA

Index

Note: Page numbers of article titles are in **boldface** type.

0733-8627/07/$ - see front matter © 2007 Elsevier Inc. All rights reserved.
doi:10.1016/S0733-8627(07)00052-1

emed.theclinics.com

Moving?

Make sure your subscription moves with you!

To notify us of your new address, find your **Clinics Account Number** (located on your mailing label above your name), and contact customer service at:

E-mail: elspcs@elsevier.com

800-654-2452 (subscribers in the U.S. & Canada)
407-345-4000 (subscribers outside of the U.S. & Canada)

Fax number: 407-363-9661

Elsevier Periodicals Customer Service
6277 Sea Harbor Drive
Orlando, FL 32887-4800

*To ensure uninterrupted delivery of your subscription, please notify us at least 4 weeks in advance of move.